Manual Of Artificial Limbs: An Exhaustive Exposition Of Prothesis...

George Edwin Marks

MANUAL

OF

ARTIFICIAL LIMBS

COPIOUSLY ILLUSTRATED

*Artificial Toes, Feet, Legs, Fingers, Hands, Arms,
for Amputations and Deformities, Appliances
for Excisions, Fractures, and other
Disabilities of Lower and Upper
Extremities, Suggestions on
Amputations, Treatment
of Stumps, History,
etc., etc., etc.*

AN EXHAUSTIVE EXPOSITION OF PROTHESIS

A. A. MARKS

701 BROADWAY, NEW YORK, N. Y., U. S. A.

1914

PREFACE

MANUAL OF ARTIFICIAL LIMBS is the title given to this book to distinguish it from the Treatise and all other publications which it succeeds and supplants. It is in no sense a catalogue, although containing the information usually given in catalogues; but it is a true manual of the subject of prothesis and the most exhaustive work ever produced on that topic. Prothesis or prosthesis is defined by Webster as "The process of adding to the human body some artificial part in place of one that may be wanting."

The Manual thus treats of all losses and impairments of the extremities, whether caused by accident, disease or birth, shows what they are and clearly describes how they may be repaired by artificial methods.

The Manual is divided into chapters, each devoted to a distinct phase of the subject or to a particular part of the leg or arm under discussion.

The illustrations are designated by letters and numbers for convenience of reference. For example, partial foot amputations are discussed in Chapter III, and the illustrations in that chapter all have the letter C and are numbered in order, 1, 2, 3, etc. Amputations of different sections of the legs and arms are similarly divided and the illustrations numbered in the same manner. This gives definiteness and avoids confusions with earlier publications.

The need of the Prothesist becomes more and more urgent every day. Losses of limbs by accidents and injuries of every kind are constantly multiplying, and the demands made upon the thoughtful and skillful maker of artificial limbs and other surgical apparatus increase in the same proportion.

The successful maker cannot confine himself to the narrow methods of former times. Specific treatment is now called for in almost every case, the peculiarities of each requires closer study, separate methods must be devised by which complicated cases can be treated more skillfully and reparation more complete. These are advanced methods, called for by the progress of the science and necessitated by the importance of the work required. The skillful maker thus occupies a much more prominent position than can be filled by those who persist in clinging to archaic systems. It has been said by those most competent to judge that the house of A. A. Marks through persistent endeavor, broad enterprise, attentive study and a real sense of the importance of the work has earned and occupies the foremost position in its branch of industry.

3

While the loss of a limb is a serious personal deprivation, it is no longer regarded as a grievous or irreparable one. There are many thousands of people who walk, work and mingle with other people without disclosing their own loss and without suffering. The absence of a leg or an arm, therefore, is now regarded, and quite rightly, as one of the minor misfortunes. Testimonials substantiating these statements, and explaining and endorsing the principles presented in this Manual for the construction of artificial limbs, will be found in copious numbers in Chapter XXXVII.

TABLE OF CONTENTS

5

CHAPTER IV

CHAPTER V

CHAPTER VI

CHAPTER VII

CHAPTER VIII

CHAPTER XVII

CHAPTER XVIII

CHAPTER XIX

CHAPTER XX

CHAPTER XXI

CHAPTER XXII

CHAPTER XXIII

CHAPTER XXIV

CHAPTER XXV

CHAPTER XXVI

CHAPTER XXVII

CHAPTER XXVIII

CHAPTER XXIX

CHAPTER XXX

CHAPTER XXXI

CHAPTER XXXII

CHAPTER XXXIII

CHAPTER XXXIV

CHAPTER XXXV

CHAPTER XXXVI

INTRODUCTION

In reviewing "Manual of Artificial Limbs" and introducing same to the reader privilege is taken to advert briefly to the House itself and its enviable history.

The house of A. A. Marks was founded for the purpose of relieving and helping the maimed and deformed. Established in the year 1853 it has had a continuous existence of more than half a century and has become the leading house of its kind in the world.

Its manufacturing plants, the factory and office in New York City, and the mills in Connecticut, occupy more ground and employ more help than any establishment elsewhere in the world devoted to the manufacture of artificial legs or artificial arms. The business is a large one, conducted in a large way and by men thoroughly familiar with every detail of artificial limb manufacture; men who have brought to it the widest practical knowledge and years of the most attentive study and effort.

Their specialty is the making of artificial legs and arms with rubber feet and hands, of which they are the inventors and patentees. The spring mattress rubber foot and the rubber hand with ductile fingers are the most recent improvements. That the house has grown from a small shop to a vast manufacturing establishment with a hundred thousand correspondents located in all parts of the world is due not only to the intelligent way in which its business has been conducted, but to the inherent merits of its products. These are described at length in the pages which follow and the descriptions are supplemented by innumerable letters from grateful clients.

Modern skill has brought no more useful aid to humanity than the artificial limb which transforms a helpless member of society into a useful one.

The firm does not claim that every maimed and crippled person can be restored to the full use of his extremities by its apparatus. It is reasonable, however, to claim that its skill and facilities enable the firm to help the maimed better and more thoroughly than any other establishment in the world, and as the house has helped so many in the past there is abundant encouragement for the maimed of the future.

This book has been prepared not as an exposition of the firm's business, but as a guide and help to those seeking alleviation.

The firm manufactures limbs for simple amputations as well as for the most complicated and difficult ones. It has developed special types of limbs for groups of special cases, many of which are of utmost complexity; it has fitted and helped persons with delicate and tender stumps, also many with stumps of awkward shape and difficult forms; it has applied artificial limbs and appliances to persons with one sound limb as well as to those who have been deprived of both, and the volume of testimony it has on view received from its clients, filled with gratitude, stimulates it to continued endeavors.

The book is destined to be an authority on the important subject of prothesis, a book of interest and concern to the surgeon and physician as well as to the maimed. It contains not only a description of multifarious devices but much general matter both descriptive and critical, and in a way didactic, bearing close relations to the work of the surgeon.

It is a matter of highest gratification and pride that in all the exhibitions in which the firm of A. A. Marks has been represented it has received forty-six first and highest awards, always in competition with others. But the freely proffered expressions of regard and satisfaction from its clients, from the men and women who have been helped and whose lives have been aided and bettered through the use of its apparatus, are more stimulating, and the very highest measure of praise one can hope to receive. Numerous as are those that are printed, they constitute but a fragment of the kind and grateful words that have been uttered in its favor during its career.

The book will reach many readers. To them let us say one word. The firm of A. A. Marks has helped others. It surely can help you.

JAMES LAW, M. D.

CHAPTER I

HOW WE WALK

ON NATURAL FEET.—No two persons walk exactly alike. Everyone carries his mannerisms in his steps. The way in which he lands on his heel, rolls on the sole, lifts on the ball, throws himself to the right or the left, the uniformity and regularity of each joint's action, the angle at which the hip is checked, the range of articulation permitted in the knee and the angular motion of the ankle,—all form a part of his individuality and make it possible to distinguish a friend from a stranger long before his features have come within the reach of vision. All sorts of forces—heredity, early habits, occupation, disease, injuries, and age—influence the movements of the leg and foot. A man in good health walks differently from an invalid, a farmer can be distinguished from a merchant, a bookkeeper from a railroad conductor, the sprightliness of youth, the infirmities of age are reflected in every step that is taken. Yet there are certain facts connected with walking that are common to all and which can be ascertained by observation and study. These facts are so universal that they become laws governing locomotion; they form a necessary part of the limb-maker's education, and unless he is familiar with them and applies them thoughtfully to the construction of artificial limbs, he is not competent to work out the problems that are continually arising.

As this work is designed as a text-book on artificial limbs, it is essential, at the outset, to present the cardinal facts relating to natural walking, in order that the application of them to artificial aids may be clearly understood and appreciated.

Kinetoscopic photography affords the most valuable aid to an investigation of the actions of the knee and ankle joints when performing their functions. It shows that when a man walks slowly, say two miles an hour, the knee flexes but slightly and the ankle considerably. When walking three miles an hour, the knee joint acts through a greater range and the ankle joint through a lesser one. When walking moderately fast, say four miles an hour, the knee action becomes considerable and the ankle action scarcely perceptible. When walking rapidly, say five miles an hour, the knee action is increased and the ankle becomes practically rigid. When running the knee increases its activity, and the ankle reverses its action and throws the man forward by the ball of the foot.

The ratio that exists between the range of motion of the knee and that of the ankle is in proportion to the speed with which one moves. An impulse is had to walk slowly or rapidly, or to change from one gait to another. The proper muscles and tendons instantly respond to the mind, and the required speed is attained. If the co-operation between the mind and muscles be disrupted the person becomes a paralytic and his steps are unreliable. The same may be said of a person walking on an artificial leg with ankle motion that is not under control.

Three miles an hour is the ordinary gait of a person occupied in

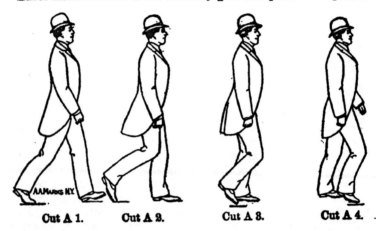

Cut A 1.   Cut A 2.   Cut A 3.   Cut A 4.

commercial life. Successive photographs of a man with natural legs, walking at this gait, show that there is but very little motion in the ankle joint; and limited as that motion is, it is of a character that cannot be imitated by mechanical means. The walker throws his left foot forward, barely touching the heel to the

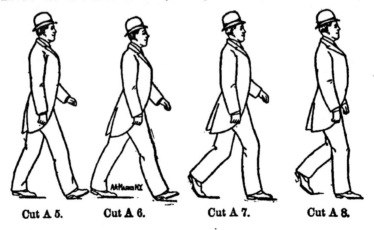

Cut A 5.   Cut A 6.   Cut A 7.   Cut A 8.

ground, as shown in Cut A 1; instantly the right foot under control of the tendo-Achilles extends and the heel is raised from the ground, throwing the weight of the body on the ball, supplying the impetus that urges the body forward. As the body is carried forward, the ball of the left foot reaches the ground at about the time the body is vertically over it, as shown in Cut A 2. At this point the right foot is in the act of leaving the ground, and, as shown in Cut A 3, is passing the left which, still being flat on the ground, performs no function, except that of supporting the body, as shown in Cut A 4. The right leg is carried a little further forward when a slight amount of flexion is admitted in the left ankle joint, as shown in Cut A 5. But this is for a very brief period, as Cut A 6 shows that the tendo-Achilles instantly contracts and the foot extends and the entire body is lifted and thrown on the ball, and when the weight of the body is placed on the heel of the right foot, there is a slight flexion in the knee joint which permits the sole to reach the ground. At this time, the knee joint of the left is flexed and the foot of that leg is raised, as shown in Cut A 7, and when the weight of the body is practically over the right foot the knee is extended, so as to support the weight securely, as shown in Cut A 8.

A study of these successive photographs shows that in making a complete step the soles of both feet are not on the ground at the same time, and at times when the weight of the body is placed equally on each foot, the heel of the advanced foot and the toes of the rear foot are only those parts that are on the ground. It also shows that propulsion is obtained by rising on the ball of the rear foot.

On Artificial Feet with Ankle Joints.—Similar photographs of a man walking with one or a pair of artificial legs with ankle joints set to act at a constant range of motion, show that he walks fairly well at a slow gait, but at a speed of three or more miles an hour his step becomes perceptibly awkward, and the effort required to overcome the too liberal motion in the ankle is fatiguing. So far as the knee joint is concerned the motions of the artificial and natural legs are approximately the same, but the motions of the ankles are very different. The sole of the foot is flat on the ground for a considerably longer period with the artificial ankle joint than with the natural. As the walker advances and strikes the heel of the artificial foot on the ground, almost immediately the front of the foot drops and the entire sole rests on the ground and remains there during the interval through which the body is passing over it.

Having made plain the movements of the natural foot in walking, and contrasted them with the movements of the artificial foot articulating at the ankle, we now propose to carry the contrast to the spring-mattress rubber foot attached rigidly to the leg socket.

On Spring-Mattress Rubber Feet without Ankle Joints.—As the walker advances on the rubber foot he touches the heel to the ground. He applies his weight, and the sponge rubber in the heel compresses sufficiently to allow him to roll on the bottom of the foot; the moment the body is carried a little in advance, he rises on the ball very much the same as he does on the natural foot. There is no effort required to lift on the ball, as the weight of the body, being in advance of its center of gravity, overcomes that apparent obstruction; not a muscle or tendon is brought into play; the weight of the body does the entire work.

These studies and comparisons of the movements in walking bring out very clearly the essential fact that with the artificial ankle joint the interval that the plantar surface rests on the ground is very much greater than that of the natural foot, while with the sponge rubber spring-mattress foot it is approximately the same, and, by compelling the walker to rise on the ball, produces a very natural action, giving greater assistance in walking and dispensing with a vast amount of mechanism.

It is apparent also that the value of mental force in controlling the actions of the natural ankle joint cannot be overestimated. When these forces become inert, as they necessarily do in artificial joints, the embarrassments that follow are the same as with paralytics, locomotor ataxia, etc. The injured are obliged to walk cautiously, the affected foot is placed almost entirely by the sense of sight, and the step is made with meditation and progress must necessarily be slow.

If an artificial leg with ankle articulation be applied to a person who desires to walk at a gait faster than two miles an hour, he will find himself not only greatly hindered, but required to put more energy into the natural foot and leg in order to overcome the influence of the articulating ankle in retarding his progress. The rubber foot without ankle joint will assist rather than hinder rapid walking, and will not hinder slow walking when desired.

CHAPTER II

ARTIFICIAL FEET, THEIR CONSTRUCTION AND RELATIVE MERITS

THE RUBBER FOOT.—With an experience of eight years in manufacturing artificial legs with wood feet, articulating at the toes and ankles, A. A. Marks in 1861 invented the sponge rubber foot hereinafter described, to protect which the United States Government issued letters patent in 1863. Like all great inventions it passed through various stages of development.

The perfected form consists of a wooden core, carved to size and shape to secure the best results. The faint lines in Cut B 1

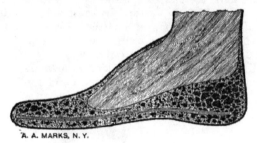

A. A. MARKS, N. Y.

Cut B 1.

represent the core, which reaches to the ball of the foot, localizing the toe movement. The distance from the core to the floor at the heel is considerably greater than at any other part; this is done to obtain the proper degree of compressibility at the heel; the core is entirely surrounded with sponge rubber of great porosity which will yield under the weight of the wearer sufficiently to make the step realistic. Less rubber is placed at the ball so as to provide phalangeal support and make the wearer feel that there is a supporting medium at the front of the foot; ample, to steady him when standing, to keep him from limping, and to act as a lever to urge him forward when walking. A spring mattress is floated in the foot below the core, covering the entire distance from the back of the heel to the tips of the toes; it is shown by the lines running lengthwise in Cut B 1. The spring mattress is formed by a series of composition strips embedded in strong sail duck, each having a pocket of its own, see Cut B 2; the strips occupy the pockets *a a a a*.

THE SPRING MATTRESS.—Is a device for giving additional resiliency for both the toes and heel. Every movement of the foot

21

when in action applies pressure to the springs at the heel, ball, or
on the sides. The counteracting tendency of the strips aids in
forcing the foot back to its proper shape as soon as pressure is
removed.

Cut B 3 represents the rubber foot with the weight applied at
the ball as it is when the wearer is being urged forward, while walk-

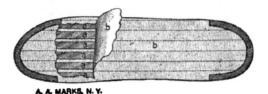

Cut B 2.

ing. The spring mattress is now forced upwards at the ball and
the sponge rubber is compressed above and below the mattress.
This pressure pulls the mattress forward in the foot. These movements—the yielding of the spring, the compressing of the rubber,
and the pulling of the spring mattress forward—form a very
powerful resultant force that brings the foot back to its normal
lines as soon as the foot is relieved of weight.

The condition of the foot when under heel pressure, as it is when
the wearer places the artificial limb forward and applies his weight

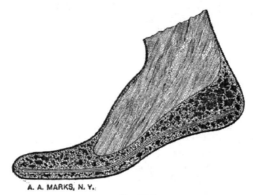

Cut B 8.

upon it, is somewhat the same. The spring mattress is forced
upward, the sponge rubber is compressed above and below, the heel
becomes flattened, and the mattress being pulled lengthwise, all
combine to force the foot to its shape as soon as pressure on the
heel is removed. The compression of the heel permits the toes and
the front part of the foot to reach the ground while the shaft of
the leg is obliquely back of the vertical line.

Cut B 4 represents the foot on an inclined surface. On account
of the yielding quality of the rubber, the up-hill side of the foot

will compress and accommodate itself to the incline and allow the foot to remain on its base. This is accomplished without complicated mechanical lateral articulation.

The spring mattress not only forces the parts of the foot back to their proper shape, but obviates the exertion required to operate the antiquated articulated wooden foot.

The impression that one receives on the new spring-mattress foot is both pleasant and agreeable. This is especially the case to one who has worn an artificial leg with wooden articulating foot.

It can readily be seen that any motion in the ankle that cannot be controlled by the will must be mechanical in appearance as well as in action. The approach to nature is made more positive by their omission.

It is the experienced man, the man who has experimented with many kinds of artificial limbs, who is capable of appreciating the

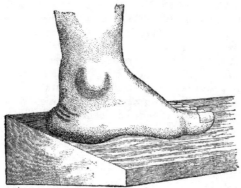

A. A. MARKS, N. Y.

Cut B 4.

principles involved in the rubber foot. He comprehends the reason why the wearers of artificial limbs with rubber feet walk further, faster, and with less fatigue, than those walking on ankle-jointed wooden feet.

The contrast between the two kinds is most striking in running. With the rubber as with the natural foot the entire plantar surface is never on the ground. It is the heel-and-toe touch to the ground that distinguishes the walker from the runner. This is extremely difficult with the ankle-jointed foot. When standing the immovably attached rubber foot furnishes a large base on which to balance; hence, a man with two artificial legs with immovably attached feet can stand restfully and safely without assuming awkward and unnatural positions, for he is not required to maintain his equilibrium on a point.

The rubber foot with spring mattress provides the laborer a substantial substitute with which to support and brace himself when working at the bench, on the road, on the farm, or at whatever occupation he may be engaged. There are no uncertain or treacherous movements to hamper him or make his position uncertain.

A painter who wears a Marks rubber foot says he can climb a ladder, stand on a scaffold, balance himself at any elevation with absolute safety. With an ankle-joint leg he would feel tottlish, and, when on his ladder, would have to depend more on the grasp of his hands than on his foot; but, with the rubber foot, his base is substantial and reliable.

A farmer who toils in the field can plod along over stony or muddy ground on a rubber foot with safety. The accumulation of mud on his shoes does not cause his toe to drop and trip him. Uneven surfaces will not throw him from his balance or violently jar his stump. We have thousands of testimonials on these points.

CONTRASTS.—There are two kinds of rubber feet. One is known as the sponge rubber foot; and the other as the pneumatic rubber foot. We will endeavor to make clear the difference between them.

When rubber is cured so that it possesses a great number of small air cells, the same as a sponge, it is called sponge rubber, and a foot made in this way is known as a sponge rubber foot.

A foot made of a sheet of rubber cast into the shape of a foot, possessing one or a limited number of large chambers into which air is pumped until sufficient pressure is obtained to maintain shape and possess resiliency is called a pneumatic foot.

THE SPONGE RUBBER FOOT.—Is composed of a vast number of cells, each charged with air created by the volatilization of a chemical while the rubber is being vulcanized. Each cell is surrounded by a wall of rubber possessing a sustaining power sufficient to maintain itself should it become deflated. In fact, if all the cells become deflated the foot would keep its shape on account of the presence of the sustaining walls, therefore the shape and resilience of the sponge rubber foot are not dependent upon the air in the cells.

THE PNEUMATIC FOOT.—Having but a limited number of large air chambers into which compressed air is forced, is wholly dependent upon the presence and retention of the compressed air for its stability. The sponge rubber spring-mattress foot receives no injury from puncture. The pneumatic foot will collapse and lose its sustaining power the moment the air chamber is penetrated. A protruding nail or peg in a shoe will puncture a pneumatic foot and put it out of service until the puncture is patched and the foot pumped up again with air.

The sponge rubber spring-mattress foot never has to be recharged with air.

THE WOOD FOOT.—Is now somewhat antiquated. It no longer has the merit it was formerly thought to possess—the rubber foot has practically supplanted it: The wood foot is articulated at the ankle and at the toes. The mechanical methods employed in its manufacture are as numerous as the makers who supply them. Nearly every maker has a method of his own, yet all are essentially the same. Some admit of a large range of ankle articulation, while others limit it so that there is but very slight motion. Some have side motion; others, equally as conscientious, condemn that motion and employ only front and back motion. Being convinced by most careful study and experimentation that an artificial leg is improved in proportion to the abridgment of its mechanical movements, we dissuade all from using the side motion. Some manufacturers employ rubber for springs in the ankle and toes; others prefer steel. One method has little advantage over the other.

THE ANKLE-JOINT RUBBER FOOT.—Cut B 5 represents an ankle-jointed rubber foot after our preferred plan. Cut B 6 represents

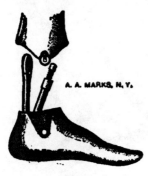 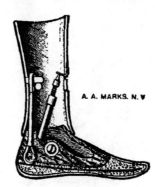

Cut B 5.   Cut B 6.

the ankle articulation in sectional view. The axis on which the foot moves consists of a bolt that passes through the foot at the ankle, connected with steel strips riveted to the lower sides of the leg. A steel spiral compression spring, one end of which is placed in a cylinder and the other, receiving a piston, is placed in the ankle in such manner as to act on the rear part of the foot, impinging against the front interior part of the socket, forcing the heel downward and the front of the foot upward. The articulation at the ankle is limited by the check cord placed in the rear. It is made of the strongest flexible material. This method of articulation can be used with wooden feet as well as rubber ones. When rubber is used it is not necessary to have a mechanical articulation at the base of the toes as the rubber itself will furnish that motion. Cut B 7 represents the ankle at extension, the foot flat on the ground when the leg is thrown forward and weight applied. Cut B 8 represents the ankle at flexion and weight applied to the toes.

THE FELT FOOT.—Is so seldom used that it is only referred to here in order to make our descriptions complete. Its use is to be strongly condemned. Felt possesses no stability. It is an absorbent of moisture and lacks resiliency, and is therefore wanting in the most essential qualities that should characterize the material used in the construction of an artificial foot.

ANKLE JOINTS WHEN PREFERRED.—While many years of observation and study have convinced us that the best results are obtained from artificial legs with rubber feet rigidly attached, it is nevertheless true that some persons form prejudices that cannot be removed even by the most logical arguments. Another class, who may be put in the same group, are those who, for a long period, have worn artificial limbs with articulating ankles; and have become so inured to them that a change, no matter how beneficial it might ultimately prove, would subject them to annoyance. We care not to antagonize those who think and feel this way; we are therefore prepared

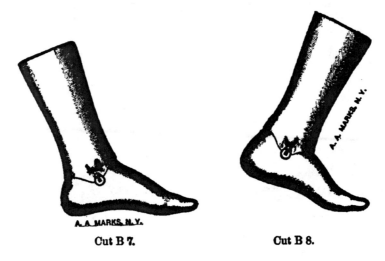

Cut B 7.   Cut B 8.

to construct artificial legs for them that are similar in construction to those they have worn and have become accustomed to.

We frequently hear of persons who are inclined to patronize us on account of the reputability of the house, but who hesitate in doing so on account of their doubts as to whether they themselves would make a success with artificial legs without ankle articulations. The idea of the rubber foot is acceptable, but rigidity at the ankle is doubtful. The element of doubt hinders their entering into any experiment the success of which is entirely at their risk.

We are disposed to meet any such person on a basis of equity and will furnish him with an artificial leg with rubber foot rigidly attached at the ankle with the understanding that, if after reasonable trial he feels that he would prefer the ankle joint, we will apply one for him without extra charge.

As we regard rubber feet rigidly attached at the ankle better for general purposes, we make limbs that way unless otherwise instructed.

Prices are the same whether rubber feet are permanently attached or made to articulate, whether feet are of wood, metal, or rubber.

CHAPTER III

PARTIAL FEET AMPUTATIONS

SINGLE-TOE AMPUTATIONS.—The loss of a single toe, particularly if it be the great one, may or may not be the cause of inconvenience and discomfort, yet the application of an artificial part is often found necessary, both as an aid in walking and as a protection to the amputated surface.

If one or more of the interplaced toes are removed and the hiatus has been filled up by the union of the adjacent surfaces, there can be no gain whatever in applying artificial ones. If the great toe (see Cut C 1) or the small toe be removed, and the am-

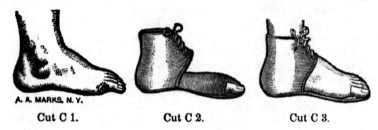

A. A. MARKS, N. Y.

Cut C 1.   Cut C 2.   Cut C 3.

putated surface is tender and painful to the touch, an appliance similar to that represented in Cut C 2 can be advantageously applied.

This appliance consists of a duplicate of the removed part, made of suitable material and secured to a plate shaped as the sole of the foot. It is held to the foot by an incasement of leather, laced down the front; when applied it is ready for the shoe, as shown in Cut C 3. This simple arrangement protects the amputated surface, assists in walking, fills the shoe, and prevents unsightly wrinkles in the leather.

AMPUTATIONS AT BASE OF TOES.—It is necessary to apply an artificial part when all the toes have been removed, as shown in Cut C 4. It must be so constructed that it can be held in place and avoid pressure on the scarred surface. Shoes stuffed with cotton or with pieces of cork should never be used; such expedients, having no support on the under sides, will eventually encroach on the amputated surfaces and permit the shoe to bend near the ends of the stumps.

An appliance illustrated in Cut C 5 is suitable for such an amputation; it is shown applied in Cut C 6. It can be made of wood or metal as may be required, and shaped to receive the foot in a comfortable manner; tender points are protected by recesses provided for them. Cut C 6 shows this apparatus applied and ready for the shoe. Usually the mate to the shoe worn on the natural foot can be used without alteration; in cases where more room is

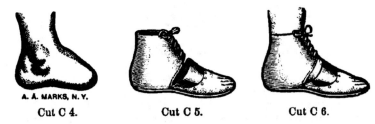

A. A. MARKS, N. Y.

Cut C 4.   Cut C 5.   Cut C 6.

needed, almost any shoemaker can supply it by ripping off part of the upper and substituting a larger piece.

INSTEP AMPUTATIONS.—These are termed tarso-metatarsal and medio-tarsal by the surgical profession, and are frequently designated by the names of the surgeons who first performed them, as Chopart, Lisfranc, Hays, Hancock, and many others. These amputations are performed with the object of sacrificing as little of the foot as possible, and retaining the heel and a part of the foot as a base on which the patient is supposed to be able to walk or stand. Although a person with the front part of his foot removed may be able to get about with an ordinary shoe, it is not long before he discovers that something is lacking and his locomotion impeded by the absence of the removed part. He may pack the vacancy in his shoe with cotton, cork, or other material, and may re-enforce the sole with a steel plate; but he soon finds that only partial relief has been obtained, and that there is an imperative demand for a substitute for the ball of the foot which will enable him to rise on and elevate his heel from the ground. Something is needed having great strength and that can be firmly secured to the remaining part of foot and leg.

The construction of artificial feet for this class of amputations has taxed the ingenuity of artificial-limb-makers for many years. The absence of space between the bottom of the heel and the floor presented an obstacle to the construction of a helpful and durable appliance until aluminum was employed. It may be useful to review some of the devices used for such cases.

Cut C 7 represents a stump resulting from a partial foot amputation.

ILL-ADVISED PROTHESIS.—Cut C 8 represents the way in which many manufacturers have endeavored to supply the want. The appliance consists of a leather shoe inclosing the stump and part of the ankle, the front of which is made of wood, rubber, or cork with a metal plate at the base, running from heel to toe, calculated to make the sole firm and unyielding at the ball. This apparatus gives a natural appearance to the amputated member, but fails to support the wearer in a helpful or substantial way. The stump will soon crowd forward, coming into unpleasant contact with the appliance; the steel plate will bend or break and the shoe will yield where the stump terminates, creasing the shoe and making it rocker-shaped; consequently it utterly fails in supplying the want, because of the lack of firmness with which it is held to the remaining part; the heel, moreover, will yield to the constantly contracting tendency of the tendo-Achilles and become displaced.

Cut C 9 represents another ill-advised apparatus. It consists of a sheet of metal formed to receive the remaining plantar surface

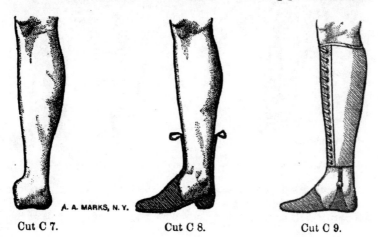

A. A. MARKS, N. Y.

Cut C 7. Cut C 8. Cut C 9.

of the foot; bent up on either side, hinged at the ankle to steel straps thus providing a joint for ankle articulation; the steel straps run up the sides of the leg and are held in position by a leather corset, shaped to inclose the leg. The front of the metal sole is secured to a part of a foot. The main objection to this device is the insecurity of the attachment; weight applied to the ball of the foot will cause the ankle to flex and permit the amputated surface of the stump to rub against either the front or the bottom plate, causing abrasions; a heel cord placed at the back connecting the leg section with the foot plate will not be effective in holding the appliance in its proper position at all times and checking the action of the ankle articulation at the proper angle.

OBJECTIONS.—A glance will show that the legs illustrated in Cuts C 8 and C 9 must prove inadequate. When weight is applied to the ball of the foot the heel of the artificial part will remain on the ground, while the heel of the stump will lift away. The wearer will walk flat-footed and will press the delicate cicatrized surface against the attachment. These conditions will not only cause suffering but defeat the object of the artificial foot.

It might appear that an appliance constructed on the plan shown in Cut C 5 could be secured so firmly to the remaining part of a Chopart stump as to enable the wearer to rise on the ball. If this were possible the method of treatment would be greatly simplified; unfortunately, however, the severity of the compression needful to hold the appliance in place when weight is thrown on the ball, will stop the flow of blood in the heel, causing great pain, endangering the health of the entire leg.

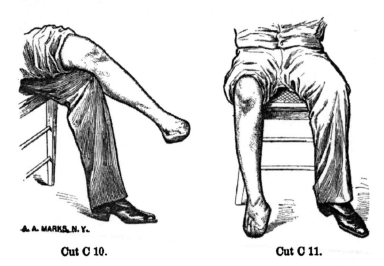

Cut C 10.   Cut C 11.

It is important to emphasize the fact that it is absolutely useless to apply any form of foot to a partial foot stump unless the artificial part is held so firmly that the wearer may rise on the ball of the

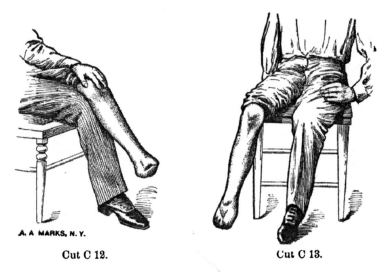

Cut C 12.   Cut C 13.

foot, and not only support his weight while in that position but carry such additional weight and resist such strains as his habits or occupation demand.

Cut C 10 represents an amputation a little forward of the instep.

The wisdom of the application of apparatus C 5 in this case is doubtful. It might prove adequate in the case of a person who does little walking and no lifting, and who places little demand on the front part of the foot; but for a laboring man, who has to lift and carry articles of weight, it would be a disappointment. It will be better considered, therefore, among instep amputations that require the placing and distribution of the strain above the ankle joint.

Cuts C 11, C 12, C 13, and C 14 show instep amputations after the Lisfranc, Hancock, and Chopart methods. Cut C 15 shows an

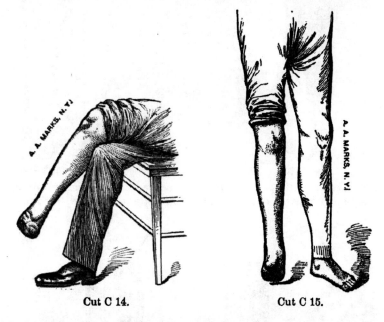

Cut C 14.   Cut C 15.

amputation of the instep with all the tarsals removed, a part of the astragalus and the entire os-calcis retained and kept in their normal relations, a very unusual occurrence.

The remaining plantar surfaces of each of these amputations are of a character to permit the application of the weight of the wearer on them.

Cuts C 16 and C 17 show instep amputations in which the heels have retracted slightly, but not so much so as to prohibit the application of weight to the remaining plantar surfaces.

PRACTICAL PROTHESIS.—The only artificial limb that has ever been devised that adequately meets the needs of any of the above instep amputations is illustrated in Cut C 18. A half leg, or front, including the core of the foot, is made of aluminum, without articulation at the ankle. The rear half is made of leather, shaped to incase the leg and the aluminum shell and hold the appliance in place, as shown in Cut C 19. The sole of the foot, including the toes, is made of rubber with a spring mattress as described in Chapter II. Comfortable bearings are provided by proper fittings

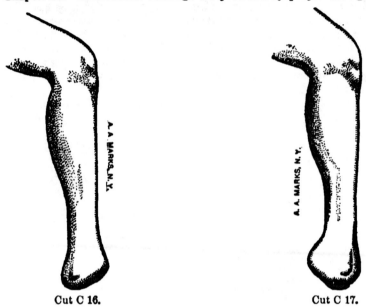

Cut C 16.   Cut C 17.

and suitable linings. The pressure needed to secure firmness is distributed over the entire leg from the ankle to the knee; with this

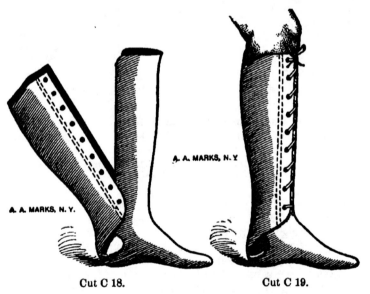

Cut C 18.   Cut C 19.

leg the wearer can rise on the ball of the foot without endangering the amputated surfaces or straining the ankle joint. The shinbone is protected by the aluminum shell on the front, and, when dressed, presents an appearance very close to nature. When there is a tendency for the heel to retract, the leather sheath at the back is re-enforced with metal shaped to hold the heel down to its proper place.

This artificial leg can be worn without inconvenience or pain. The wearer walks gracefully, striking the heel first, then rolling on

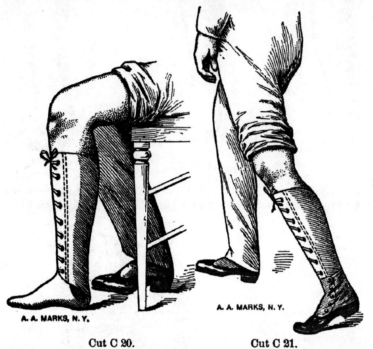

Cut C 20.   Cut C 21.

the sole until the ball is reached, and then rising on the ball he receives assistance in walking. Cut C 20 shows the leg applied and the wearer seated. Cut C 21 shows the leg applied with the shoe on and the wearer walking with the weight on the ball of the foot, similar to the position taken by the natural foot when in the act of throwing the body forward.

The method of meeting instep amputations, as just described, possesses many merits aside from those to which attention has been called.

RETRACTED HEELS.—Cuts C 22, C 23, C 24, show amputations in which the heels are retracted so that the amputated surfaces are directly under the legs, where the weight must be applied if the bearings are to be at the ends. These are unfortunate conditions. An artificial leg cannot be applied to a stump under such conditions that will permit any pressure on the scarred extremity; the weight, therefore, must be placed immediately below the knee or about the thigh.

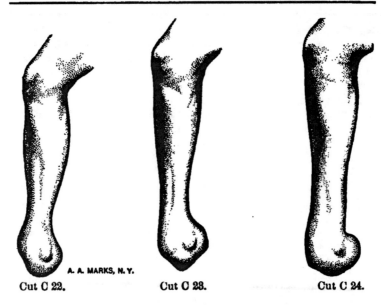

Cut C 22.　　　　Cut C 23.　　　　Cut C 24.

A limb constructed on the plan shown in Cut C 25 is adaptable for some stumps with retracted heels; the rear half is made of

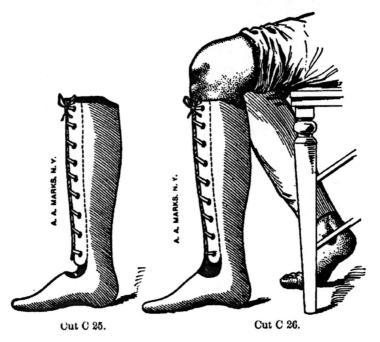

Cut C 25.　　　　　　　　Cut C 26.

metal, the front of leather, capable of being laced. This permits close fittings about the heel and tends to force it back to its proper position. If the sides of the leg are sloping, the fitting can be such as to apply all the weight on the leg immediately below the knee. Cut C 26 shows the leg applied and the wearer seated.

If the sides of a leg do not slope sufficiently to prevent settling into the artificial leg socket, it is necessary to introduce an annular top and possibly knee joints and thigh support. The annular top can be applied to a leg constructed as described; it then has the appearance of Cut C 27. It can also be applied to a leg constructed

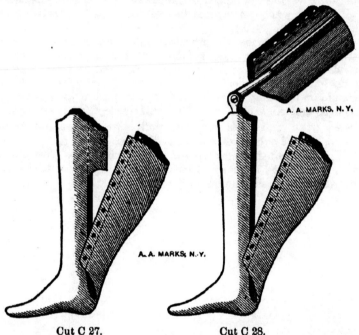

Cut C 27.   Cut C 28.

on the plan of C 25. Knee joints and thigh support can likewise be applied to a leg constructed on the plan of either C 18 or C 25. Cut C 28 shows such additions applied to C 18 leg. When the annular top is employed the support is calculated to be localized immediately below the knee. The leg is opened from the rear and the stump inserted; the annular top is laced firmly and the leather sheath is pulled over the entire apparatus and laced in front. When the knee joint and thigh support are required, as shown in Cut C 28, the lower section of the leg is made of aluminum, with the rear sheath of leather. The thigh part incases the natural thigh and holds it with sufficient firmness to carry the weight above the knee and so prevent the leg from slipping in the socket.

ALUMINUM SOCKETS.—The utilization of aluminum in the construction of artificial legs for instep amputations is especially advantageous. It can be worked to a very slight thickness, thus adding but little to the diameters of the large stump that it incases. A wood socket would require a thickness of at least half an inch on each side, thus making the leg conspicuously bulky and objectionable.

During the past few years we have made many experiments looking to the general application of aluminum in the construction of artificial limbs for upper amputations, but have met with disappointment except in ankle-joint and partial-foot amputations. The characteristics of aluminum are low specific gravity and comparative strength. Its weight is the least of all metals (one-quarter that of silver). Its strength is comparable with that of copper. It will not corrode when exposed to fresh water or to a moist atmosphere.

We desire to correct the prevalent impression often expressed in the remark that aluminum is "lighter than cork and stronger than steel." As a matter of fact aluminum will sink in water, whereas cork or wood will float; it is therefore heavier and although aluminum is strong, it has but a fractional part of the strength of straight-grained wood. Its use in artificial legs is, therefore, narrowed down to sockets for long and large stumps, where the minimizing of bulk is an important feature.

We hold United States patents on artificial limbs with aluminum sockets, and if we could make satisfactory use of that metal for general purposes we would unhesitatingly do so.

CHAPTER IV

ANKLE-JOINT AMPUTATIONS

TIBIO-TARSAL STUMPS.—Amputations through the ankle articulations with or without the maleoli, flaps formed of heel tissues, provide stumps that can be fitted with artificial legs in an advantageous way. Surgeons call these amputations tibio-tarsal or Symes, and if the os-calcis is retained and secured at the extremity of the tibia, it is known as Pirogoff's.

Usually ankle-joint amputations produce stumps that admit of weight being taken on their extremities. If cicatrices are on the

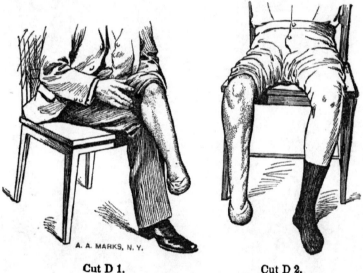

Cut D 1.   Cut D 2.

bearing surfaces or nerve complications are present, they become non-end-bearing and artificial limbs must be applied that permit no pressure or contact on the tender extremities.

END-BEARING.—Cuts D 1 to D 6 show end-bearing tibio-tarsal stumps, with flaps favorable for the application of pressure and with cicatrices well away from the bearing surfaces. Cut D 7 illustrates an artificial leg suitable for any of these types; Cut D 8 shows it applied with the wearer seated. Cut D 9 shows a Pirogoff stump with a suitable leg, patterned after style D 7. Cut D 10 shows the leg applied and the foot covered with stocking and shoe. Cut D 11 shows the wearer fully dressed. In walking his step is

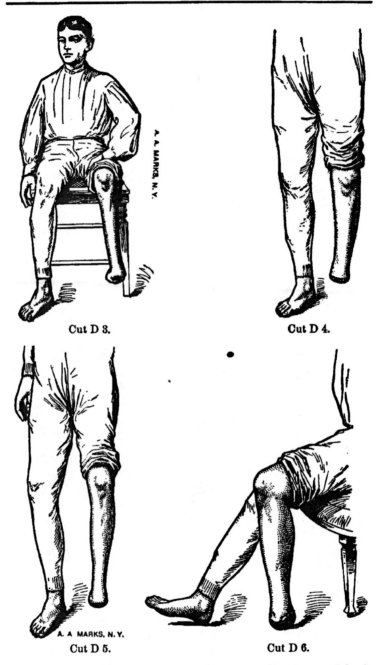

Cut D 3.   Cut D 4.

Cut D 5.   Cut D 6.

graceful, the foot imitates nature, there is no limping, and he is amply equipped to engage in any occupation, even the most laborious.

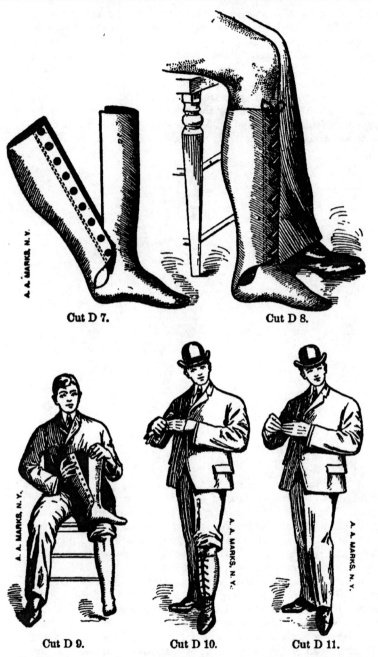

Cut D 7.   Cut D 8.

Cut D 9.   Cut D 10.   Cut D 11.

CONSTRUCTION OF SUITABLE ARTIFICIAL LEG.—The construction of
D 7 style is simple.   The front, which is the resisting part, and the
core of the foot, are cast in aluminum, the interior surface being

formed to receive the anterior surface of the leg from the knee down. It is so fitted that pressure will be distributed over the front area, the shin bone and tender parts of the leg being protected and not allowed to bear pressure. The rear part is of leather, shaped to fit the calf and the back of the leg. It is secured at its lower end to the aluminum socket, and when the stump is in place it incases the whole apparatus from the knee down, holding the leg in place with firmness, the pressure being regulated by lacing. The foot is of sponge rubber, re-enforced with spring mattress as explained in Chapter II. Weight is taken by the end of

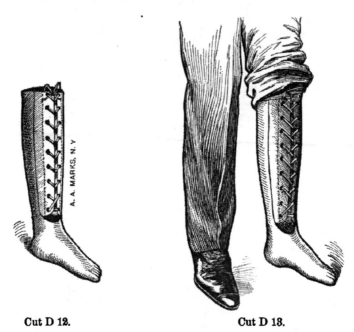

Cut D 12.   Cut D 13.

the stump resting on a surface of proper shape, covered by a suitable pad. The strains resulting from rising on the ball of the foot are not permitted to come on the stump; they are distributed over the leg, about the sides of the shin from the knee to the ankle. A stocking and shoe are drawn over the foot, and the apparatus is a counterpart in appearance to the sound leg.

This style of leg for ankle-joint amputation has received the most complimentary comments; it has given great satisfaction to those who have worn it; and it has been quite generally adopted.

Occasionally conditions require the construction of a limb in a manner reverse to that just described, the stump is admitted from the front instead of the rear. In such cases limbs are built on the plan illustrated in Cut D 12. The construction is practically the same as D 7, except that the metal socket is placed at the back and the leather lace in front. The shin bone is protected by a padded loose fly-piece over which the lacing passes. Cut D 13 illustrates the leg applied.

If the end of the stump is small and has no prominences on the side, the socket and core of the foot, which are integrally one piece, are carved from a block of wood the grain of which curves on the line of greatest strains. When the end of the stump is large and it is desired to incase it in a socket of minimum thickness, aluminum must be employed for reasons given.

PARTIALLY END-BEARING.—If only a part of the weight of the wearer can be borne on the end of the stump the top of the socket must be made annular and fitted so that it will impinge against the sloping part of the leg below the knee. Cuts D 14 and D 16

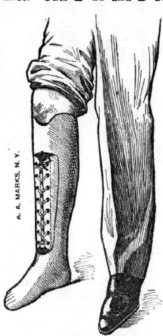

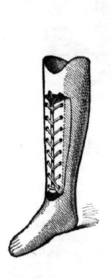

| Cut D 14. | Cut D 15. |

illustrate suitable legs for the same and Cuts D 15 and D 17 show them applied. It is obvious that a stump, being inserted from the top of the socket of either, will not enter further than the top of the socket will permit, and this is just far enough to limit pressure on the end or to avoid it altogether. When pressure can be taken on the end, it is regulated by the thickness of the pad placed in the bottom of the socket on which the end of the stump rests.

A socket that admits the stump from the front, as in Cuts D 12 and D 14, is objectionable when the end of the stump is very large. The material necessary for strength is on the sides of the stump and increases the diameter of the ankle. It also affords but little protection to the sharp or sensitive shin bone. Styles D 7 and D 16 are not open to this objection, but give a smooth, unbroken

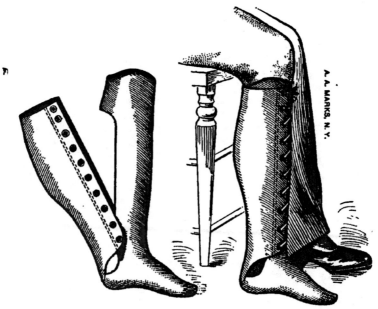

Cut D 16.   Cut D 17.

front, which can be neatly dressed; they are lighter and stronger than D 12 or D 14, because the strain resulting from rising on the ball of the foot is carried forward from the point of contact to a point on line with the front of the leg: and as this point is usually halfway between the ball and the heel the strain is one-half of that applied in D 12, which throws the strain from the ball to the rear of the heel. For this reason the material on the sides of the stump and on the rear of the leg has to be as thick again as the material on the sides and front of the D 7. Hence the difference in weight.

SENSITIVE ENDS.—There are tibio-tarsal stumps that are so sensitive at the extremities that no pressure whatever can be tolerated either on the ends or at the sides of the ends. Notwithstanding this condition, artificial limbs can be applied that will be helpful and comfortable. Cuts D 18, D 19, and D 20 represent stumps of this character.

If the surfaces immediately below the knee are sufficiently sloping to offer resistance, D 14 or D 16 leg can be used, the pressure being placed on the sides of the upper half of the leg immediately below the knee. The stump from calf down hangs in space.

When a leg and stump are nearly uniform in size, the sides being parallel or nearly so, an artificial leg with knee joints and thigh piece must be used. Cut D 21 represents a leg suitable for such a case. Cut D 22 shows the same with knee flexed and sheath un-

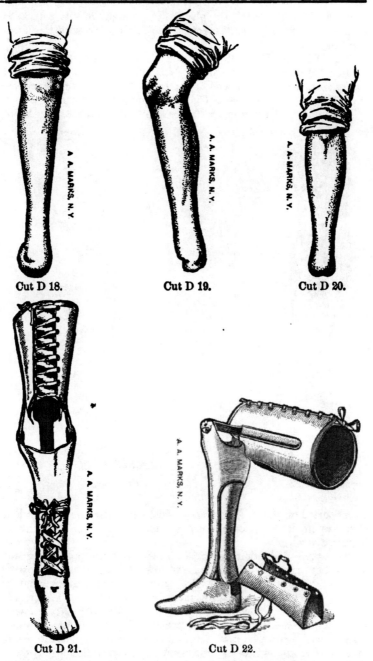

Cut D 18.   Cut D 19.   Cut D 20.

Cut D 21.   Cut D 22.

laced. The lower section is made of wood or aluminum, as the conditions of the stump demand. The rubber foot is attached in the usual way, and the leather sheath passes from the rear to the front, holding the stump in place. The weight of the wearer is supported by side joints connecting the thigh parts with the lower portions.

Cuts D 23 and D 24 illustrate the front and side views of a leg constructed in a similar manner. It is fitted to receive the leg and stump from the front instead of the rear; it contains no important advantage in construction, but is preferred by some persons.

Side joints and thigh supports are essential when stumps cannot

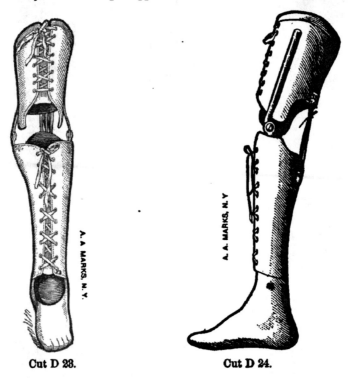

Cut D 23.   Cut D 24.

be supported on the sloping surfaces just below the knees, and when they are liable to become sensitive and irritable on account of impaired vitality.

PEG LEGS.—Ankle-joint stumps should never use peg legs except when they need disciplining or shrinking. Some stumps with extremely sensitive ends, on which pressure cannot be immediately applied, give promise of improvement in course of time. There are also stumps that are œdematous—made up with soft, flaccid tissue which will pass away in a brief period. In such cases, an inexpensive peg leg can be used to advantage. One may stump about on a peg leg applied to a stump reaching to the ankle joint, much the same as one who uses a peg leg on an upper amputation, but, having no foot, its functions are limited to that of a support.

CHAPTER V

BELOW-KNEE AMPUTATIONS

LONG TIBIAL STUMPS.—An amputation at any point above the ankle and below the knee produces a tibial stump, so termed by the surgical profession, because the tibia or shin bone has partly been saved.

ENLARGED NON-END-BEARING.—Cut E 1 illustrates a stump reaching close to the ankle joint. The extremity, as is usual in long stumps, is poorly protected and incapable of bearing pressure, and,

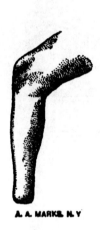

A. A. MARKS. N. Y.

Cut E 1.

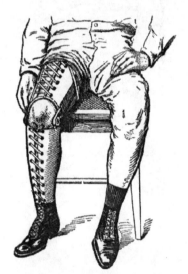

Cut E 2.

on account of a slight enlargment at the end, an artificial leg must be made so that the stump can be placed in the socket from the front or rear instead of being inserted at the top. Cut E 2 represents an artificial leg especially adapted to stumps of this description; it is shown applied and the wearer seated. It has a socket that incases the rear half of the stump, with a front of leather that can be laced. The rubber foot with spring mattress is constructed as described in Chapter II, and at the top of the socket are steel joints connecting the thigh supporter. The fitting of the leg avoids any weight or pressure on the extremity of the stump or near the end, and no pressure is applied at any point below the junction of the middle and lower thirds. Above this it is graduated

45

to the knee, where the greatest amount of pressure is applied, the interior sloping surface below the knee carrying most of the weight. The anterior prominences of the shin bone and the exterior prominence of the fibula are given ample room, so that no contact is applied; the interior sloping surfaces below the knee carry most of the weight, the supporter above the knee carrying its share.

No Pressure at the Popliteal Space.—It is most important to avoid pressure at the back of the knee in long stumps. The popliteal space is the vascular area of the leg, and any undue pressure will interfere with the circulation and impoverish or strangulate the end of the stump.

The absence of ankle articulation in a leg for a long tibial stump affords an opportunity to give ample space for the end without

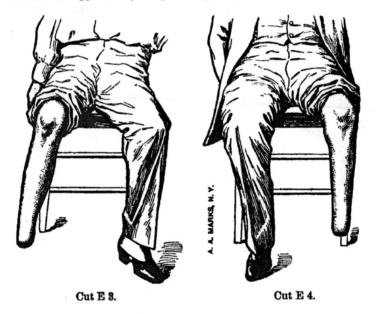

Cut E 3.	Cut E 4.

visibly increasing the external dimensions of the ankle. The rubber foot with spring mattress and yielding heel and toe provides every requisite for easy, lifelike, and noiseless walking without complicated connections. The absence of such connecting parts avoids the necessity of making the leg an inch or two longer than the natural one as is often necessary to obtain space for ankle mechanism used in other systems.

Artificial legs with wooden articulating feet for stumps that reach to any point in the lower third of the leg are impracticable. The ends of long tibial stumps are sensitive, easily irritated, and poorly nourished, and the slightest contact will cause abrasion, frequently necessitating reamputations,.

Tapering Stumps.—Cuts E 3, E 4, E 5, and E 6 illustrate long tibial stumps. Legs for such amputations must be constructed so

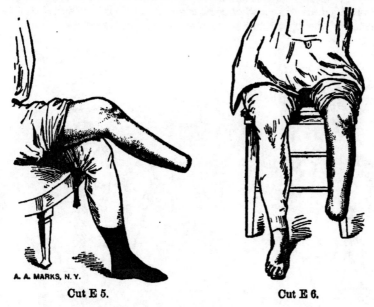

Cut E 5.   Cut E 6.

there will be ample room for the extremities.   In other words, the
ends are suspended in space.   As these stumps are tapering to the

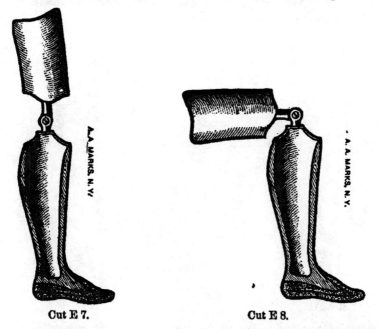

Cut E 7.   Cut E 8.

ends they can be inserted from the tops of the sockets.   The socket
is hollowed out near the bottom of the heel and an abundance of

room provided, allowing a wholesome circulation of air; the exterior diameters of the leg are not large enough to be conspicuous.   The

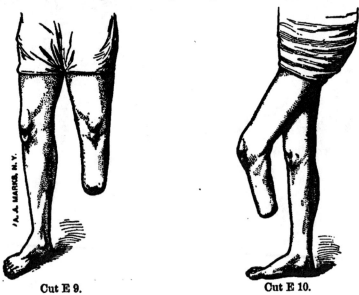

Cut E 9.   Cut E 10.

leg socket and foot core are connected by an aluminum sheath riveted to each part in the most secure way.

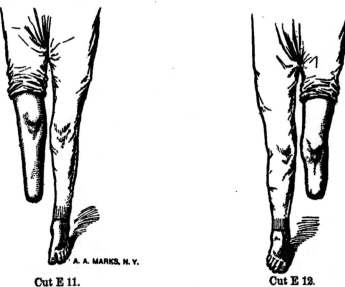

Cut E 11.   Cut E 12.

The rubber foot is attached to the core and the leg is finished so the exudations from the extremity of the stump cannot possibly impair the strength of the connected parts.

Cuts E 7 and E 8 show sectional views of a leg for a long tibial stump; the foot and leg parts are so secured that they

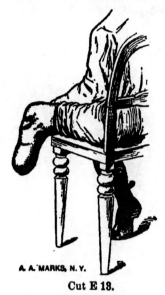

Cut E 13.

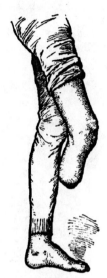

Cut E 14.

are practically one. This method of construction admits of

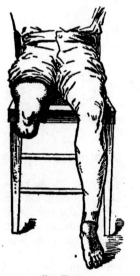

Cut E 15.

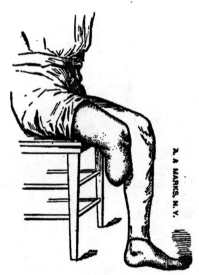

Cut E 16.

excavating the socket well into the foot so as to provide ample air space. Substantial legs for such stumps cannot be made

with ankle articulations, for cords, springs and bolts require
space needed by the stumps. As metal becomes corroded by the
exudations of the stumps, wood is the only material which will
withstand these destructive agencies.

ORDINARY AND SHORT TIBIAL STUMPS.—No difficulties attend the
fitting of an artificial leg to a tibial stump reaching to any point

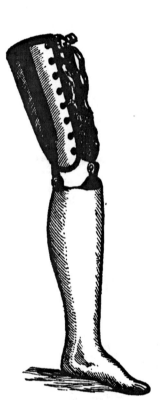

Cut E 17.

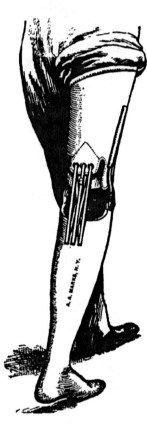

Cut E 18.

between the junction of the middle and lower thirds and the knee,
when the knee joint is mobile to not less than two-thirds of the
normal range. Cuts E 9 to E 16 are typical below-knee stumps of
a variety of lengths and conditions relative to flaps, cicatrices, etc.
The location of the cicatrices and the character of the flaps have
little importance in non-end-bearing stumps.

ARTIFICIAL LEG FOR TIBIAL STUMP.—A leg suitable for a stump of
two inches or more in length, with the knee articulating through a
range of 90 degrees or more, is shown in Cut E 17. Cut E 18 shows
it applied with the wearer standing. Cut E 19 shows it with the
wearer seated. The action of the knee joint is clearly presented.

CONSTRUCTION.—The leg consists of four parts: the foot, the leg, which fills the space between the foot and the knee; the knee joints, and the thigh piece or that part that incases the natural thigh. As the foot has been explained in Chapter II it now remains to describe in detail the other parts.

SOCKET.—The socket that receives the stump is made from willow or basswood, which is excavated to accommodate the stump. Bearings are permitted at places of toleration. No pressure whatever is put on the vascular parts of the stump or on sensitive or prominent bones. The end of the stump is usually required to hang

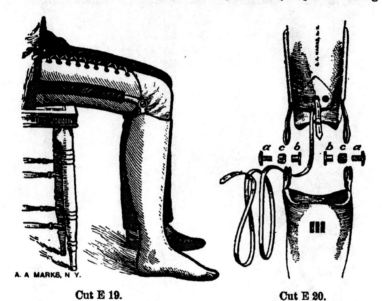

A. A MARKS, N Y.

Cut E 19.   Cut E 20.

free in space. The exterior of the leg is shaped to as near the natural form as the stump will admit. It is strongly banded and covered. The surface is enameled with a waterproof preparation having a soft flesh tint. Knee joints are of the ginglymoid pattern, and as recently improved have very durable wearing surfaces. The thigh piece is made of substantial leather shaped to the contours of the thigh.

KNEE CONNECTION.—Cut E 20 represents the upper section of the leg and the lower section of the thigh piece, with the knee joints disconnected at their articulations; *aa* are the screws that hold the bolts *bb* in place; *cc* are the bushings that work on the bolts and receive the wear; a lacing is used to regulate the action of the knee. The mechanical parts of the knee joints are completely illustrated in Cut E 21.

STEEL JOINTS.—Side joints, sometimes called hinge or ginglymoid joints, are used in legs for amputations below the knees. They are more durable and substantial when one of the parts is placed between the lips of the other and the two connected with bolts and screws.

It is unmechanical and not lasting to place one section of a joint by the side of the other, holding them together by a screw, as is done by some manufacturers. Such joints wear irregularly side-wise and have a wabbling motion after limited service. This would not occur if the lateral strains on the upper sections could be kept the same at all times; but lateral pressure, causing unequal wear at the bearings, is brought about by contracting the thigh by lacing, in order to compress an emaciated thigh or distending it to

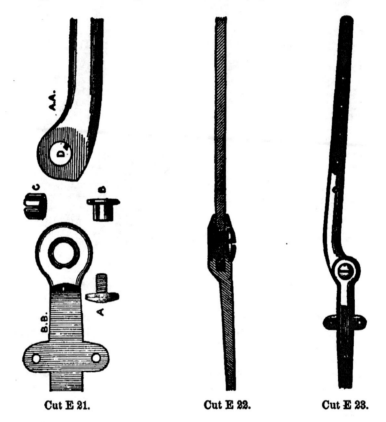

Cut E 21.   Cut E 22.   Cut E 23.

accommodate an enlarged one. These difficulties are only avoided by having one of the elements of the joints work between the lips of the other.

The greatest wear on any joint is on the bolt that holds the parts together, and as the attrition is the greatest when the wearer's weight is directly over the knee and becomes less as the knee is flexed, the bolt must necessarily wear irregularly. As the wearing surface on the bolt was formerly limited to the thickness of the section that worked on it, the wear was necessarily very rapid.

The object of the improved joint is to increase the wearing surface as much as possible and to make the wearing parts independent and removable. They can then be highly tempered and the non-wearing parts left untempered, so that the supporting parts will not become friable.

The wearing surfaces are increased more than double. They cover the entire surface of the bolt, and the inferior surfaces of the holes in the lips of the lower part. Cut E 21 shows the mechanism very clearly. AA is the upper part; BB the lower part; C is a long bushing which passes through the two lips of the lower part and the one of the upper; the lug D holds the bushing immovably fixed to the upper part. The bolt B passes through the long bushing and becomes immovably fixed to the lower part by means of a stop pin, which is fastened to the hub of the lower part, and fits a recess made in the head of the bolt. The screw A holds the bolt in place and clamps the joint.

A glance at the section, Cut E 22, will show how these parts work together. Every movement of the joint causes the long bushing to revolve about the surface of the bolt and in the lips of the lower part. This mechanism prevents any wear from taking place on either the upper or lower parts, and distributes what does take place over the entire area of the bolt. The bushing and bolt are made very hard, and can be removed and replaced with new ones at any time that may be desirable. Cut E 23 shows a side view of the entire joints and ready to be attached to the leg.

TEST.—A pair of these joints, subjected to a practical test equivalent to that of being worn by a man weighing two hundred pounds, walking an average distance of three miles every day for six consecutive years, failed to develop sufficient wear to cause noise. The joints are made from the most suitable steel, forged from solid material faced and slotted with absolute accuracy, drilled, reamed, and countersunk in templates, the parts being fitted to a nicety and thoroughly tested before being placed on a leg.

THIGH PART.—The thigh part of the leg is made of durable oak-tanned russet leather, formed to the shape of the thigh, and suitably lined inside. There are several methods by which it is made to compress the thigh; buckles and straps are sometimes used; metallic clamps are occasionally preferred; but the greatest number of limb-wearers find the lacing method the most satisfactory, as it permits uniform adjustments and is neat and durable.

LACING METHODS.—Cut E 24 shows the double-eyelet method. A row of eyelets is placed on each front edge, and a strong buckskin lacing passed through them. This method has been in vogue for many years and is still preferred by many wearers.

Cut E 25 shows the lacing system more generally used at the present time. A row of hooks is placed on one edge and a row of eyelets on the other. On removing the leg the loops of the lacing are simply slipped off the hooks, the string remaining in the eyelet holes. When the leg is put on, the loops are put over the hooks and the cord is tightly drawn. Some wearers wish hooks on each edge.

the same as on shoes. When this is wanted it should be specified
in the order.

Cut E 26 shows a device for rapid application. A row of studs
is placed on one edge of the thigh piece, and a row of eyelets on
the other; a separate piece of leather has also a row of eyelets and a

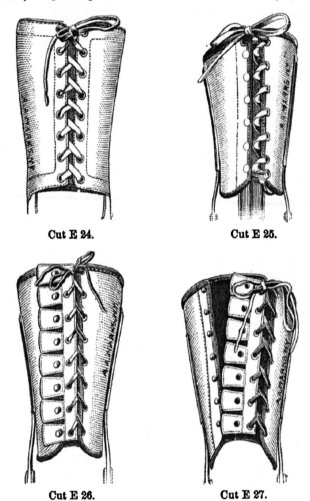

Cut E 24.   Cut E 25.

Cut E 26.   Cut E 27.

row of studs. This is laced to one side of the thigh piece and
buttoned to the other; the lacing can be adjusted once for all. On
removing the leg one side is unbuttoned, and the other remains
laced, as shown in Cut E 27.

CHECK STRAP.—The lacing at the back of the knee checks the
knee action and is regulated by the wearer. It is a very strong
leather thong, passing from the thigh piece to the leg part, as in
Cut E 20. The more the thong is tightened the less becomes the

motion in the knee, and the more weight will be placed on the ball of the foot and less at the heel.

The stump, in all cases, is inserted into the leg socket; the thigh piece is drawn around the thigh and laced tight enough to hold the leg firmly in place. The stump enters the socket comfortably. Bearings are only admitted about the sloping part immediately below the knee; the anterior surface of the tibia is always accommodated by a channel; the bony prominence of the fibula is provided for by a cavity; and the end of the stump hangs free in space, receiving no pressure whatever, either on the sides or at the end, except when conditions will permit.

SENSITIVE STUMPS.—In cases of extreme sensitiveness the weight can be carried entirely above the knee, and the stump is only

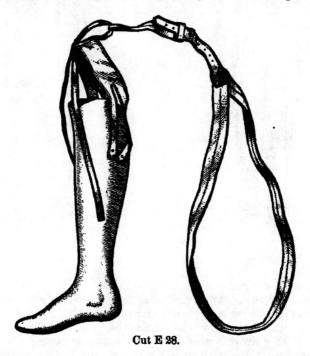

Cut E 28.

permitted to perform the function of moving the lower leg forward and backward.

NON-END-BEARING AND END-BEARING.—Weight can rarely be applied to the end of a tibial stump, and only when the end is protected by bone flap or periosteal flap and well covered with muscle tissue. When such favorable conditions exist an end-bearing pad is placed in the socket of the leg, the thickness of which is adjustable, so as to increase or decrease the amount of pressure on the extremity. The wearer, when dressed either with or without the end-bearing pad, is able to walk, run, sit, or lie down. Every posture will have the semblance of nature, every movement will be made with surprising naturalness. The loss of the natural leg is absolutely concealed, and the substitution by the artificial restores the wearer to his usefulness.

THIGHLESS LEGS.—Artificial legs for tibial stumps are sometimes made without knee joints and thigh pieces, dependence being

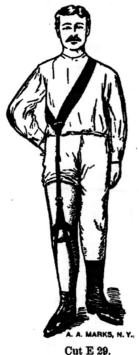

Cut E 29.

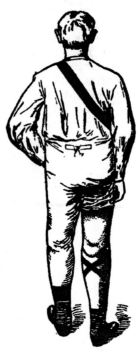

Cut E 30.

placed upon the socket when supporting the weight of the wearer, and resisting such lateral strains as may occasionally be brought upon the leg. Such a leg is shown in Cut E 28. From the knee down its construction is much the same as leg E 17. The socket is made of wood excavated to receive the stump properly. The foot is of sponge rubber with spring mattress, and the leg is covered substantially and finished in flesh-colored enamel. Straps attached to the leg in the region of the calf are made to pass around the thigh immediately above the knee cap. If these do not hold the leg firmly in place auxiliary straps are attached, to pass over one or both shoulders.

Some manufacturers advocate the use of thighless legs whether the stumps are long or short, and pay little attention to the character of the extremities. They attach more importance to the absence of thigh constriction than they do to the danger of abrasions on the stump or injury to the extremity.

While it is true that there are many cases in which thighless legs are applied and worn with evident satisfaction, it must be clear that the absence of a thigh supporter entails a sacrifice of efficiency and protection. Metal knee joints and thigh supporters perform the very important functions of protecting stumps, avoiding side strains, injuries from concussions, and the tearing of cicatrices. Cut E 29 shows a thighless leg applied, the wearer standing; Cut E 30 the rear view of the same, Cut E 31 the side view, and Cut E

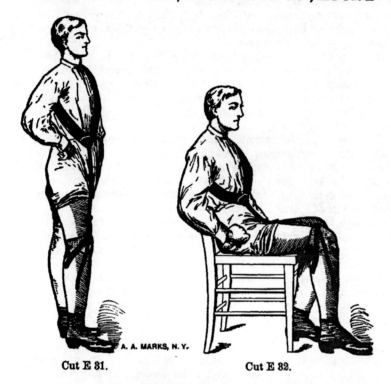

A. A. MARKS, N. Y.

Cut E 31.   Cut E 32.

32 the wearer seated. These cuts show the operations of the leg and the action of the suspenders.

DANGERS.—When the wearer is standing with his weight on an artificial leg of the thighless type the stump has to carry all his weight. This usually comes upon the sloping parts immediately below the knee. If the wearer makes a misstep and recovers himself by his artificial leg the stump will receive a strain; if he carries a heavy weight his stump must resist a force that tends to push it further into the socket; and unless the sides of the stump are sufficiently sloping to oppose this there will be danger of injury to the flap and cicatrix.

One of the chief objections to the thighless leg is the difficulty that arises when the stump changes in size, as it so often does. If the stump becomes emaciated the socket of the artificial leg must be filled up to compensate for the loss of flesh, and if the emaciation is not uniform there will be considerable difficulty in padding the inner surfaces of the socket so as to avoid pressure on delicate parts.

One should never experiment with the thighless leg unless the stump has been accustomed to wearing an artificial leg for a considerable length of time, and has become so thoroughly disciplined that further changes are not likely to occur. Those who insist on wearing thighless artificial legs, who have worn them from choice, and who have their stumps sufficiently disciplined will be accommodated in their wishes.

SLIP SOCKETS VERSUS WOOD SOCKETS.—Rival manufacturers have said and published much about the slip or sliding socket and considerable curiosity has been aroused among limb-wearers as to the merits of the idea. As the slip socket applies almost exclusively to artificial legs for tibial stumps, the subject may be introduced and discussed at this time.

We have given the matter much thought and subjected it to a most rigid investigation. We have, moreover, submitted the scheme to many tests and have conferred with several hundred persons who had worn slip sockets. Our investigations were planned to determine whether the scheme had sufficient merit to warrant us in adapting it to our work.

We have long been aware that a well-fitting socket of wood or any smooth hard material will never chafe the stump, even if the stump is permitted to move in it. On the other hand we have known that any socket made of a yielding material like leather will, from the constant pressure and heat of the stump, change in form and cease to be comfortable. Perspiration and other exudations from the stump have deteriorating effect on any material that permits absorption. All exudations from the stump becomes putrid in a very short time and cause offensive odors and bring effete matter in contact with the skin. This almost invariably infects the stump and causes unhealthy conditions. A hard highly polished surface is more pleasant for the stump than any form of soft yielding cushions.

The slip-socket idea is somewhat antiquated. In 1866 the United States Patent Office issued letters patent No. 55,645 to Daniel Gilson, covering the principle of the slip socket, consisting of a leather socket molded on a cast of the stump, then placed inside the artificial leg, and held in place by springs. Its object was to obviate the movement of the stump in the socket and to localize all the motion between the stump socket and the socket of the artificial leg. It was very soon found that the stump socket, being tightly held to the stump at all times, constricted the blood vessels and caused much trouble. The inventor, being conscientious, abandoned the manufacture of legs on that plan.

Quite recently, however, the slip-socket feature has been revived, and some insignificant modifications made on the original Gilson model, mainly in the mode of suspending the inner or slip socket. The idea has been extensively advertised and a considerable number put in use. We have records of many of these cases, and we feel it a duty to the maimed community to disclose the effects a slip socket has had on many stumps.

It must be remembered that in order to carry out the principle of the slip or sliding socket the stump must remain under constant pressure, great enough to avoid any motion or friction between the stump and the socket. All the slipping and sliding due to the intermittent application of weight, as in walking, takes place between the slip socket and the socket of the artificial leg. Few stumps can tolerate this constant pressure without the blood vessels becoming strangulated; we therefore do all we can to dissuade clients from risking such a dangerous experiment.

SLIPPING OF THE STUMP DESIRABLE.—There is nothing so pleasant to a wearer of an artificial limb, no matter what kind of a leg he is wearing, as to be able to lift his stump from its bearings and give it a chance to rest and recover, exactly as one does when standing on natural legs. He throws his weight on one leg for a while and then on the other, and in this way both legs in their turn become rested. Every wearer of a wood-socket limb invariably does this. It is a source of comfort and relief; but it cannot be done with the slip socket, which clings to the stump like a leech.

The socket that is made to fit the stump so that pressure will be uniformly distributed over all its parts, is neither scientific nor tolerable. Every stump has parts that will bear pressure and parts that will not stand any at all. Parts where blood vessels and nerves are clustered, where the bones are close to the surface and poorly protected by tissue, must be prevented from impact. A flexible socket has a tendency to assume the shape of the stump and distribute the pressure uniformly, bringing as much on the forbidden parts as elsewhere. Therefore the flexible socket is a dangerous one to wear.

A socket that fits properly will never chafe the stump, no matter how much it may slip, slide, or move in it. This is a fact ascertained by most careful, thoughtful, and conscientious investigation, and cannot be successfully controverted. We know from very ample experience and inquiry that there is no socket so pleasant to wear, so light, so cool, and so healthful for the stump as the wooden one, when properly and scientifically fitted. No material has ever given such permanently good results as wood.

AN INSTANCE.—Mr. Frank M. Talbot met with a railroad accident in 1890 which crushed his leg. Amputation was made below the knee, leaving a stump four inches in length. He obtained an artificial leg with wooden socket, which he wore for some time with efficiency. His stump, following the usual course, emaciated, and instead of having the leg refitted he was prevailed upon to order a new leg with a slip socket. He wore the leg for a while, but gradually the end of his stump became congested and painful. He went to his slip-socket leg-maker for relief, but was told that his stump was diseased and nothing but medical or surgical treatment would help him. The stump grew worse; he called in a physician, who by medication brought it to a healthy condition, but put him on his back for a while. Shortly after he resumed wearing the slip-socket leg, the trouble recurred. He came to New York, and under the impression that his stump was diseased, consulted several prominent surgeons. All agreed that the stump had been strangulated by the artificial leg, and unless the cause was removed the bone would soon become infected and re-amputation would be necessary.

Mr. Talbot called upon us, and on examination we found the end of the stump swollen and as blue as indigo. An abscess was forming. We told him that his trouble was due to pressure upon the blood vessels, and advised him to abandon the slip socket, and wear a wooden one, so fitted that it would not constrict the blood vessels nor permit any of the tender parts of the stump to take pressure. He yielded to our advice, and we made and applied a leg with wooden socket and our patent rubber foot. It was remarkable how quickly his stump recovered. As soon as the pressure was removed from the vascular parts, circulation was restored and the stump became healthy. This was eleven years ago and the stump at this writing is in a healthy condition, without the slightest indication of a recurrence of his trouble. We can cite hundreds of cases similar to this and will gladly furnish additional data to those desirous of investigating further.

WATERPROOF LEGS.—There are some occupations that require limb-wearers to stand in damp and wet places, exposing their artificial legs to moisture, much to their injury. Farmers, miners, builders, woodsmen, raftsmen, trappers, oystermen, fishermen, watchmen, sailors, stablemen, chauffeurs and a thousand others are of this class.

Our method of constructing artificial legs enables us to meet the requirements of these people as they have never been met before. The foot is of sponge rubber with spring mattress, it is permanently secured to the leg and the whole is covered with suitable material coated with a waterproof preparation. This method is secured by Letters-Patent July 9, 1912.

BATHING LEGS.—Persons who indulge in aquatic sports can use artificial legs of this kind; with them they can wade, bathe, or swim in salt or fresh water exactly as persons in possession of their natural limbs and without disclosing the fact that their limbs are other than those provided by nature. Cut E 7 is a sectional view on which waterproof legs are constructed. It will be seen that there are no parts that can be affected by moisture. The entire lower leg is capable of withstanding the severest strains and exposure.

SHORTENED THIGH.—Complicated conditions in tibial amputations frequently present themselves and require specially designed artificial limbs. Cut E 33 illustrates a case in point. The injury to the patient, necessitating the amputation of the leg below the

knee, fractured the thigh and dislocated the hip. The femur
became lapped and deflected and its head was permanently displaced. This occasioned a shortening of the thigh of several
inches. In the artificial leg the shortening of the thigh was com-

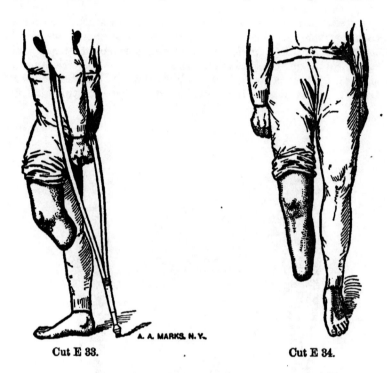

Cut E 33. Cut E 34.

pensated for by lengthening below the knee. A leg constructed
on the plan of E 17 is suitable for cases of this character. Its
thigh piece is made to extend well up to the body and take in the
gluteal folds and the entire external surface as far as the crest
of the ilium, thus giving the necessary support to the fractured
part.

Cut E 34 illustrates a case of shortened thigh of the left leg
while the right was amputated. It resulted from a railroad accident which crushed the right foot and ankle and fractured the
opposite thigh. The right foot was amputated at the junction of
the lower and middle thirds. Despite every effort to bring about
the correct union of the fractured femur of the left leg, the bones
slipped, resulting in a shortening of the thigh by several inches.
An artificial leg constructed on the plan of E 17 was applied. The
leg from the knee down was as much shorter than the left as the
thigh of the left was shorter than the right.

In both these cases the artificial legs necessarily caused a disparity in the lengths of the legs from the knees down, but the
differences were not noticeable, even when the wearers were seated,

except when closely scrutinized. In other respects there were no inconveniences experienced.

In ordering an artificial leg every peculiarity of the sound leg as well as the partly amputated one should be brought to the attention of the manufacturer.

THE LATERAL ADJUSTING SOCKET.—Changeable stumps are more frequent than generally known. By changeable stumps we mean those that remain large for a period and then became small and then large again. This characteristic is inherent in some stumps and cannot be controlled by any method of treatment. An artificial leg capable of being endured on a stump of this kind is

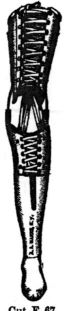
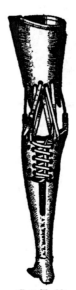

Cut E 67.   Cut E 68.

usually made large enough to receive the stump when it is at its largest dimensions, and when at its smallest additional socks are worn, or linings are put in the socket. There is some inconvenience and annoyance incurred in this way of adjusting.

Some manufacturers make sockets of leather, with lacings down the front, or rear, or both and claim that by drawing these lacings up or letting them out, the required adjustment can be made. It is easily seen that this method admits of adjustment from front to back only; the distance from side to side remains the same; the steel side joints, necessarily moving on the same axis, will not admit of any change in that direction. This is opposite to what it should be; if the distance from front to back is lessened there is increased pressure on the shin bone as well as on the blood vessel back of the knee. The shin bone cannot endure pressure and the blood vessels back of the knee, if constricted for a length of time, will suffer from interference with the circulation, and trouble in the end of the stump will follow.

The Marks lateral adjustable socket admits of the adjustment in the right direction; this is made possible by giving the side joints an additional hinge so that they will move sidewise as well as front and back. With this hinge, and a socket slitted front and back, it is possible to draw the sides of the socket closer together or set them further apart, and still have the centers of motion in the knee joints work on the same axis.

This method of constructing artificial legs with provisions for

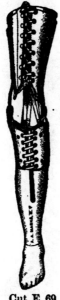

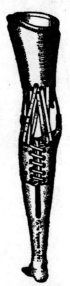

Cut E 69.   Cut E 70.

lateral adjustment has been applied to changeable stumps since 1909. It has stood this thorough test and proved its efficiency in many cases. Patented July 9, 1912.

Cuts E 67 and E 68 present front and rear views of a leg with socket wide enough to accommodate a large stump, and cuts E 69 and E 70 present the same leg front and rear views with the socket made smaller by drawing together the sides, thereby accommodating the same stump when it has become smaller.

CONTRACTED KNEE JOINTS.—Another class of leg stumps are those which are sufficiently long to control the knee movements of the artificial leg, but being partly contracted, the extension of the knee is somewhat limited, so that the use of the ordinary type of E 17 leg is impossible, while the contraction is not sufficient to make the knee joint inoperative in controlling the artificial leg.

Knee joints of tibial stumps become contracted either from the results of the injuries that occasioned their amputation, or, more frequently, from neglect in permitting the stumps to remain in semi-flexed positions during the convalescent periods. Cut E 39

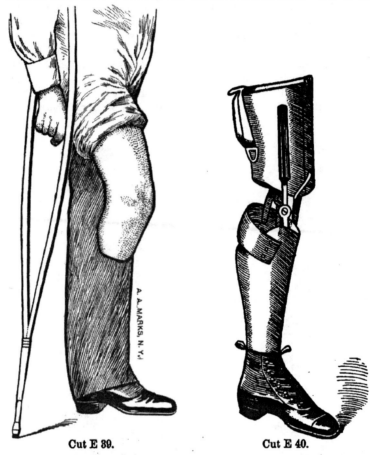

Cut E 39.   Cut E 40.

illustrates a partially contracted knee of a tibial stump which is capable of full flexion but of limited extension.

An artificial leg on the plan of E 17 with a slight modification of the socket, as shown in Cut E 40, meets the requirements of the case. By referring to Cut E 41 it will be seen that the stump is received in the socket while in a semi-flexed position. The socket is so made as to bring constant and gentle pressure upon the hamstrings every time a step is taken. The object of this is to induce the breaking up of the contraction and eventually restore full knee motion. The artificial leg is provided with a lacing attachment that passes over the rear part of the stump. As the stump improves in extension this lacing strap is tightened and greater pressure brought upon the stump.

Although a stump may be contracted to a considerable angle a leg of this character can be worn and the wearer enabled to get about in an advantageous way, concealing his loss, walking in a graceful manner, and dispensing with the use of crutches.

We know of no more practical method for breaking up the contraction in the hamstrings than wearing an artificial leg of this type. The wearer is permitted to engage in his usual occupations while the work of restoration of the knee motion progresses. When the knee has become corrected and the stump can be extended to a straight line, the socket on the artificial leg can be removed and the regular socket, similar to that shown in Cut E 17, applied at a very slight expense.

Cut E 41 shows the leg applied to a contracted stump and the wearer walking. Cut E 42 shows it with the wearer seated. The

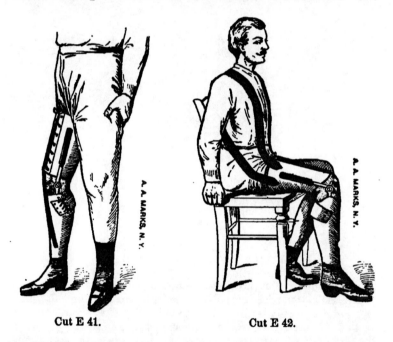

Cut E 41.   Cut E 42.

contraction of the hamstrings does not interfere with walking, standing, or sitting.

Cut E 43 illustrates a tibial stump with a contraction of the hamstrings considerably greater than in the last case, so great as to prevent the knee from extending beyond a right angle with the thigh. Cut E 44 represents an artificial leg suitable for this case.

A knee-bearing leg might be considered the more suitable, but when the fact is remembered that there is an angular motion in the knee, with the possibility of improvement, it is better to apply a leg that will keep up the action of the knee and bring a constantly increasing tension on the hamstrings. A leg constructed on the plan of that represented in Cut E 44 is made for this purpose.

HYPERTROPHIED TIBIAL STUMP.—Amputations through the tibia are sometimes necessitated by hypertrophy, with induration of the foot and ankle, as in the case of elephantiasis. Such cases usually

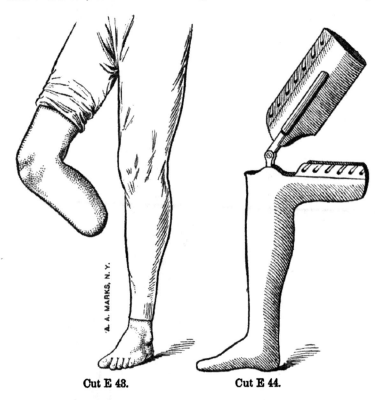

Cut E 43.   Cut E 44.

produce stumps that are much larger at their extremities than above, the extremities incapable of bearing pressure, and the sides able to tolerate only limited compression. Cut E 45 shows a stump of this character. It requires an artificial leg constructed upon the plan of E 46, with the rear open so as to receive the stump, the stump and socket are incased by a sheath holding the parts together. Cut E 46 represents a side view of an artificial leg suitable for such cases. Cut E 47 presents the front view with leg applied.

In all the complicated cases previously described, the method of constructing artificial legs with rubber feet and spring mattress is especially advantageous. Great strength is obtained, durability is secured with minimum weight and bulk about the enlarged extremity.

ANCHYLOSED KNEE TIBIAL STUMPS EXTENDED.—Some tibial stumps are rigid when extended. That is, they cannot be flexed, owing to anchylosis of the knees resulting from the injuries that

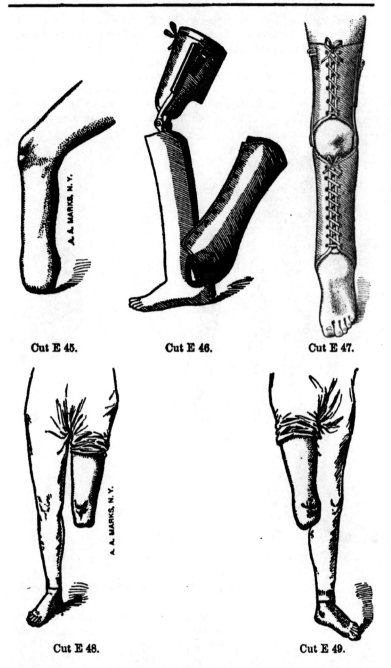

Cut E 45.   Cut E 46.   Cut E 47.

Cut E 48.   Cut E 49.

caused the amputations, impairment of the knee tendons, calcareous deposits in the articulations, and many other causes. If there is an absence of mobility in the knee and the stump is extended, an artificial leg must be constructed so that the artificial knee articulation will be independent of the natural knee and operate on the sides of the stump approximately at the points where the natural articulation takes place. Cuts E 48 and E 49 represent tibial stumps extended, with knee joints anchylosed.

It will be observed that in Cut E 48 the sides of the stump and thigh are approximately parallel, or in other words they do not slope sufficiently to offer any sustaining surfaces. An artificial leg

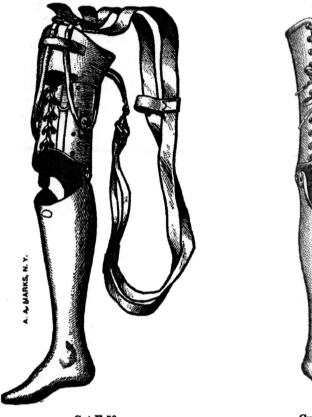

Cut E 50.   Cut E 51.

constructed on the plan of Cut E 50 is intended for a stump of this character.

The top part of the thigh piece is annular and permits the stump and thigh to enter until the gluteal folds, the ischium, and the perineum come in contact with the top border of the socket, where the entire weight is applied, the same as if the amputation had been made in the middle of the thigh. Cut E 49 represents a stump the sides of which are tapering sufficiently to offer some opposition, sustaining in part the weight and lessening the amount of pressure on the top border of the socket. An artificial leg constructed on the plan of E 51 will meet the requirements of this case. Both of the above artificial legs are made to articulate at the knees.

The legs from the knees down are constructed practically the same as the E 17. The thigh piece is leather and wood; the rear of wood and the front of leather arranged for lacing, so that the required pressure will be brought upon the thigh to hold it in place. Leg E 50 differs from E 51 in the top of the socket, it being annular with continuous border. It is held securely to the body by the lacing front, assisted by suspenders passing over the shoulders.

The knee joints of these legs are of the hinge style as illustrated in Cut E 21. Articulation at the knee is limited by a check cord

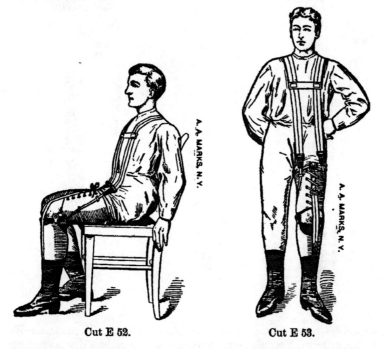

Cut E 52.   Cut E 53.

connecting the thigh and calf sections. Cut E 52 shows the leg applied, the wearer seated; and Cut E 53 shows it with the wearer standing. It will be seen that the knee articulation approximates very closely the action of the opposite leg and permits the wearer to stand, walk, sit, or kneel.

PEG LEGS.—Peg legs suitable for tibial stumps are of three kinds. The simplest and least expensive is shown in Cut E 54. It consists of two wooden branches, one running up on the outside of the thigh, well up on the body, the other on the inner side reaching nearly to the crotch.

These branches unite below the point of bearing and continue to the ground, terminating in a rubber tip. A padded shelf is placed between the branches on which the knee rests when in a flexed position. The leg is held in place by leather straps passing around the thigh and body.

Cut E 55 shows a peg leg without knee joint or thigh support suitable for a tibial stump. The socket is shaped to receive the

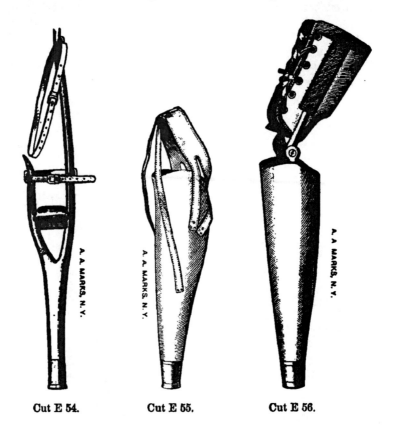

Cut E 54.   Cut E 55.   Cut E 56.

stump from the knee down in a comfortable way. The base terminates with a rubber tip, and straps necessary to hold the socket on the leg are connected with the leg and passed around the thigh immediately above the knee cap. When necessary, suspenders are attached to help carry the weight.

Cut E 56 shows a peg leg suitable for a tibial stump constructed practically as E 17, except that there is no rubber foot, a rubber tip taking its place.

PEG LEGS SHOULD NOT BE USED PERMANENTLY.—Peg legs are worn as temporary expedients, for disciplining stumps, or to bridge over an impecunious period. We know persons, however, of ample means who have reached advanced years, who from childhood have constantly worn peg legs, and doubtless will continue to do so, as long as they live.

It is quite possible to stump around on peg legs and do much hard work with them. They are immeasurably better than crutches, but they are very far from rendering the services that can be obtained from artificial legs with sponge rubber feet. The foot is an essential factor in helpful easy walking, and a means of opposing strains required in carrying heavy weights, ascending or descending stairs or elevations, and in walking long distances.

We disparage the use of peg legs, as we are keenly alive to the fact that they are inadequate to meet the demands that must be put upon them. Any form of peg leg that will keep the knee joint in a flexed position is liable to weaken the tendons of the knee, impair the knee movement, and limit its range of motion. They should, therefore, be used only as expedients.

FERRULES FOR PEG LEGS.—Cut E 57 represents an aluminum peg-leg ferrule and rubber tip. Cut E 58 represents the aluminum ferrule separate, and Cut E 59 represents a pure gum rubber tip

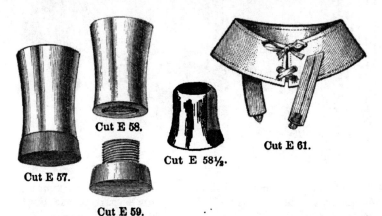

Cut E 58.

Cut E 58½.

Cut E 61.

Cut E 57.

Cut E 59.

separate, which screws into the ferrule. Cuts represent one-quarter size. The ferrule is permanently fastened to the peg leg, and the rubber tip screws into it.

RUBBER TIP.—When the rubber tip wears down so that the metal ferrule touches the ground, it should be removed and a new one put in. The base of the rubber tip is 2 1-2 inches in diameter and the threaded shank is 1 1-2 inches in diameter.

SUSPENDERS.—Suspenders for artificial legs for tibial stumps are of many kinds. Most persons with long and healthy stumps do not use suspenders at all, and a very small number retain them after they have become accustomed to their artificial legs.

As an aid for the beginner, however, we deem it advisable to put suspenders on every leg made for tibial amputation, whether the stump is long or short.

Cut E 60 shows a double suspender for a tibial stump leg. It consists of two-inch elastic webbing connected with the back of the thigh piece and running well up to the shoulder, where two non-elastic straps, each 1 1-2 inches wide, are attached which branch so as to pass over the shoulder. They are connected with the upper part of the thigh piece in front, and adjusted by clamp buckles with snaps.

Cut E 61 presents a simple yoke suspender preferred by women. It is made to fit the body immediately above and upon the hips.

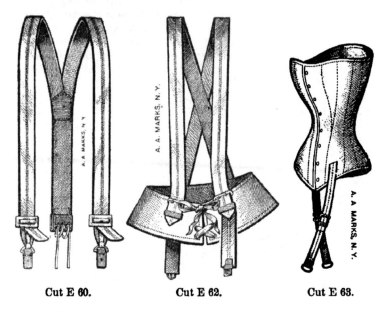

Cut E 60.   Cut E 62.   Cut E 63.

It is seldom necessary to use shoulder straps. Straps running down from the belt connected with the upper part of the thigh piece are usually ample.

Cut E 62 shows a yoke suspender similar to the last, but provided with shoulder straps. Elastic straps buckled into the attachments connected with the thigh piece are used to fasten the yoke to the leg. This method is necessary for small hips and in cases where entire support from the hips or pressure about the loins or over the abdomen cannot be tolerated.

The corset style is frequently preferred by women. It consists of strong elastic straps secured to the lower part of the corset, one in front and one at the back as shown in Cut E 63; they are buckled into straps secured to the upper part of the thigh piece.

CHAPTER VI

KNEE-BEARING STUMPS

DEFINITION.—When the knee joints of tibial stumps are contracted at right angles, or when the stumps are so short that they are unable to control the artificial knee joint, they are termed knee-bearing stumps, and require artificial legs constructed to receive them in flexed positions.

It is sometimes problematical to determine whether a stump should be placed in this class or in the class requiring legs constructed on the plan of E 17. The conditions to be considered in deciding the question are as follows: First, anchylosis or immobility of the knee joint when flexed. Second, length of the stump projecting back of the thigh when at right angles. If this is less than two inches the knee-bearing leg must be selected. Third, remediless contraction of the flexors, limiting the angular

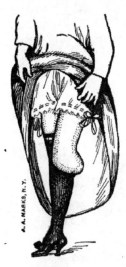

Cut F 1.

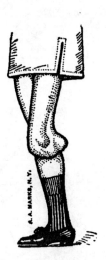

Cut F 2.

range of motion to one-half the normal range, no matter how long the stump may be. Cuts F 1 to F 4 show typical knee-bearing stumps.

KNEE-BEARING LEGS.—Cut F 5 shows a leg suitable for stumps of above character. The socket and leg part are made of wood covered with rawhide and enameled. The socket is excavated to receive the stump and thigh in a comfortable way, and the

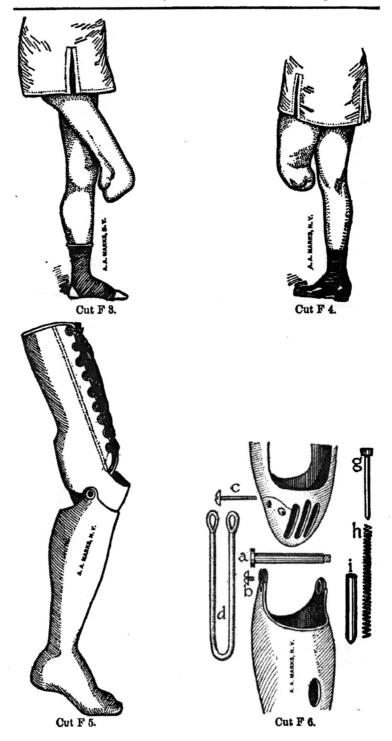

Cut F 3.

Cut F 4.

Cut F 5.

Cut F 6.

part from the knee down is hollowed out to reduce the weight. The exterior dimensions are as close to those of the natural leg as conditions will admit. The foot is of rubber with spring mattress as previously described.

BOLT JOINT.—Cut F 6 shows the knee mechanism with the parts separated: *a* is the knee-bolt which holds the leg and thigh sections together, forming an axis for the knee. It is flanged on

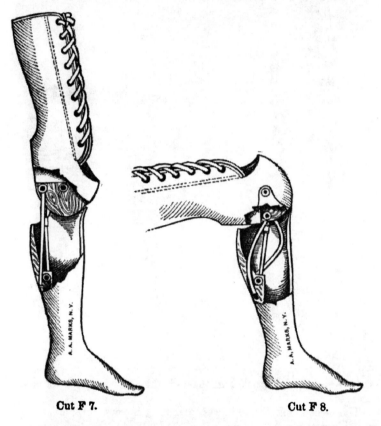

Cut F 7.   Cut F 8.

one end and threaded on the other. When the bolt is passing through the metal ear which is riveted to the lower leg the head sinks into its bed and the threaded end screws into the ear riveted to the opposite side. The set screw *b*, placed into the flanged end, prevents the bolt from moving and working out; *c* is the check cord screw; *d* the check cord; *g* the spring piston; *h* the spiral spring; *i* the cylinder. The relations and functions of these parts can be understood from an examination of Cuts F 7 and F 8, which show the leg with the knee extended and fully flexed.

The action of the spring holds the leg at flexion when the wearer is seated, and urges the leg forward when walking. The range of articulation can be regulated by means of pads placed between the lower end of the check cord and the bridge under which it passes. These pads can be reached through the opening in the calf of the leg. The upper loops of the check cord rest in

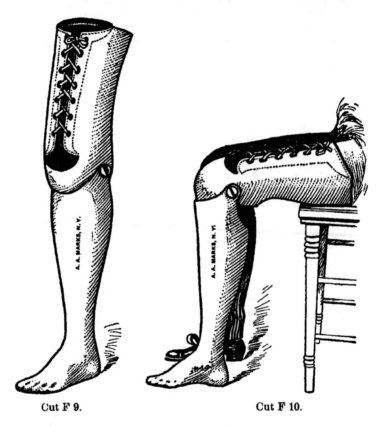

Cut F 9.   Cut F 10.

their respective channels and through them a steel screw is passed and set.

The mechanism of the knee-bearing leg is very durable, and will stand severe use for years.

SIDE JOINT.—The center of motion being placed below the natural knee, causes a disparity in the lengths of the two thighs; only noticeable, however, when the wearer is seated and subjected to close scrutiny. The durability of the knee-joint mechanism in style of leg shown in Cut F 5 fully compensates for excessive length of thigh, moreover, this mechanism admits of the minimum width of the knee. The choice of style remains with the wearer; if he prefers the wide knee to the long thigh, and is willing to sacrifice durability, he can have the leg constructed with side joints, as represented in Cut F 9, the center of knee motion of which is brought to the sides of the knee by means of hinge joints, of the style shown in Cut E 23, page 52. The knee-check cord is practically the same as that represented in Cut F 6. Cut F 10 shows the leg applied, wearer seated with knees flexed.

PEG LEGS.—Peg legs for knee-bearing stumps are of three kinds; and will be considered in their order: Cut F 11 shows the cheapest form of peg leg for a knee-bearing stump; its construction is of

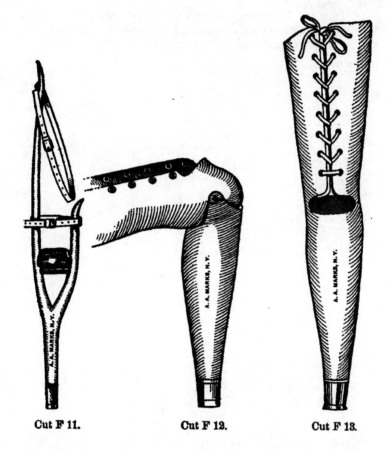

| Cut F 11. | Cut F 12. | Cut F 13. |

bent wood with metal ferrule, rubber tips, and leather strappings. Cut F 12 shows a peg leg with knee joint suitable for a knee-bearing stump.

Cut F 13 shows a peg leg without knee articulation for knee-bearing stump. The upper parts, F 12 and F 13, made of wood and leather, fitted to receive the stump, which is held in place by lacing.

The ends of peg legs are terminated by metal ferrules and rubber tips as described in Cuts E 57, E 58, and E 59, page 71.

INCOMPLETE RESTORATIVES.—For reasons heretofore given, we do not advocate peg legs for knee-bearing stumps and only furnish them when they are especially ordered. It is far better for a person to procure a complete artificial leg with rubber foot, with spring mattress, one that will possess all the elements necessary for helpful and convenient walking, even if he has to deny himself in other ways in order to obtain one. A peg leg is a makeshift, and will in all probability weaken or destroy what knee motion remains.

SUSPENDERS.—Suspenders suitable for knee-bearing legs are substantially the same as those employed for tibial stump legs. The details are given in the preceding chapter.

CHAPTER VII

DISARTICULATED KNEE STUMPS

END-BEARING AND NON-END-BEARING STUMPS. — Amputations through the articulations of the knees call for careful prothetical consideration. Stumps resulting from such amputations may be end-bearing or not; when they are covered with tissue flaps, free from cicatrices and nervous complications, they are end-bearing; if they are cicatrized, and sensitive, pressure must be applied elsewhere; if they are tapering to the ends or are broadened at the

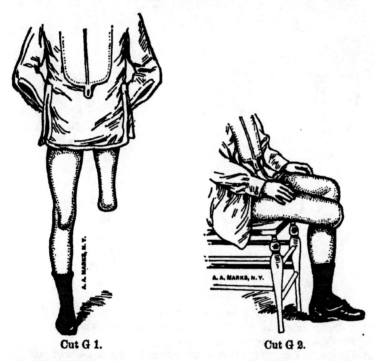

Cut G 1.   Cut G 2.

extremities they must be treated accordingly. The presence of the patella, securely united in the intercondylar space, will improve the character of the stump, but if it is not united it is doubtful if the end will tolerate any weight whatever.

FITTINGS. — Artificial legs for knee-joint amputations must admit of placing pressure only on parts capable of enduring it. Tender, delicate, sensitive, and irritable spots must be guarded, and non-end-bearing stumps must be provided with limbs that will take the weight at the ischial and perineal regions; if the sides of the stumps are sloping a share of the weight can be distributed over those parts. Sensitive condyles, bony prominences, and fascia must be properly cared for.

PECULIARITIES OF STUMPS.—Cut G 1 shows a type of stump resulting from knee-joint amputations; the nodulous extremity due to the presence of condyles, together with ample coverings, provide desirable conditions. An artificial leg suitable for this stump is so fitted that the weight is carried on the end, which rests on a padded surface at the lower end of the socket, and held securely in place by the leather lacing. The shoulder suspension is greatly simplified when condyles are present in the stump. Cut G 2 shows

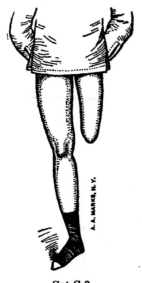
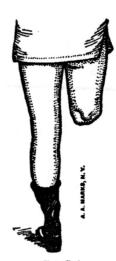

Cut G 3.   Cut G 4.

a side view of a stump favorable for end pressure. Cut G 3 shows a stump reaching to the knee, patella present and without cicatrices, thus admitting of end pressure.

. Cut G 4 shows a thigh stump reaching to the knee and extremely well protected, with cicatrices at the rear and well away from the end; bunches of sensitive tissue hanging from the extremity prevent the application of weight at that point. Cut G 5 shows a thigh stump reaching to the knee with an end incapable of bearing pressure; the condyles and all the natural coverings of the bone were removed in the operation. Bunches of tissue and ganglia were gathered at the end back of the stump. The muscle tissue puckered considerably and the presence of cicatrices on and about the end prevents the application of weight there. Cut G 6 shows a stump reaching to the knee, condyles present, the extremity covered with integumentary folds, deep fissures and cicatrices, preventing the application of weight upon the extremity.

MOST FAVORABLE CONDITIONS.—These examples develop the following points: Stumps extending to the knee with nodulous extremities, capable of bearing weight, are the most favorable of all knee-joint stumps. They result from amputations through the

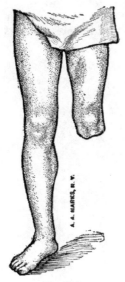

Cut G 5.

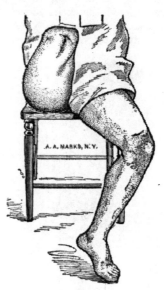

Cut G 6.

knee articulations, the condyles remaining untrimmed, or, if trimmed, the ends protected by bone and muscle flaps; the natural coverings to the bones permitted to remain on the articulating surfaces; the patellas, if present, firmly united to the end of the femur; flaps well carried to the posterior and the cicatrices some distance from the ends. Stumps possessing these favorable conditions can be efficiently accommodated with artificial legs that will minimize the pressure about their upper borders and simplify the mode of suspension.

A stump reaching to the knee, with a nodulous extremity and incapable of bearing weight on the end, is capable of operating an artificial leg, but the means of attachment are necessarily more extensive and more severe than when the weight can be borne on the ends.

Inability to bear weight on the extremities of knee-joint stumps is not always due to surgery.

Sloughing, bone degeneration, hyperæsthesia, etc., frequently occur despite the most careful precautions of the operator.

SUITABLE ARTIFICIAL LEGS.—The foregoing cuts illustrate stumps that can be advantageously fitted with artificial legs constructed upon plans of those shown in Cuts G 7 or G 8, according as the stump is tapering or straight, or whether the end can endure weight or not. The thigh of either leg is made partly of wood and partly of leather. The rear section is of wood, excavated to receive the stump in the most comfortable way. The front portion is of leather arranged for lacing as shown. If the stump is tapering to the end there will be no advantage in having the front laced, the entire socket can be better constructed of wood.

Cut G 7 illustrates a leg made to place a large amount of the weight of the wearer directly on the extremity of the stump. Cut

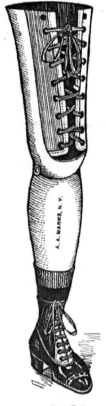
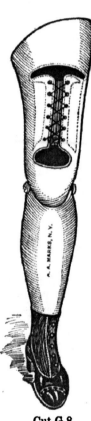

Cut G 7.   Cut G 8.

G 8 shows a leg with annular top designed to hold the end of the stump away from the bottom of the socket, all the weight being distributed over the sides, above the knees and about the top borders of the socket. In both these styles every requirement for the comfort of the wearer and the efficiency of the leg is considered.

The stump socket of either leg is of proper size and shaped to receive the stump and carry the weight of the wearer.

Both upper and lower sections are made of selected kiln-dried wood, carved to the shape of the stump with external proportions as near those of the natural leg as the conditions will admit. The lower leg is excavated to reduce weight. The foot is of rubber as heretofore described, and both leg and thigh are coverd with suitable material properly enameled. The knee mechanism is the same as that illustrated in Cuts F 6 and F 7.

Suspenders for legs for knee-joint amputations are the same as those applied to thigh amputations, and are fully treated in the following chapter.

We point with pride to many thousand persons who walk on artificial legs of either the above type with efficiency and naturalness and who voluntarily bear witness to the excellence of the manner in which they have been fitted out, and their increased capabilities to perform their full share of work.

CHAPTER VIII

THIGH OR FEMORAL STUMPS

DEFINITIONS.—Thigh or femoral stumps are those that reach to any point above the knee joint; they are designated upper-, middle-, or lower-third thigh stumps, according to their lengths, in relation to the three divisions of the thigh.

LONG OR LOWER-THIRD THIGH STUMPS.—When a stump reaches to a point in the region of the lower third, it is commonly termed

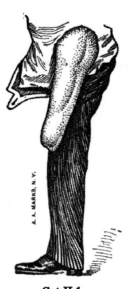

Cut H 1.

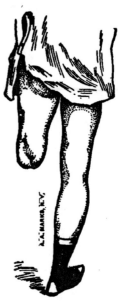

Cut H 2.

a long thigh stump, a few of which are illustrated in Cuts H 1 to H 4.

Artificial legs suitable for such are illustrated in Cuts H 5 and H 6.

In cases of long and flabby stumps the number G 7 leg, see page 82, can be applied to advantage.

STUMPS OUT OF LINE.—Persons walking on crutches for a considerable length of time permit their stumps to incline forward. The flexors in the groin become contracted and the extensors yield to the influence, and the stump assuming the position, when hanging at ease, of that shown in Cut H 1, and occasionally that shown in Cut H 3. This condition should not cause anxiety on the part of the wearer, as it can be controlled and corrected by a suitably attached artificial leg.

CONSTRUCTION OF LEGS.—The thigh and leg sections of H 5 are constructed of wood of choice character. The socket is hollowed

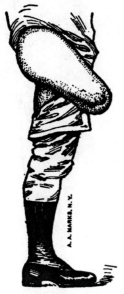

Cut H 3.

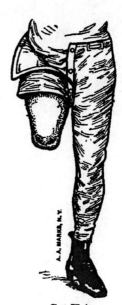

Cut H 4.

out to receive the stump properly, and to receive the weight of the wearer where it can be tolerated.

The outside dimensions both above and below the knee are dressed down to the curves and dimensions of the natural leg as far as conditions will admit. The lower part excavated to minimize weight, both sections are covered with rawhide and enameled, the foot is of sponge rubber with spring mattress as heretofore described. The manner in which the knee joint is constructed is substantially the same as shown in Cut F 6, and described on page 74.

VARIETY OF MIDDLE-THIRD THIGH STUMPS.—Thigh amputations through or above the middle thirds produce stumps that admit of the simplest form of knee-joint mechanism, called the T joint, explained further on.

Cuts H 7 to H 14 show thigh stumps of a variety of lengths with flaps and cicatrices of many characters.

END AND NON-END-BEARING.—As a rule thigh stumps are incapable of taking weight on their extremities, and as there is but little advantage in putting pressure on that point, and as the risk of doing so is very great, we rarely consent to construct limbs

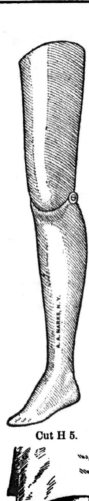

Cut H 5.

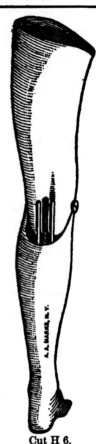

Cut H 6.

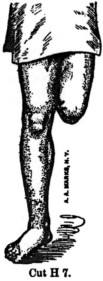

Cut H 7.

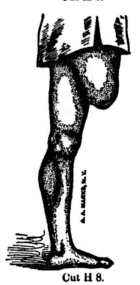

Cut H 8.

in that way and only do so when we are positive that the ends of the stumps will not be injured. Cut H 15 shows the usual type

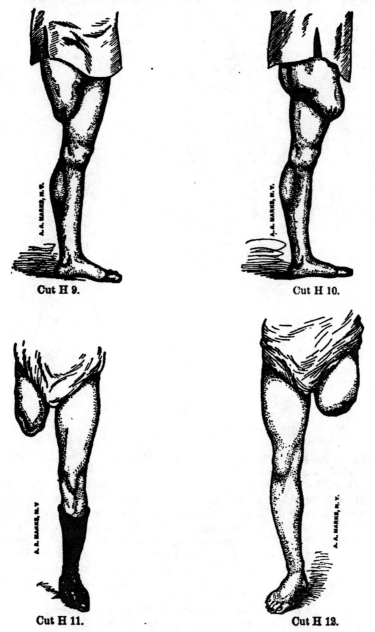

Cut H 9.   Cut H 10.

Cut H 11.   Cut H 12.

of artificial leg for a thigh stump. The thigh and leg sections are made of tough, light, bass or willow wood, shaped to the size and contours of the natural leg so far as conditions will permit. The thigh is excavated to receive the stump in the best way, permitting pressure only at admissable places. The end of the stump, together with a few inches of the thigh, are, as a rule, required to hang in space, all the weight being applied to the upper borders of the thigh socket and along the sides of the stump immediately adjacent to the body. When weight can be prudently applied to the end a cushion is provided for that purpose. The lower section of the

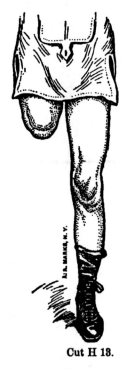 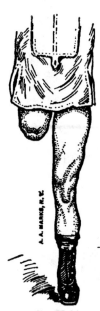

Cut H 13.   Cut H 14.

leg is excavated to reduce weight. The whole is covered with rawhide and elegantly finished with a flesh-tinted enamel.

A rubber foot with spring mattress as heretofore described, is properly attached at the ankle. Cut H 16 represents the rear view showing the knee mechanism with parts together, and Cut H 17 represents the working parts of the knee separated. Cut H 18 shows the T joint, the spring, and their connections; *a* is the T joint which is secured to the knee block located at the lower end of the stump socket. The two arms work in journals made in the leg section; *bb* are the cap screws that hold the T joint to its place; *cc* the caps; *d* the spring piston; *e* the spiral spring; *f* the cylinder; *g* spring cover, and parts of the spring together; *iii* represent the steel screws used to hold the T joint firmly to thigh. The joint *a* has the shape of an inverted T, hence its name, T joint. It is made of gun metal forged from one piece, turned, drilled, and finished on the lathe. When the leg and thigh sections are placed together the arms of the T joint rest in boxes and are held by two hardwood caps, *cc,* which are secured by long steel screws, *bb,* which depend for their security on steel nuts, imbedded in the front part of the leg.

THOROUGH CONTROL.—The wearer has thorough command over this joint; the pressure of the caps on the joints can be regulated

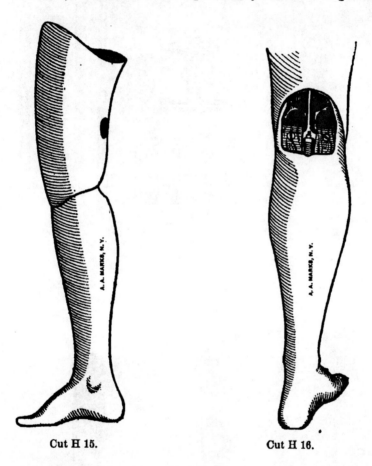

Cut H 15.   Cut H 16.

by the screws, and thus any desired tension on the articulation be made.

KNEE SPRING.—The small steel lever with ball on the end, projecting from the back of the joint, operates in the cavity of the hardwood piston *d;* the piston is inserted in one end of the steel spring, *e,* which has its lower part encased with leather *g,* and then placed in a drawn metal cylinder *f.* The lower convexed end of the cylinder is received on a bridge placed in the interior of the leg in the region of the calf.

HELPS KNEE MOTION WHEN WALKING.—The operation of the spring is twofold; it urges the lower leg forward in walking, and

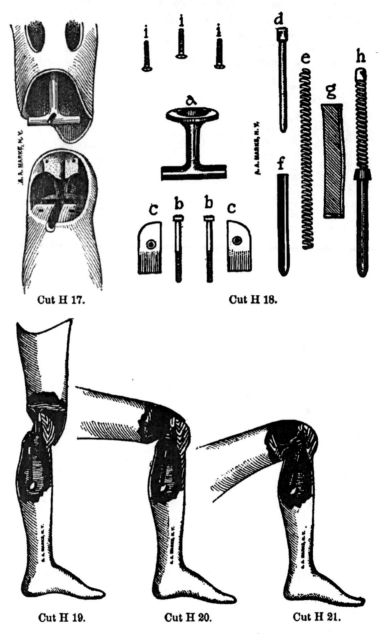

Cut H 17.   Cut H 18.

Cut H 19.   Cut H 20.   Cut H 21.

holds it at full flexion when sitting. This is done in the following manner: When the leg is extended, the point at which the spring pressure is applied is on the end of a steel lever projecting an inch back of the center of motion in the knee. This urges further extension, as shown in Cut H 19, the lever revolves with the joint; and when the leg is partly flexed, as shown in Cut H 20, it has been carried to a neutral point where the spring neither urges flexion nor extension; but when the knee is further flexed, as shown in Cut H 21, the lever has passed forward of the neutral line and the spring forces the ball upward, urging greater flexion; and when the flexion is at its limit the leg is kept in that position by the spring. Thus the objection to the usual spring knee articulation is removed, that of the tendency of the leg to fly out when the wearer is sitting and unguarded.

SPRING STRENGTH CAN BE REGULATED.—The power of the spring in the knee can be increased or diminished. If it is desired to increase it, a little packing can be tamped in the cylinder, or a longer spring can be substituted; and if it is desired to diminish it, a coil or two of the spring can be cut off or a shorter one substituted. If the wearer does not want the spring he can take it out and discard it. When the leg is together and in working order, the knee movement is arrested by the striking of the vertical shaft of the T joint against a pad placed in the knee, which can be increased or diminished by the wearer, and the range of articulation in the knee made less or greater, as may be desired.

The center of motion of this knee is placed considerably back of the center of gravity of the leg in order to secure the knee against treacherous bending.

KNEE LOCK.—The knee lock is a device placed in the knees of artificial legs to keep them from flexing, or from flexing beyond a fixed limit. When the wearer wishes to sit the knee can readily be unlocked. It is not very often that knee locks are required, therefore they are only placed in artificial limbs when conditions demand.

Cut H 22 shows an artificial leg with knee lock for thigh stump; *a* is a sliding bar that can be moved upwardly or downwardly. When down the leg is incapable of moving at the knee, or is permitted to move only through a limited angle, as shown in Cut H 23. When the sliding bar is pulled up, the lock is out of action, and the knee can be bent at right ankles as represented in Cut H 24.

This device is found to be of value to those who have short, weak, or deflected stumps, and is also used to advantage by equestrians. We have a patron, a baptist clergyman, who finds the knee lock indispensable when performing the rites of immersion; because of the buoyancy of the lower leg the knee without the lock would flex the moment he enters the baptismal font. Knee locks are used to advantage by persons who are required to walk through obstructions, such as underbrush, heavy grass, snow, etc.: without the locks these obstructions are likely to flex the knees inopportunely. Hip joints and waist belts are occasionally attached to the thighs of these legs.

HIP JOINTS.—The knee lock, hip joint, and waist belt can be combined to advantage in legs applied to stumps that are deflected, abducted, or that in any way incline out of the normal lines. The knee lock places the knee beyond the influence of the partly flexed stump, and the hip joint places the leg beyond the influence of

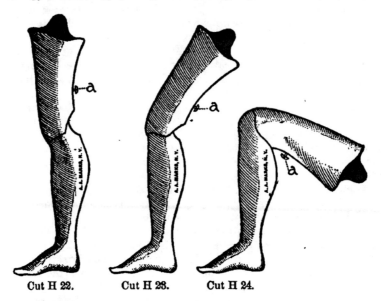

Cut H 22.   Cut H 23.   Cut H 24.

the abducted stump. As these auxiliary parts complicate the construction of the leg, add weight, and more or less hamper graceful and natural walking, it is not considered desirable to add them unless the conditions of the stump or the occupation of the wearer demand.

WATERPROOF AND BATHING LEGS.—Persons wearing artificial legs on thigh stumps frequently find it desirable to use their artificial legs while they are bathing or swimming in salt or fresh water. It is embarrassing to those who have but one leg to be viewed with curiosity while hopping or walking with crutches or hitching on hands and knees on the shore. This embarrassment often prevents them from indulging in the exhilarating and health-giving river, lake, or ocean bath.

An artificial leg especially designed for swimming and bathing purposes is constructed practically the same as those heretofore described, differing only in the fact that they are absolutely waterproof, the knee to articulate or not, as the wearer may elect. As the wearing parts of waterproof legs are made of composition instead of steel, they are not as durable as those made for ordinary purposes; they are therefore only made when especially ordered.

LEGS WITHOUT KNEE JOINTS.—We have on a number of occasions been required to construct artificial legs for thigh stumps without knee joints. Cut H 25 shows an artificial leg of this type. The entire structure, including the foot core, is carved from a single piece of wood, slightly curved at the knee so as to represent the natural leg when partly flexed, for better accommodation when sitting. The foot is of rubber with spring mattress as described. The leg is covered in the usual way and enameled or waterproofed if it is to be used in watery places.

PEG LEGS—Peg legs are occasionally used on thigh stumps. They are practically artificial legs without feet. As already stated we do not advocate the use of peg legs, as they are of limited effi-

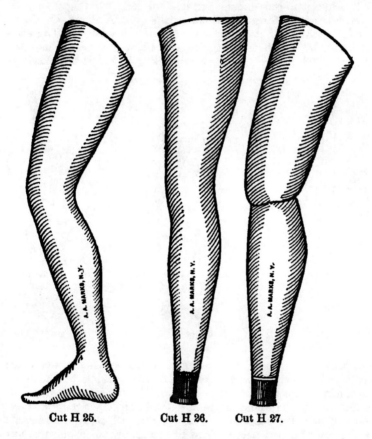

Cut H 25.   Cut H 26.   Cut H 27.

ciency. The foot is a very important part of an artificial leg. It assists in balancing, aids in walking, and restores the appearance.

Years ago before artificial legs with rubber feet and spring mattress were so generally used, the peg leg was more in evidence, but lately it is worn more as a means of disciplining the stump or as a makeshift to bridge an impecunious period.

Persons are able to stand, stump about, and perform a limited amount of labor on peg legs, which are unquestionably better than crutches, but their restoration is not complete until they are wearing artificial legs with spring mattress rubber feet. Cut H 26 shows a peg leg for a thigh stump. It is made of suitable wood, excavated to receive the stump and reduce weight. The outside has the contours of nature as closely as the conditions will admit, the end terminating in a metal ferrule and rubber tip, as illustrated on page 71, Cuts E 57-58-59. Cut H 27 shows a peg leg with knee joint, for a thigh stump. It is constructed in all parts the same as H 15, heretofore described. The absence of the foot and the substitution of a rubber tip is the only difference.

SUSPENDERS.—Suspenders suitable for legs for thigh amputations, as well as for amputations in the knee joint are of various kinds to suit the habits and demands of the wearers. The style of suspender which is most generally adopted is that illustrated in Cut H 28, termed the roller suspender. While it has excellent

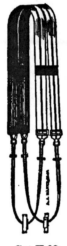

Cut H 28.

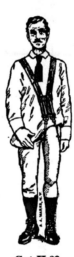

Cut H 29.

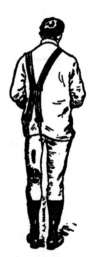

Cut H 30.

features it has limited application. It can be used to advantage on stumps reaching to any point from the middle of the thigh to the knee, but for shorter stumps and for hip-joint amputations a method that will hold the limb to the body more firmly is necessary. The roller suspender is the product of many experiments and years of experience, assisted by the kindly suggestions of our patrons.

The shoulder straps are usually of two-inch non-elastic webbing. A strip of webbing is attached to the right strap, and forms a loop through which the left strap passes. A piece of webbing stitched to the back of both straps holds them together. The front lower ends of the shoulder straps are received into buckles, and the back lower ends are terminated by snaps; each hooks into the ends of the leather roller cords which pass around rollers attached to

either side of the leg. Any degree of pressure upon the shoulders
can be obtained by means of the clamp buckles, and when obtained,
the buckles are clamped and are never disturbed, unless the pressure
on the shoulders needs further adjustment. When it is desired
to remove the limb, the suspenders are detached by unsnapping
both front and back.

Cut H. 29 shows a front view of a person wearing a pair of
roller suspenders.

Cut H 30 gives the back view, and Cuts H 31, H 32, and H 33
side views.

These cuts show the relative positions of the rollers, as well as
the effect of the loops in holding the shoulder straps in place and

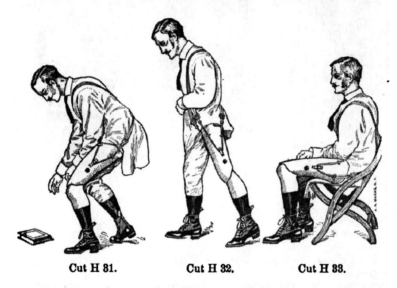

Cut H 31.   Cut H 32.   Cut H 33.

in directing the leg. Elasticity is obtained by two pieces of
elastic webbing attached to the backs of the shoulder straps a
little below the shoulder blades.

The operation of the suspenders is illustrated in Cuts H 29-
30-31-32-33. All the traveling of the suspenders due to changes
of position takes place about the rollers on the sides of the thigh,
instead of on the shoulders of the wearer, whether the person is
standing, stooping, walking, or sitting.

STRAIGHT SHOULDER STRAPS.—Cut H 34 shows a style of suspender especially adapted to an artificial leg for a short thigh
stump. It is the style very generally used before roller suspenders
were devised. The shoulder straps are of fine elastic webbing, 2
inches wide.

The front straps are of two-inch non-elastic webbing; each front
strap passes through a metal link attached to the lower end of
the elastic shoulder strap. After passing through the metal link
the front straps are received into a two-prong buckle. The sus-

penders are attached to the leg by means of leather tags and metal
D's screwed to the back and front. The metal D admits of side
motion, thereby insuring direct pull.

BELT ATTACHMENT.—Cut H 35 represents a belt and suspender
combined. The shoulder straps and belt are preferably of non-
elastic webbing. The straps running from the belt to the leg are

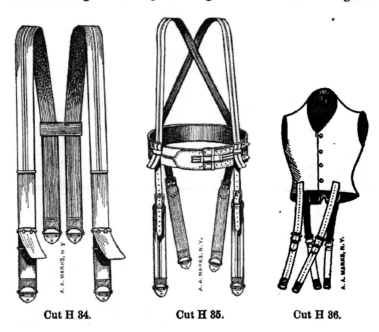

Cut H 34.   Cut H 35.   Cut H 36.

made of elastic webbing, 2 inches wide or less, as the case may
demand.

VEST METHOD.—Cut H 36 illustrates the vest method. It is made
of strong muslin, fitted to the person and worn under the shirt.
Elastic straps are attached to the lower border and buckled into
straps that are secured to the leg. In order to obtain the best
results, the vest must be made and fitted by a tailor. Persons who
desire to have their artificial limbs constructed from measurements, and choose the vest suspender, are required to have vests
made at home, and if sent to us, we will attach the straps and
make the proper connections with the leg without additional charge.

SUSPENDERS FOR WOMEN.—For obvious reasons the means of suspending artificial limbs to women differ from those employed with
men. When shoulder straps are used they must pass over the
shoulders and not press upon the breasts. Yokes, girths, or bands
must pass around the waists so as to place the burden all or in
part on the hips.

YOKE METHOD.—Cut H 37 shows a combination of the roller
straps with the yoke; rollers or pulleys are secured to the sides of
the thigh, and leather cords pass around them. The yoke is made

to fit the loins and hips, adjustable by lacing in front or on the sides, as may be preferred; the shoulder and roller straps are also

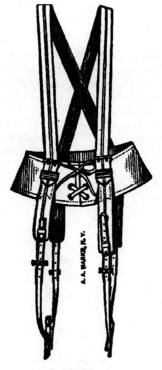

Cut H 37.

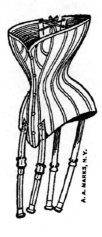

Cut H 38.

adjustable, so as to bring the proportionate weight about the shoulders and hips without displacing the yoke.

CORSET METHOD.—As many women pride themselves on their trim waists and neat-fitting garments, it is especially desirable that means of leg suspension should be light and neat. Straps securely sewed to the corset, extending downward and connected with the artificial limb, admit of the neatest adjustment. Cut H 38 shows the corset method, which can be easily adjusted by the wearer.

CHAPTER IX

HIP-JOINT AMPUTATIONS

REQUIREMENT.—An amputation at the hip joint or close to the body requires an artificial leg identical in construction to either of the patterns heretofore described for thigh stumps, with the exception that some modifications are introduced in the knee and the means of suspension is more complex.

MUSCLE STUMP.—Cuts I-1 and I-2 illustrate front and side views of amputations at the coxo-femoral or hip articulation, leaving a stump composed entirely of muscle tissue. A muscle

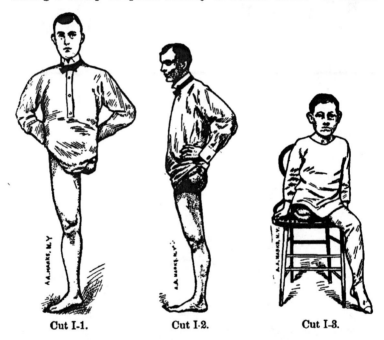

Cut I-1.   Cut I-2.   Cut I-3.

stump is capable of performing some functions, although limited, in the management of an artificial leg, and may be considered as more desirable than no stump at all. Cuts I-3 and I-4 represent a hip-joint amputation in which there is no protruding stump by which the artificial leg can be directed. The amputated surface at the base of the pelvis is capable of bearing pressure.

LEG APPLIED.—Cuts I-5 and I-6 show a leg applied to hip-joint amputation having muscle stump. The means by which it is suspended consist of a waist belt, shoulder strap, over each shoulder, flexion and extension elastic straps, a metal hip joint

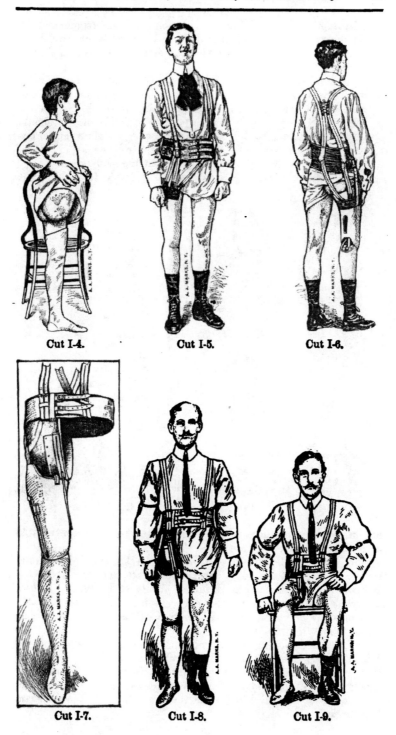

Cut I-4.   Cut I-5.   Cut I-6.

Cut I-7.   Cut I-8.   Cut I-9.

substituting the natural hip articulation, and an attachment by which the knee can be locked and made immovable, or capable of having but limited motion, these features have all been explained in the preceding chapter.

The hip joint is important as it keeps the artificial leg directly under the wearer. The waist belt with its elastic straps front and rear assists in flexing and extending the leg at the hip. The leg is held firmly to the body when standing or walking; it should be especially noted, that it is not advisable to allow any knee motion while the wearer is learning to control the leg. During this period the knee motion is only for sitting convenience.

Cut I-7 shows a leg with pelvic socket suitable for a hip-joint

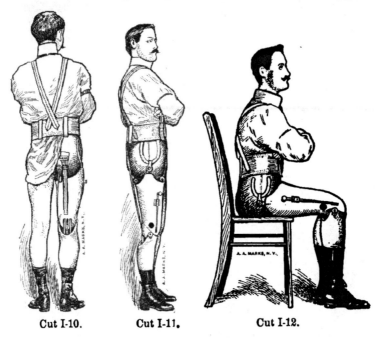

Cut I-10.   Cut I-11.   Cut I-12.

amputation where there is no protruding stump to control the artificial hip motion.

Cuts I-8, I-9, I-10, I-11, I-12, show the leg applied and the wearer in many positions. The pelvic socket takes in a part of the pelvis and holds the artificial leg firmly to its place no matter what positions the wearer may assume. The hip joint is controlled by throwing the body forward or backward of the center of gravity of the leg.

Artificial legs for hip-joint amputations support the amputated side in a very comfortable and natural manner. The leg, having little or no stump to control it, is thrown forward by means of a side motion of the body. Persons with reasonable perseverance soon learn to control legs under these conditions in an advantageous way.

CHAPTER X

BOTH-LEG AMPUTATIONS

The triumphs of artificial limb-making are shown to advantage in the restoration to active life of those who have had both of their lower extremities removed. When such persons are enabled to get about freely, walk gracefully, and engage in such labors as their callings in life require, a great and beneficial work has been accomplished, and the strongest possible evidence is presented to show that the mind of the prothesist has not been passive during

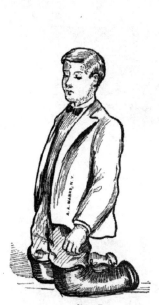

Cut J 1.

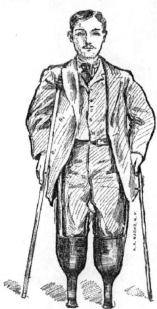

Cut J 2.

the past half century. The problems these cases present are profoundly difficult, thought and effort have never been given to more laudable purposes than to their solution. The amelioration of the conditions of these unfortunate persons commands the highest talent and the most humane impulses.

ANCIENT METHODS.—But a short time ago the loss of both legs was regarded as irreparable. The person who met with that misfortune was either consigned to a wheel chair, or obliged to hitch himself about on his knees or haunches. Cuts J 1 to J 4 show some of the various methods employed by those deprived of both their limbs. Formerly these methods were the only means for

locomotion the subject could employ. But at the present time
the methods are used preliminary to obtaining and wearing arti-

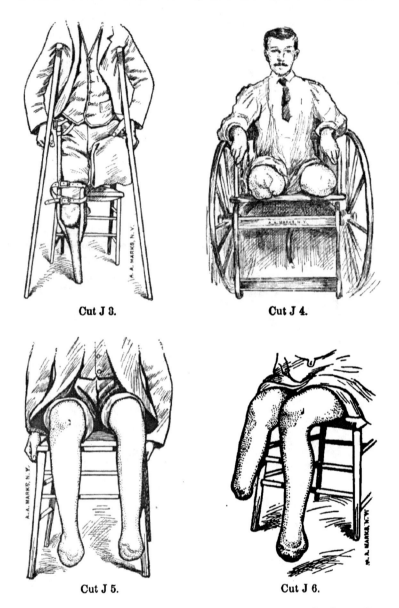

Cut J 3.   Cut J 4.

Cut J 5.   Cut J 6.

ficial legs. When these methods are contrasted with those that
are shown later on, the progress and developments that have been
made in the adaptation of artificial legs will be in plain view.

BOTH FEET PARTLY AMPUTATED.—Cut J 5 shows a case in which

both feet were removed at the insteps; a pair of artificial legs constructed on the plan of Cut C 18, page 32, was applied.

LOWER INSTEP AND LEG AMPUTATIONS.—Cut J 6 shows an amputation of the left foot at the instep and of the right leg at the junction of the lower and middle third. Artificial legs C 18 and E 17 were applied.

BOTH FEET AMPUTATED AT THE ANKLES.—Cut J 7 shows a double ankle-joint amputation with the extremities incapable of

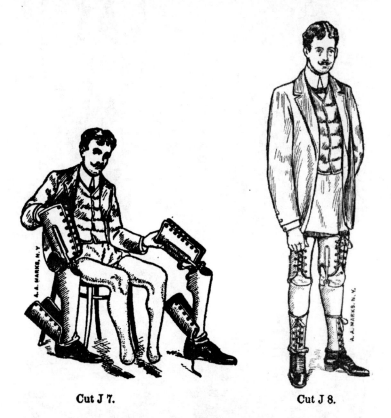

Cut J 7.   Cut J 8.

bearing pressure. A pair of artificial legs, constructed on the plan of D 21 and described on page 43, was applied. Cut J 8 shows the same case with the legs applied and the wearer standing. In this particular instance the amputations resulted from frostbite, and the extremities of the stumps were very sensitive and with impaired circulation. It was therefore necessary to avoid interference with circulation and to secure the absolute freedom of the extremities from contact.

ANKLE JOINT AND KNEE AMPUTATIONS.—Cut J 9 shows an amputation of the left foot at the ankle after the Pirogoff method, and the right leg at the knee joint after the Gritti operation;

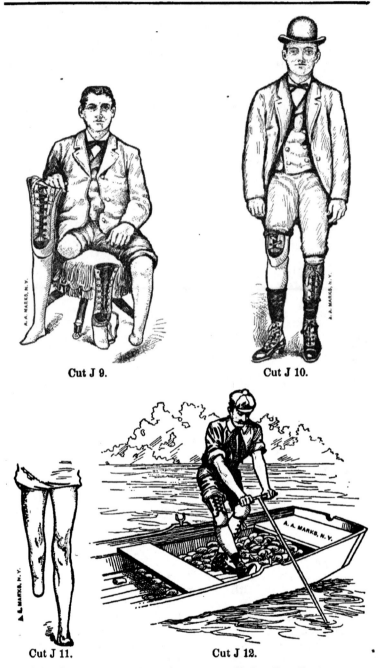

Cut J 9.   Cut J 10.

Cut J 11.   Cut J 12.

artificial legs D 12 and G 17 were applied. Cut J 10 presents
the wearer with artificial legs applied and attired as in daily life.
UPPER INSTEP AND LEG AMPUTATIONS.—Cut J 11 shows an am-

putation of left foot at the instep and the right leg at the middle
third. Artificial legs C 18 and E 17 were applied. Cut J 12

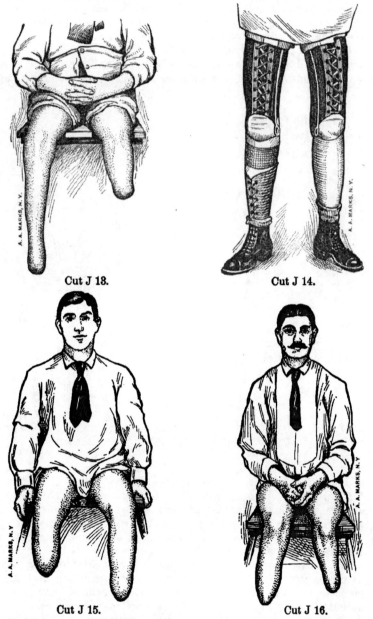

Cut J 13.

Cut J 14.

Cut J 15.

Cut J 16.

shows the wearer with the legs applied, engaging in his occupation as oysterman. This person has been employed in that industry for many years, and finds himself unhampered in his work.

Cut J 13 shows an amputation of the right foot at the instep and of the left leg immediately below the knee. The right foot was poorly nourished, and sensitive at the extremity, so much so as to completely prohibit any pressure. Cut J 14 illustrates the same case with D 21 and E 17 legs applied.

BOTH-LEG AMPUTATIONS.—Cuts J 15 to J 21 illustrate amputations of both legs at various points between the knees and ankles, covering many lengths, characteristics of flaps, and situations of

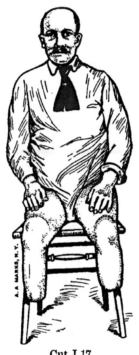

Cut J 17.

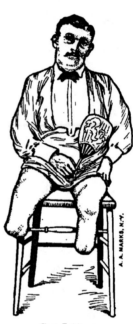

Cut J 18.

cicatrices. Artificial legs suitable for any of these amputations, as shown in Cut J 21, are constructed on the plan of E 17. Cut J 22 shows the legs applied. The freedom with which wearers of legs for double amputations can get about, the naturalness with which they can sit, lie down, stand, walk, ascend elevations, ladders, ride bicycles, skate, and engage in almost any occupation are shown in Cuts J 22 to J 32.

PRACTICAL RESULTS.—Persons wearing two artificial legs are so thoroughly in control of their means of locomotion that they go about much as other people. They readily resume their former occupations, no matter how arduous they may have been. Cut J 28 illustrates a case of double-leg amputations with artificial legs E 17 applied. A short time after obtaining the legs the wearer resumed his work of baggage master, lifting heavy trunks, carrying them about, and putting them on trains as one would

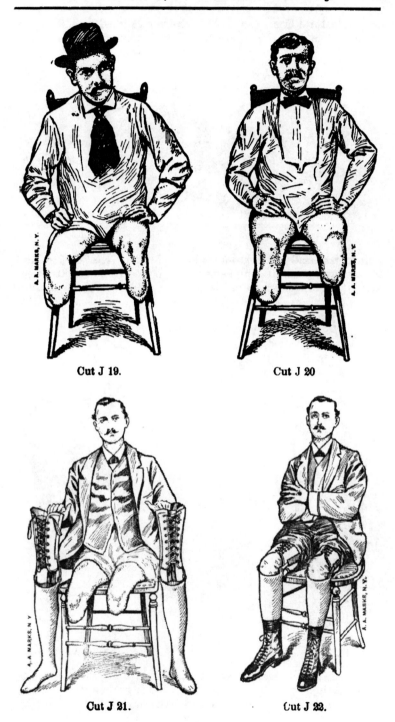

Cut J 19.   Cut J 20

Cut J 21.   Cut J 22.

do with natural legs. Cut J 29 portrays a railroad man with two artificial legs operating a switch. He dismounts, attends to the

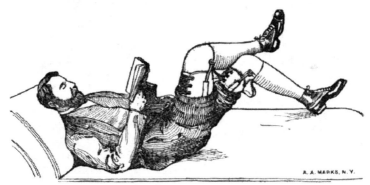

Cut J 23.

switch, frequently gets aboard while the train is in motion, and performs the work of a brakeman. He moves about quickly, steps over ties, and appears to be on as firm footing as if he had never

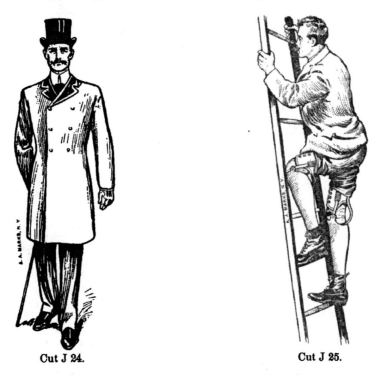

Cut J 24.   Cut J 25.

been deprived of nature's extremities. Cut J 30 shows a young man wearing two artificial legs, plan E 17; he is a conductor on a railroad, performing his duties in a thoroughly efficient manner.

He walks through the train when it is running at its greatest
speed, collects tickets, and punches them. The cars jolt, pitch,

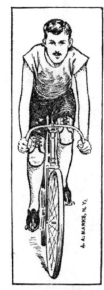

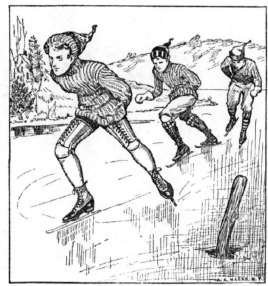

Cut J 26.   Cut J 27.

and sway, but he retains his balance with no perceptible effort
or awkwardness.

At stations he alights, watches passengers, gives signals, and
boards his train. It never occurs to anyone that his lower ex-

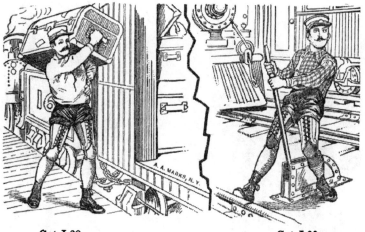

Cut J 28.   Cut J 29.

tremities are not real, and his actions never betray that fact.
With wooden articulating feet it would be extremely difficult for

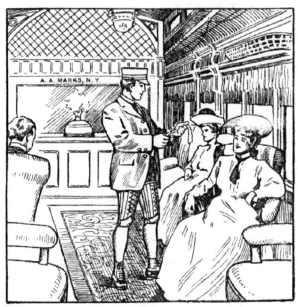

Cut J 30.

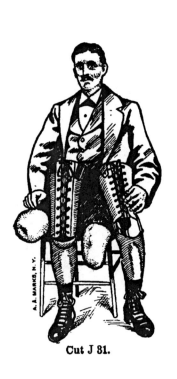

Cut J 31.

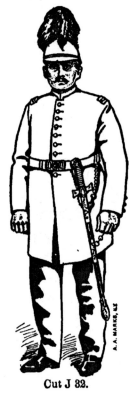

Cut J 32.

him to discharge such duties. He would feel unsafe, tottlish, and unsteady, but with rubber feet with spring mattress, rigidly attached, he has sound footing, and is capable of the most difficult feats of balancing.

BELOW-KNEE AND KNEE-JOINT AMPUTATIONS.—Cut J 31 represents a case with both legs amputated; the right disjointed at the knee, and the left amputated three inches below the knee; Nos. E 17 and G 7 legs were applied. This man when in street

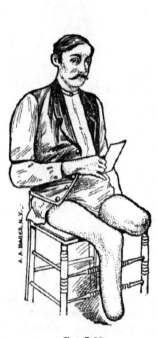

Cut J 33.

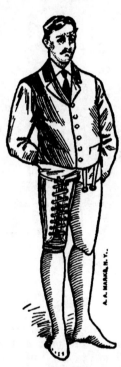

Cut J 34.

attire presents the appearance of a person with natural extremities. He walks naturally, and never consents to use a cane. He is a member of the Knights of Pythias, and takes pride in parading with his lodge. Cut J 32 shows him in his uniform.

BELOW-KNEE AND ABOVE-KNEE AMPUTATIONS.—Cut J 33 represents amputations of both legs, the right below the knee and the left above the knee. Cut J 34 represents the same case, with E 17 and H 15 legs applied.

. Cut J 35 shows a similar case; the right stump only five and one-half inches from the body, and the left one and one-half inches below the knee. E 17 was applied to the left side and H 15 to the right. The subject was restored to not only a natural appearance, but to the ability of walking without the aid of

canes or crutches, and so naturally that he has associated with
persons for long periods without betraying the fact that his lower
limbs were artificial. This young man has walked half a mile

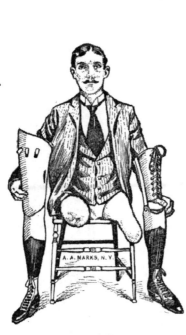

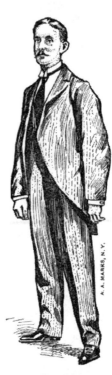

Cut J 35.   Cut J 36.

in eight minutes without great effort. He works at the bench
during the day, and the evenings are frequently spent at the
billiard table. Cut J 36 shows him as he appears on his artificial
legs, and in street attire.

ENGAGING IN FORMER PURSUITS.—We have many patrons wearing
E 17 and H 15 artificial legs for double amputations who exhibit
remarkable skill in performing feats that require sound footing.

Cut J 37 shows a person with two artificial legs as above described in a rowboat, illustrating the manner in which he can
brace himself while pulling a strong oar.

Cut J 38 shows another similarly equipped at the pool table,
balancing himself on one foot while making a difficult shot.

Cut J 39 represents another with thigh and leg amputation, on
a ladder, at a great distance from the ground; his footing is
sound, his arms are free; he can hold a paint can in one hand,
while he applies a brush with the other.

Cut J 40 represents another riding horseback, securely seated
in the saddle, and feet in stirrups. The spring mattress rubber

feet are used in all of these cases, and sound and reliable footing are due to the excellent feature obtained by that means.

BOTH LEGS AND BOTH ARMS AMPUTATED.—Cut J 41 represents a case in which both legs and both hands were amputated. A

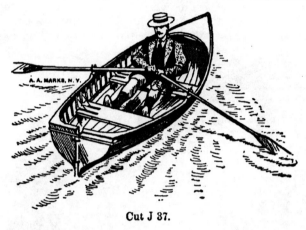

Cut J 37.

pair of artificial legs, and a pair of artificial arms were applied. The wearer became able to walk about in a very natural way; his artificial arms enabled him to feed himself at the table, write,

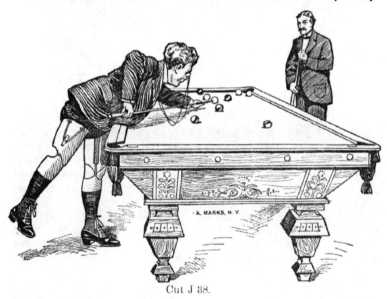

Cut J 38.

and perform such work as does not depend upon delicate finger movements and the sense of touch.

BOTH LEGS AMPUTATED ABOVE THE KNEES.—No matter how extensively a person may be dismembered, prothetic science is capable of rescuing him from a life of helplessness. Only a brief period has elapsed since it was considered rash to apply a pair of artificial legs to a person who had both of his natural legs amputated above the knées. Attempts to substitute such a large portion of the body depending on short thigh stumps for support, resulted in failures, and until modern ideas were introduced and appropriate means for attachments were devised, failure followed

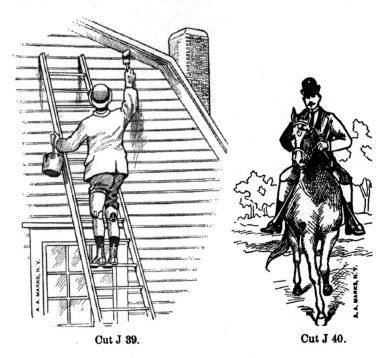

Cut J 39.   Cut J 40.

every effort. In 1864 the first pair of artificial legs was applied to double thigh amputations; the subject was a soldier of the Civil War. Although he was able to sit, stand, and walk on his artificial legs, the effort was so great that the wearer soon tired of them and abandoned their use, and became the occupant of a wheel-chair, dependent on his family.

In 1879 Mr. Marks made his second attempt, and succeeded admirably. The subject was a young man with two thigh stumps that reached nearly to the knees. This man soon acquired the art of balancing, and became so adept that he could walk about the house without the aid of canes or crutches, but when in the street he found it necessary to use a pair of canes. He has worn the pair of legs made in 1879 up to the present time. He is engaged in active business pursuits, and has reared and supported a large family.

Since the above date we have applied upwards of a hundred **pairs** of artificial legs to double thigh amputations. The **manner**

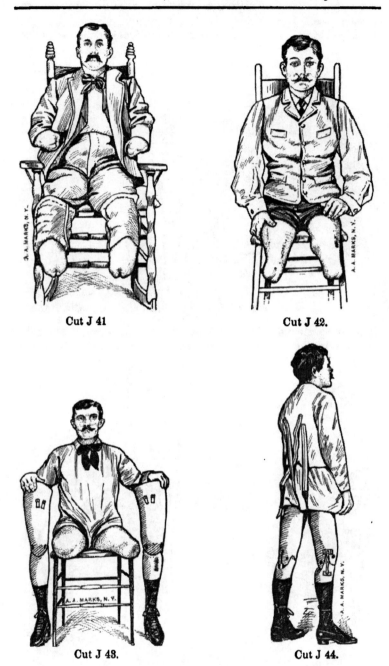

Cut J 41.   Cut J 42.

Cut J 43.   Cut J 44.

in which these limbs were constructed, the way in which they were
applied and adjusted, and the methods employed to give better
control of the movements have varied according to the conditions

of each case. Each double thigh amputation presents problems of an individual character, and as there are seldom two alike,

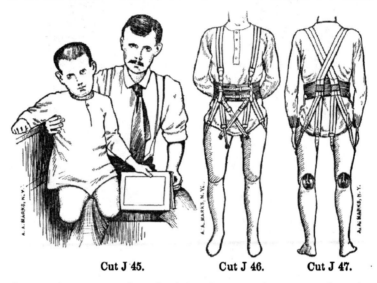

Cut J 45.   Cut J 46.   Cut J 47.

these problems must be solved by the manufacturer. The solution lies in the hanging of the legs, the method of suspension,

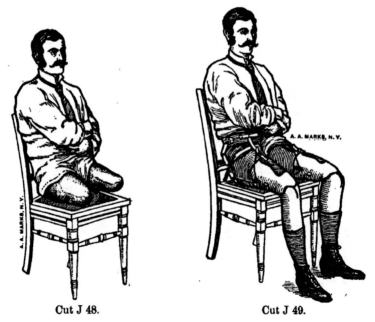

Cut J 48.   Cut J 49.

limiting the motion of the knees, and the absolute rigidity of the ankles. We cite a few cases.

Cut J 42 represents double thigh stumps, produced by amputations made to remove deformed parts. A pair of artificial legs of suitable construction was applied. The great lengths of these stumps gave such control over the artificial limbs that it was not necessary to apply hip joints or knee locks. The subject was a musician. In a brief time he was able to walk naturally, resuming his profession, and now has a national reputation as a clarionetist. He walks on the stage, plays the instrument, acknowledges encores, and retires in the usual stage manner.

Cut J 43 represents a double knee joint amputation. A pair of suitable artificial legs are shown in the same cut. Cut J 44

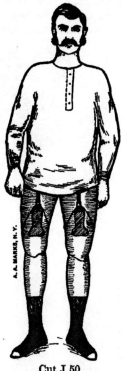
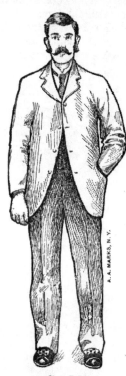

Cut J 50.   Cut J 51.

shows the artificial legs applied, and the wearer in the act of walking.

Cut J 45 represents a child who had both legs amputated above the knees on account of a railroad accident. A pair of artificial legs with knee locks was applied to advantage. The child has, for a number of years, walked on the artificial legs very satisfactorily. He has been enabled to walk to school and indulge in childish pastimes. The manner in which the artificial legs were held in place is shown in Cut J 46, front view, and Cut J 47, rear view.

Cut J 48 represents a double thigh amputation, the result of a railroad accident. Cut J 49 shows the application of a pair of artificial legs with the wearer seated. Cut J 50 represents the same person standing, and in Cut J 51 he is attired as he appears when walking. This case is one of the most remarkable on record. The stumps only extended to about the middle of the thighs, but through the energy of the wearer and the efficiency of the artificial legs, he was able, in a brief time, to walk about in a very natural way, and go up and down stairs; he uses no canes about the house. The artificial legs H 15 were applied with hip joints and automatic knee locks, but after a brief time the wearer dispensed with the locks and found that he could control the artificial knee joints without danger of treacherous flexing. Under earlier systems this case would have been considered hopeless, and the thought of applying artificial limbs would never have been entertained.

CHAPTER XI

ARTIFICIAL FEET AND LEGS FOR DEFORMITIES, PARALYSIS, EXCISIONS, ARRESTED GROWTH, SHORTENED LEGS, ETC.

Deformities of the feet or legs may be due to causes congenital, traumatic, or pathological. Appliances for such cases frequently partake of the character of artificial legs and call for the skill of the prothetician.

No matter how greatly distorted, deformed, or weakened one or both legs may be, there is reasonable hope that some appliance can be used that will aid locomotion, hide the affected parts, and restore a fair degree of symmetry to the person.

SHORT LEG.—The most frequent leg abnormity is that of shortening, due to hip-joint troubles in infancy, or to paralysis.

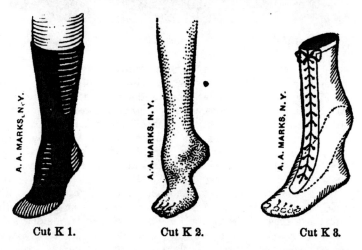

Cut K 1.   Cut K 2.   Cut K 3.

Cut K 1 represents a case of shortened leg caused by hip dislocation. The front of the foot is dropped downwardly to enable the subject to walk on the ball of his foot.

TALIPES-EQUINUS.—Cut K 2 represents a case of talipes-equinus, leg shortened from one to three or more inches, due to paralysis. The ankle joints in K 1 and K 2 were normally strong and the knees and hips under thorough control. Cut K 3 shows an appliance suitable for either of the above cases. It is termed an extension foot, and is constructed from a wooden block, the upper surface shaped to receive the sole of the affected foot, with the front part dropped to a convenient angle (see dotted line). The

119

under surface of the block is connected with the lower part of a rubber foot. The entire structure is covered with suitable leather, the upper of which runs well up on the leg, incasing the entire foot and ankle. Cut K 4 is a shoe, to be drawn over the foot and appliance. It is usually a part of the mate of the

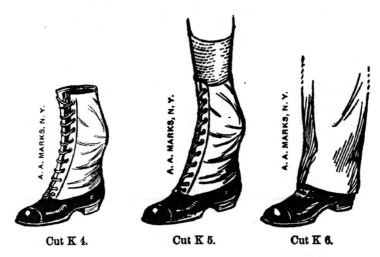

Cut K 4.   Cut K 5.   Cut K 6.

shoe worn on the opposite foot, the quarter having been removed and a larger one put on having the shape and dimensions required to fit properly. This alteration in the shoe is easily made, and can be done by any shoemaker at slight expense. The extension, when complete and covered by a shoe, is shown in cut K 5. Cut K 6 shows it covered with the trousers. Persons with these appliances walk much better than they do with the old style, thick sole and high-heel shoe. They present a better appearance and are far more comfortable.

TALIPES WITH LATERAL WEAKNESS.—Cut K 7 represents a shortened leg with talipes and loss of control over the ankle joint, there being a strong tendency for the ankle to give way sidewise. A suitable appliance is shown in the same cut. It is constructed of wood, carved from a block with naturally curved grains, or made of aluminum, as conditions require. It receives the leg and foot in a comfortable way and holds them firmly in place. The heel and toes are of rubber. Cut K 8 represents the case with appliance in place and wearer walking. In cases of atrophy of the calf, which frequently accompanies these cases, the leg structure can be carved to approximate the contours and dimensions of the sound leg. There will scarcely be an appreciable increase in weight.

TOE SUPPORT.—An appliance of above type is helpful in holding the foot in correct position, and on account of the rigidity of the ankle the wearer obtains toe support that enables him to rise on the ball of the foot when walking. This produces a natural step, avoids limping, and enables the wearer to go up and down stairs and alight on elevations. It also aids him in balancing, and, as the point of resistance at the ball of the foot is in advance of the knee joint, the tendency of the knee to flex is counteracted; this adds materially to the efficiency of the apparatus, giving the wearer a feeling of confidence and security. A person

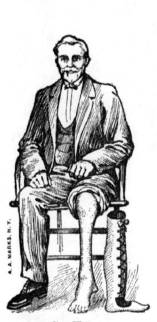

Cut K 7.

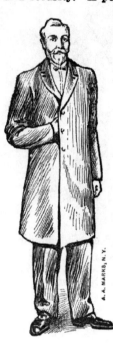

Cut K 8.

with a paralyzed leg, using ordinary braces, usually finds it necessary to press his hand against his knee joint when his weight is on the affected leg. He does this to keep the knee from flexing and precipitating a fall, but with the appliance just described firmness of the knee joint is obtained by phalangeal support in the foot, and the wearer is not dependent on pressure placed in his knee joint, or on attachments going above the knee.

Cut K 9 shows a shortened leg with hip and knee joints under control; the ankle suffered a loss of strength and required supporting.

Cut K 10 represents a leg shortened by hip-joint trouble in youth, producing a deficiency in length of about ten inches; the knee and hip joints are under control and the bottom of the foot is capable of bearing weight. Cut K 11 represents a leg, designed for each of the above cases, the natural foot is dropped to the greatest angle that can be tolerated and made to rest on an

inclined surface at the required distance from the floor. The leg
is incased by a socket made of wood and leather. Cut K 12

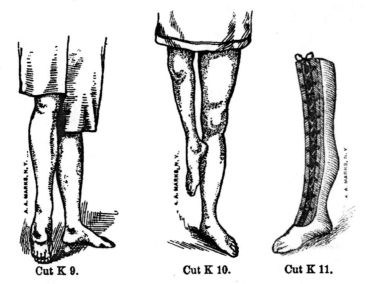

Cut K 9.   Cut K 10.   Cut K 11.

represents the appliance in place, and Cut K 13 shows the patient
properly and neatly attired.

CONGENITAL DEFORMITY.—Cuts K 14 and 15 illustrate the front
and side views of a case of congenital deformity. The foot

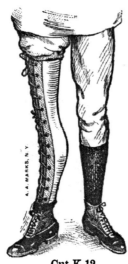

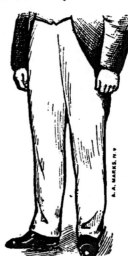

Cut K 12.   Cut K 13.

appears to be attached to the external side of the tibia immediately under the fibula. Weight can be borne on the sole only
when the foot is held in position. Cut K 16 gives a side view of

a suitable appliance constructed substantially the same as K 11. The displaced foot is held firmly in correct position and the wearer walks helpfully and quite naturally.

TALIPES-VARUS.—Cut K 17 represents a case of talipes varus, resulting from paralysis—the knee joint being involved. A suit-

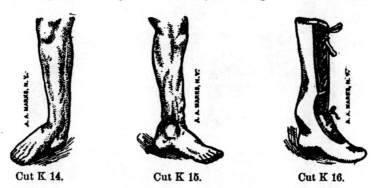

Cut K 14.   Cut K 15.   Cut K 16.

able appliance is shown in the same cut. Cut K 18 shows appliance in place and the wearer seated; with this appliance the wearer is enabled to walk acceptably.

LEG DEFORMITIES.—Cut K 19 represents a deformed right leg. From the knee down, the leg is diminutive, terminating in a

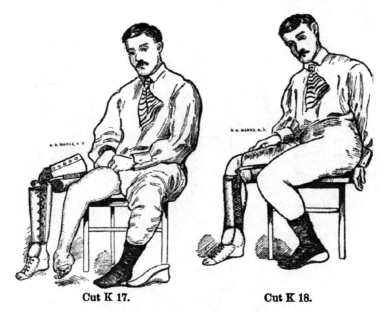

Cut K 17.   Cut K 18.

miniature foot, inclined inwardly and backwardly; the shortening due to arrested development amounts to eight inches. Cut K 20 shows a suitable leg. The deformed leg, from the knee down, is

received into the socket of the artificial leg and held there comfortably. A rubber foot, with spring mattress placed at the
required distance to restore length, fully equipped the child with
means of locomotion.

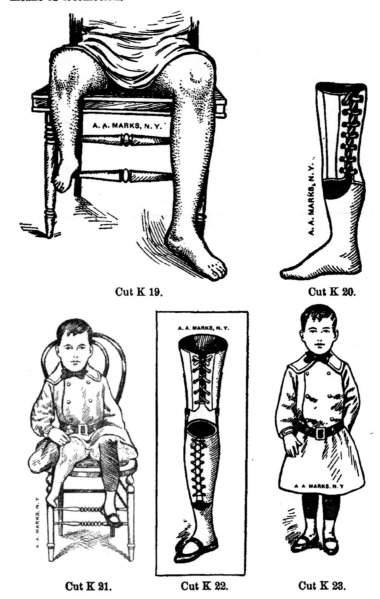

Cut K 19.   Cut K 20.

Cut K 21.   Cut K 22.   Cut K 23.

Cut K 21 represents a right-leg deformity; hip, thigh, and knee
under normal conditions; the leg from the knee down undeveloped, foot very small, terminating in a great toe growing from

the internal side. Cut K 22 shows an artificial leg devised for the case. The deformed leg is received in the socket and laced. The toe is provided with a protecting pocket, the weight is taken partly on the plantar surface of the miniature foot and partly about the leg below the knee and about the thigh. When first applied the leg only reached to the knee, but it was found that there was a weakness in the knee, with a tendency to abduct; knee joints and thigh support were added, which prevented yielding to lateral weakness. Cut K 23 shows the leg applied and the child standing. Since the application of the appliance the child has

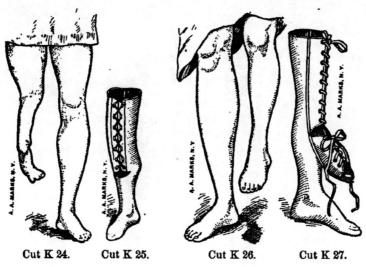

Cut K 24. Cut K 25. Cut K 26. Cut K 27.

grown rapidly in stature and weight, well developed, strong and healthy.

Cut K 24 represents a congenital deformity of the right leg, consisting of a malformed foot, miniature leg, and abnormal relations of tibia and fibula. The tibia extends to the ankle, without connecting with the foot. The fibula connects with the foot, but not with the leg, the two bones held in position by cartilage. When standing on the right foot the bones would slide by each other over an inch; there was also lateral weakness, rendering walking impossible without assistance. Cut K 25 represents an appliance constructed for the case, made of aluminum formed to receive the foot and leg in a comfortable way, terminating with a rubber foot. The weight, when standing or walking, was placed on the internal sloping surface of the tibia, immediately below the knee. The socket held the tibia and fibula in position. This appliance has been used for many years, enabling the wearer to engage in arduous labors, and capable of walking great distances without fatigue.

Cut K 26 represents a shortened and malformed leg. The shortening appears to have been located wholly in the leg between the knee and ankle. Cut K 27 represents a suitable leg. It is constructed to receive and hold the deformed member firmly in place. A rubber foot, placed under the foot-rest, gives the required length. The motion in the ankle made it possible to drop the toe to a concealable angle. Although the apparatus had the appearance of a double foot, there was no difficulty in concealing the deformity by the trousers.

Cut K 28 illustrates a deformity of the right leg. The hip and thigh are normal and an undersized foot appears to have grown

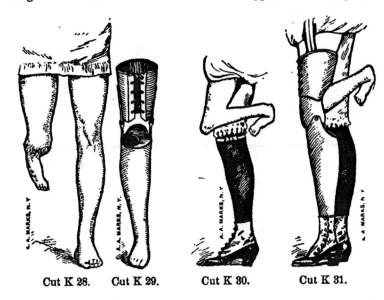

Cut K 28.   Cut K 29.   Cut K 30.   Cut K 31.

immediately from the knee. The patient was able to flex and extend the foot the same as a leg, or, in other words, he had an articulation at the junction of the thigh and the foot, the tibial section being absent. Cut K 29 represents an artificial leg devised for the case. It is similar in its general construction to that represented in Cut E 17. The socket of the leg is excavated to receive the foot, the knee joints and thigh supporter give the foot control over the artificial part.

Cut K 30 represents a deformed left leg. From the knee down it was misshapen, contracted, and distorted. Cut K 31 represents a suitable artificial leg applied. The deformed parts were placed well up and out of the way, concealed by the dress.

Cut K 32 represents a deformed lower right leg, very similar to the one just described. The knee, however, admitted of more flexion, and the artificial leg was made to receive the thigh and deformed part in one socket and was held in place by means of a leather sheath passing from the rear and lacing to the front line of the thigh, as shown in Cut K 33.

INFANTILE PARALYSIS.—Cut K 34 represents an undeveloped left leg, the entire limb considerably atrophied and the joints weak, caused by infantile paralysis. Cut K 35 represents an artificial leg especially designed for the case. The deformed leg is received in the socket and laced in place and the foot dropped to the greatest angle of toleration. The thigh piece incases the thigh

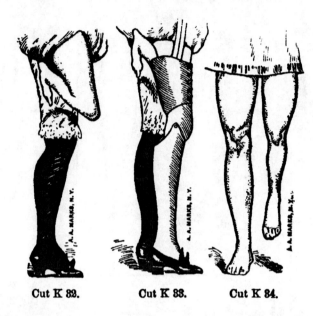

Cut K 82.   Cut K 33.   Cut K 34.

and the joints support the knee; a rubber foot is placed at the extremity. Cut K 36 presents a side view of a similar appliance with a knee lock, which is necessary in cases of loss of control in the joints.

Cut K 37 represents a deformity of the right leg; the hip, thigh, and knee normal and healthy, but the leg and foot diminutive in size, with foot rotated outwardly. Cut K 38 represents an artificial limb especially devised for the case. The undeveloped leg is received into the socket, the foot protrudes through an aperture on the external side, the knee joints and thigh piece, placed above the knee, give support and strength about the thigh. A rubber foot, with spring mattress at the lower extremity, completes the apparatus and gives the required support.

OBSTRUCTED GROWTH.—Cuts K 39 and K 40 represent cases of obstructed growth, the hip joints normal, the thighs possessing nearly the proper lengths, terminating in short and misshapen legs. Cut K 41 represents a leg suitable for either case. Both these persons were enabled to walk nearly as well as if normal conditions existed. A slight enlargement of the trousers a little above the knee (necessary to accommodate the deformed leg) is the only noticeable difference in the two sides, and that difference so slight as to be observed only by the critical eye.

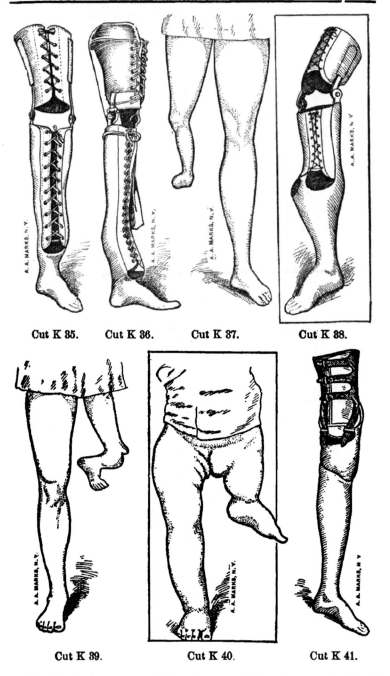

Cut K 35.   Cut K 36.   Cut K 37.   Cut K 38.

Cut K 39.   Cut K 40.   Cut K 41.

Cut K 42 represents a deformity consisting of an undeveloped femur and partially developed leg, the knee joint located very close to the hip. A suitable artificial leg is shown in same cut. The wearer walks so perfectly with this leg that his deformity is absolutely concealed.

BOTH LEGS DEFORMED.—Cut K 43 represents a deformity, both legs atrophied, talipes-varus, feet abnormally large. Amputation of both feet at the ankle joint after the Symes method was advised. This was done and the patient obtained a pair of legs, on which he walks and performs labor acceptably. Cuts K 44 and K 45 represent front and side views of a deformity of

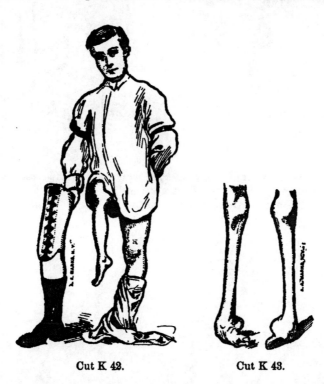

Cut K 42.   Cut K 43.

both feet. From the hips to a little below the calves normal conditions were present; at about the calves there were false joints supplementary to the knee and ankle articulations. These false joints were under poor control, not sufficient to hold the feet in proper position. We advised the amputation of both limbs through the false joints. This was done, and the child had two excellent tibial stumps on which artificial legs, style E 17, were applied and worn with comfort and efficiency.

Cut K 46 represents a case of amputation of right leg and talipes-varus in the left. A suitable artificial leg for the right side and a helpful appliance for the left are shown in the same cut; Cut K 47 shows the limbs applied and the wearer standing erect. The disposition of the leg to rotate inwardly was controlled

by the appliance and the leg was compelled to operate in the line
of progress.

Cuts K 48 and K 49 represent front and side views of a case

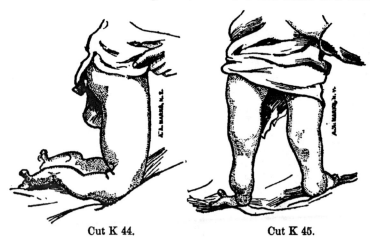

Cut K 44.   Cut K 45.

of congenital deformity of both legs, rendering walking very difficult and more largely dependent upon crutches than on feet. We
advised the amputation of both legs at the calves. The subject

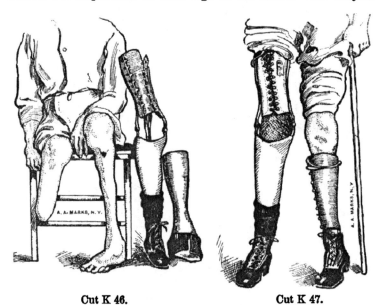

Cut K 46.   Cut K 47.

submitted to the amputation of the right leg, but decided to retain
his left, which appeared to have more sustaining power. Cut K
50 represents the case after the amputation of the right leg, and

Cut K 51 represents him with the artificial leg applied, while Cut K 52 shows him dressed. The condition of the wearer was greatly improved by the removal of the right leg and the application of

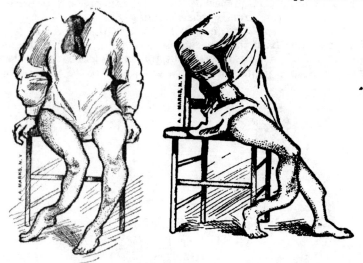

Cut K 48.   Cut K 49.

an artificial one. The improvement would have been carried further if he had submitted to a similar operation on the left side, thereby obviating the outward curve of the lower leg, which

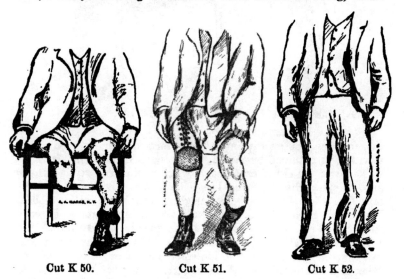

Cut K 50.   Cut K 51.   Cut K 52.

is conspicuous even when covered with trousers. Cut K 53 represents a case of paralysis of the right leg, knee slightly flexed. Cut K 54 represents the same with one of our instruments applied; wearer seated. It was constructed with knee joint, provided with automatic lock, preventing flexing with the weight directly over the leg, permitting flexion when the wearer is seated. The foot is held in proper position for standing and prevented from flexing treacherously when walking.

Cut K 55 represents congenital deformities of both legs; branches grew from the inner surfaces of both femurs. That on the right thigh was ten inches in length, on the left not more than two. The knee joints were on the inner surfaces of the ends of

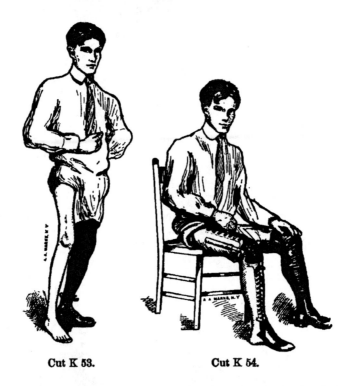

Cut K 53.   Cut K 54.

the femurs, feet everted and badly formed. In boyhood, locomotion was obtained by moving about on his haunches; later he walked with the aid of crutches, bearing on the ends of his femurs and dragging the deformed legs. For twenty-five years he submitted to these awkward and unsightly means for getting about. His attention was finally called to artificial limbs, and upon consulting well-informed persons he found that he could improve his condition by having the useless parts of the legs removed and artificial ones applied. We indicated points at which amputations could be performed to advantage. After the operations his stumps presented the appearances shown in Cut K 56. We applied a pair of artificial legs, constructed on the plan of those represented in Cut G 8. When dressed, this man had the appearance of a person with natural and well-formed legs. Cut K 57 is taken from a photograph, showing him as he appears in ordinary life.

Cut K 58 represents a case of arrested development. The child was well formed from the knees up, but from the knees down his deformity was pronounced and of a character to render walking

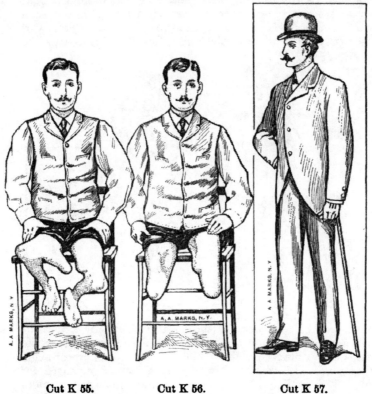

Cut K 55.　　　　Cut K 56.　　　　Cut K 57.

impossible. The child managed to get about rather awkwardly with crutches, permitting but little weight to come on his feet. As the joints in the ankles and knees were flexible, and as the feet were small, we found that we could incase the entire legs, provide knee motion, and place rubber feet at suitable distances below the deformed ones. This was done, and the lad was brought to his proper height, making a presentable appearance and walking in a very acceptable way, without the aid of crutches. He controlled the artificial knee joints by means of his feet and had little or no difficulty in balancing, walking, sitting, rising, ascending or descending steps. Attention was given to ornamentation, and when dressed his deformity was entirely concealed, as shown in Cut K 59.

DROP FOOT.—The drop foot, resulting from paralysis or arrested development, is a frequent infirmity. Usually the leg is of normal length, the knee joints contracted and weak, with loss of control at the ankles and lateral weakness or a tendency for the foot to bend sidewise, either varus or valgus. The only practical manner in which a leg of this sort can be rendered useful is by fixing the ankle joint artificially, thus providing a resistance at the ball of the foot, the concomitant for balancing, maintaining height when walking and serving as a lever for propulsion, and as a counteracting influence to the tendency of the knee to flex. Cut K 60 represents a case of this kind. Cut K 61 represents the

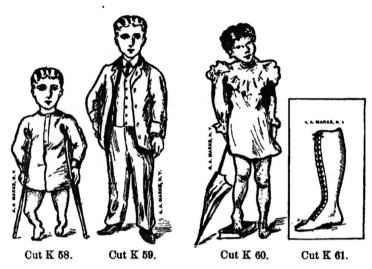

Cut K 58.   Cut K 59.   Cut K 60.   Cut K 61.

appliance we have devised for such. It is practically a form of splint, cast of aluminum to the shape of the leg and foot. The metal is carried under the entire foot, holding it at a proper angle for walking. The front is provided with leather, arranged for lacing. This appliance holds the ankle joint firmly and provides support at the ball of the foot, which is so far in advance of the center of motion of the knee that it prevents the knee from flexing when the weight of the wearer is directly over the foot. Persons with these appliances walk rapidly and quite naturally, seldom requiring any attachments above the knees.

In connection with appliances of this type for paralyzed lower extremities we may quote from the Cincinnati *Lancet-Clinic* of October 9, 1897. A prominent physician read a paper before the academy regarding the treatment of his own paralyzed leg:

"An illustrated catalogue fell into my hands, in which was pictured, among artificial legs, etc., an apparatus made of aluminum, splint-like in character, with a rubber cushion under the foot to compensate for shortening. It was made for a case of congenital dislocation of the ankle. The more I studied it, the more it appealed to me that such an apparatus could be made for my own comfort. I had reached a period when I was considering amputation and the substitution of an artificial leg for my paralyzed one. Impressed with the illustration of this apparatus, I consulted a friend upon the subject. He was as much impressed with it as I was, but advised me to obtain the opinion of our surgical friends. They were likewise impressed with it and advised that I try the conservative measure first before I resort to the radical one. I went to New York and consulted the maker. After studying my deformity for a few minutes, he stated that an apparatus could be constructed that would materially improve my condition. The appliance was made and worn for four years. But those four years! How can I describe them? Pen and words fail me. It was like a beautiful oasis in a dreary desert of years of suffering. In connection with my deformity there was a weakness of the abductor muscles, which permits of a rotation outwardly of the thigh. This has been overcome by rubber abductor muscles. The one fastened to the outer side of the apparatus crossed the front part of the right thigh, crossing to the left side of the trunk, and is inserted into the harness. The one attached to the inner side of apparatus is inserted over the right posterior part of the harness, which is suspended from the left shoulder.

"Who are my benefactors? Who are those who have given to me the comfort of four years' duration, with a bright future of many more? And, within such a short period, free from pain, caused the twenty odd years of suffering to disappear in the dim and misty past?

"Oh, for a trumpet of such power to herald to the world their name, that those who are needy may seek them! But instead, in gratitude do I raise my feeble voice and wish the cup brimful of happiness for the firm of A. A. Marks, New York City.

"'By thy deeds shalt thou be known!'"

KNEE JOINTS LOCKED.—Shortened and paralyzed legs are frequently accompanied with total loss of the power of extension and flexion in the knee joints. In such cases the mechanism of the artificial knee joints is provided with locks that hold the knees rigid when standing or walking. The joints are capable of being unlocked to admit of flexion when sitting.

Cut K 62 represents a shortened, atrophied, paralyzed leg. Cuts K 63 and K 64 show the same case, with apparatus in place. The apparatus consists of a socket that incases the leg, knee joints with locks that support the knee, thigh piece that takes the support about the thigh, and a rubber foot placed under the deformed natural foot in order to obtain the proper length.

LIMITED KNEE MOTIONS.—Cut K 65 represents a shortened leg with limited motion in the knee, the knee capable of flexion, but incapable of extension beyond the angle represented in the cut; the hip normal and the bottom of the foot capable of enduring pressure. Cut K 66 represents an artificial leg suitable for the case. It is

made with a wooden socket, fitted to receive the leg. A comfortable
shelf is provided for the foot to rest upon. Knee joints with pawl and

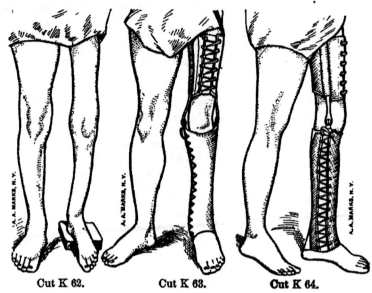

Cut K 62.   Cut K 63.   Cut K 64.

rack and thigh piece incasing the thigh are provided. The pawls
at the knee joints are operated by levers which pass up the rear of

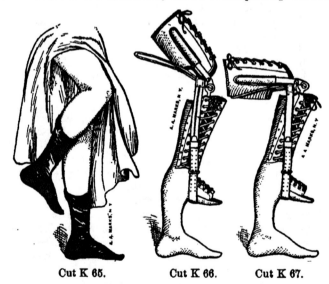

Cut K 65.   Cut K 66.   Cut K 67.

the thigh. When standing or walking, the leg is brought to the
point of greatest extension, the pawls automatically drop into the
rack and make the leg immovable at the knee. The moment the

wearer is seated, the lever will rest on the chair and force the pawls out of their racks, allowing the knee to flex (see Cut K 67). By this means the wearer is able to walk safely with rigid knee

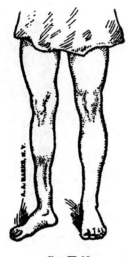

Cut K 68.

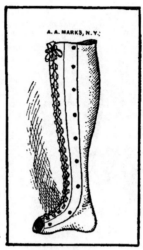

Cut K 69.

and bend the knee when sitting. The apparatus has a rubber foot with spring mattress placed at the proper distance below the paralyzed one.

UNUNITED FRACTURES.—Cut K 68 represents an ununited fracture of the tibia and fibula at a point a little above the ankle joint. Usually, in cases of this kind, it is deemed advisable to amputate, the wisdom of which we do not question. Occasionally, however, and particularly in the case here illustrated, the horror of the knife kept the patient from submitting to that alternative, and he came to us for help with a dangling foot, under no control whatever. He was young and in good health, and cherished the hope that if the fractured parts were held firmly in juxtaposition, nature might eventually, in her mysterious way, bring about a union. We constructed an aluminum socket, incasing the leg from the knee down and the entire foot, fixing the ankle. This appliance, shown in Cut K 69, was fitted when the tibia and fibula were in apposition. Weight was communicated from the bottom of the appliance to the leg immediately below the knee. No weight whatever was brought on the foot and no strains permitted to cause the bones to move out of the places in which they were held. The appliance has been worn advantageously for a number of years. The manner in which the wearer gets about, walks, and attends to his vocation is exceedingly gratifying.

Cut K 70 represents an ununited fracture of the right tibia, due to gunshot wound. All efforts to bring about a union failed. The fibula was not injured, but in consequence of failure of union in the tibia it was obliged to do the work of both bones. Being overtaxed, it gradually yielded and became curved, as shown in the cut. The dark spot immediately below the patella represents a deeply indented scar at the point of fracture. Cut K 71 repre-

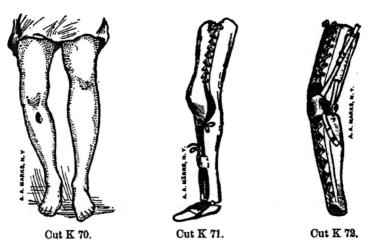

Cut K 70.   Cut K 71.   Cut K 72.

sents a suitable brace for the case, made of wood and leather. A block of wood is excavated to receive the fractured member in its most comfortable position. The leg, when placed in this splint-like appliance, is held firmly by means of lacing. As the injury shortened the leg about one inch, a block of suitable thickness was hinged to the lower extremity of the splint on which the foot rested. Owing to the proximity of the fracture to the knee articulation, it was impossible to construct the brace that would admit of knee motion. The appliance has done its work for a great many years with great satisfaction to the wearer.

FRACTURED KNEE CAPS, ETC.—Resections of knee joints, fractures of knee caps, weakening of the patella ligaments, in fact any ailment that lessens or destroys control over the knee articulation is greatly benefited by appliances similar to that represented in Cut K 72. The socket below the joint is made of wood, with a leather front capable of being laced. The upper socket is made entirely of leather. The knee joints are made with stops, so that extension cannot be made beyond the proper limit. In cases of partly flexed knees, due to knee-joint disease, this appliance can be used to advantage, requiring knee locks in addition.

CHAPTER XII

FACTS FOR CONSIDERATION

Wooden Feet Substituted by Rubber Ones.—Artificial legs, manufactured with wooden articulating feet, are more or less troublesome and expensive to keep in order, and are deficient in supplying the requisite propulsive power in walking, it is therefore often deemed advisable to remove them and substitute rubber ones. We have devised methods by which this can be done, whether the legs be constructed of wood, leather, or metal. Our charge is $20.00 in each case. We guarantee the attachment to be strong and lasting. A foot of any size or shape to meet the wishes of the wearer can be put on, and the leg can be made longer or shorter, as may be desired.

A Way to Test the Rubber Foot.—The attachment of a rubber foot to an old artificial leg is often done to test its merits. It gives an admirable opportunity for the wearer to try the rubber foot and ascertain for himself the advantages it has over those he has worn.

An experiment of this sort can only be successful when the socket of the old artificial leg fits correctly; if it does not, the leg cannot be worn comfortably and satisfactorily, no matter what kind of a foot it may have.

A cabinet maker, carpenter, or other mechanic, be his skill in his own line what it may, should not be expected to connect a rubber foot to an artificial leg with assurance of satisfactory results. The alignment, the set of the foot, the angle at which it should be placed relative to the shaft, are important factors and must be thoroughly understood and their relations to each other comprehended, or the results will be disappointing. This knowledge can only come from experience; we therefore dissuade persons from buying rubber feet and having them put on their artificial legs by home mechanics. We therefore insist that artificial legs be sent to us for such work, and for which we make no extra charge.

Ease and comfort in wearing an artificial leg depend almost entirely upon the manner in which the socket receives the stump. No matter how correctly the leg may be constructed, or with what nicety the parts operate, it is worthless if it causes pain, abrades the stump, or interferes with the circulation.

Fitting—an Art.—The fitting of an artificial leg is an art, only acquired by thought and the experience of years. A thorough knowledge of the anatomy of the stump, the effects of pressure on various points, the manner in which interference with the circulation or the displacement of tissues on the stump can be obviated must be understood, or the fitter is not qualified to be intrusted with such work.

There are a great many artificial limb manufacturers in the world, but there are a very few fitters.

ONLY ONE WAY TO FIT.—There is but one way in which a leg can be made to fit correctly, and that is to excavate a block of wood until it has the proper size and shape to receive the stump, so that pressure will be placed where it can be endured, there must be absolute freedom from contact on the blood vessels and exposed nerve areas.

A leg that puts pressure uniformly on the stump is not a comfortable one to wear, for there are many places on every stump that cannot bear any pressure whatever. There are other places that can endure any amount of pressure; a socket to be comfortable must, therefore, be made so as to apply pressure only where it can be endured.

WHEN PLASTER CASTS ARE USELESS.—A plaster cast of a stump and a plaster cast of the inside of a socket that fits the stump correctly are no more alike than the last on which the shoe is built is like the foot on which the shoe is worn. It is absurd to assume that a serviceable, comfortable socket can be made by molding a plastic material, such as leather, felt, or wax, on the cast of a stump or by molding it on the stump itself. Sockets so made are always irritating and cause pain and suffering. It is likewise an error to assume that a block of wood can be cut out to the contours of a plaster cast of a stump and fit the stump comfortably. If it were so, the fitting of an artificial leg would be reduced to a mechanical operation which could be conducted by inexperienced and inexpensive persons. If the work could be done in this way, the cost of an artificial leg might be considerably lessened.

MACHINE FITTING A FAILURE.—The irregular form turning lathe, with which all mechanics are familiar, carves a stick of wood to the exact shape of the model. Axe handles, gun stocks, shoe lasts, and many other articles are made in this way. A machine of this kind has been modified so as to excavate a block of wood so it will have the exact shape of a plaster mold of a stump. A socket for an artificial leg made in this way must be greatly modified by hand before it can be worn with comfort.

When we are reminded that the stump is bone covered with muscles, fat, blood vessels, nerves, tendons, and skin; that these coverings are not of uniform thickness: that they are soft, yielding, and easily displaced: that more pressure can be applied on the least sensitive parts, and that where the nerves and blood vessels are the most numerous less pressure can be endured, we will readily see that a socket, to fit properly and not injure the stump, must be fitted by persons skilled in the work, who know the location of the large blood vessels, the character and disposition of the nerves, and who are keenly alive to the necessity of avoiding pressure on the vascular parts. The skilled fitter does not always need the presence of the person who is to wear the leg he is fitting. Circumferences and diagrams of the stump will guide him in doing more accurate work than is possible for an incompetent fitter, though he be supplied with plaster casts, or fits directly to the stump.

WHEN CASTS ARE NECESSARY.—Plaster casts are desirable in some cases. They convey contours, locate irregularities, prominences, and tender spots on abnormal stumps, or on those that reach to the knees, ankle joints or insteps, and in such cases are quite necessary, but, generally speaking, stumps that extend to any point between the articulations do not require to be reproduced in plaster.

WOOD SOCKETS THE BEST.—The advantages of wood sockets are many. Wood is light and firm, retaining the shape it receives from the skillful fitter. No matter what conditions may exist—the tender spots of a stump are always protected, weight is applied where it can be endured, and when the socket is highly polished there is absolutely no friction. A stump may move, slip, and slide without becoming blistered or abraded.

WEIGHT.—The weight of an artificial leg varies from one to seven pounds, according to its size and the severity of the labor it is to perform. We have made artificial legs that weighed less than a pound for infants, and we have been obliged to make them seven or eight pounds in weight in order to be strong enough for active, three-hundred-pound persons. The only way to obtain strength is by the employment and proper disposition of suitable material. A small leg is not as heavy as a large one, and a strong leg must be heavier than a frail one.

RUBBER FOOT NOT HEAVY.—A leg with a rubber foot can be made from six to sixteen ounces lighter than the ordinary artificial leg with articulating ankle. The lessening of weight is chiefly caused by the absence of the metallic ankle connection.

The notions of those wearing artificial legs are varied, therefore they cannot be used as guides. One man says, make my leg as light as you can, even at the sacrifice of strength; I would rather have a light leg and renew it more frequently than to carry a heavy one. Another will say, do not make my leg too light; I have worn light and heavy ones, and I find that I can walk more steadily and step more naturally with a leg of moderate weight. The leg should act as a pendulum; the moment it is lifted from the ground it should swing forward of its own weight and not depend upon energy imparted by the stump. Still another will say, I do not care what the leg weighs so long as it is made strong: strength is the desideratum. If it weighs a pound or two more I will not object to it, as I can soon get used to that, but it must be strong and last a long time. I cannot afford to take chances on the leg breaking. The utmost diversity of opinion, therefore, exists on this subject.

The greatest demand, however, is for the lightest leg, consistent with strength.

For light, delicate women, weighing less than a hundred pounds, a full-length leg weighing three pounds without attachments is as light as it is prudent to produce. So light a leg with ample sustaining strength is almost a marvel. We know of nothing calculated to withstand equivalent strains that weighs so little. A leg weighing six pounds for a large, heavy person, who is likely to subject it to severe use, is not excessive, and should not be objected to.

Let us think, for a moment, of the weight of other instruments that are made to stand similar strains. The weight of the bicycle has been reduced from sixty to nineteen pounds, and it is generally conceded that a nineteen-pound bicycle is as light as prudence will allow. Persons marvel at a bicycle weighing so little, yet the nineteen-pound bicycle has no more work to perform and is not subjected to any more strains than an artificial leg weighing from three to six pounds. The bicycle, like the leg, has only to support the weight of the rider and resist such strains as may occasionally be brought upon it.

In constructing a leg it is essential to make it strong enough to sustain the weight of the wearer and not break under such sudden strains as it is likely to receive at times. If one slips and recovers himself with his artificial leg, some part receives a strain that is much greater than the weight of the wearer. In ascending or descending stairs the strains on the leg are greater than in walking. A leg should be made strong enough to meet these demands, and, in addition, must have a margin of strength that will enable the wearer to carry such articles and lift such weights as his vocation requires. No matter how crippled one may be, or what his station in life is, nor how delicate, there will be times when he will thoughtlessly lift, carry, push, or pull some weighty object. Should the leg break under any of these conditions, the maker would unquestionably be severely censured.

It is not wise to build an artificial leg so close to the danger line, especially for delicate persons, that when those persons become healthier, stronger, and heavier the leg will break. Conditions do not remain the same. "The weak of to-day are the strong of to-morrow." The light person frequently becomes heavy, and the careful limb maker, if he guards his reputation, will keep well on the side of safety.

The average weight of a substantial artificial leg, suitable for a thigh amputation, worn by a man weighing one hundred and fifty pounds, engaged in an ordinary occupation, may be placed at five pounds, less for a below-knee or foot amputation.

It is possible to localize the weight of a leg weighing six pounds so that it will feel lighter than one weighing half as much, improperly adjusted. Inadequate means of attaching the leg to the body will make it feel heavy. A heavy lower part, with a light thigh piece, produces an apparently heavy leg, because the weight is distant from the stump and the frail thigh piece does not hold it in place securely. On the other hand, a strong, substantial thigh piece, which properly holds the leg in place, will lessen the apparent weight considerably.

ODOR.—The contention that rubber emits a disagreeable odor is untrue. Sponge rubber has no more odor than wood; moreover, the rubber foot is incased with an air-tight material. Even if the rubber had a disagreeable odor—which it has not—it would not be possible for it to escape. On the other hand, the ankle joints of articulating feet have to be oiled very frequently, and the oil in time becomes rancid. No refined person can possibly tolerate such an odor.

TEMPERATURE.—The rubber foot will not alter its consistency on account of changes in temperature. Properly vulcanized rubber, such as is used in the manufacture of our rubber feet, will not lose its elasticity in any temperature the human body is capable of enduring. It requires 280 degrees of heat (Fahrenheit) to produce a change in rubber, and as there is no habitable place on the earth with a temperature half of that, the rubber foot is never in danger from heat; no human being could live in a temperature intense enough to harden pure rubber.

THE MASS OF LIMB WEARERS ARE OF SMALL MEANS.—The greater number of wearers of artificial limbs are in limited circumstances. It is exceptional to find a wealthy person in need of one. The wage-earner, the laborer, the man who works in the mill, the engineer, fireman, brakeman, or the miner, the private in the army, those whose occupations place them in jeopardy and who are exposed to the dangers that destroy life or mutilate the body, these make the greatest number of limb wearers. This being so, it is the more important that artificial limbs should be durable and as inexpensive to wear as possible. The first cost, the purchase of the limb, should be the only important item to be provided for. An artificial leg constructed with delicate machinery, or parts subject to friction, may be attractive to look at, but is ill-suited to the wants of the man who has to support himself and his family by daily toil. The loss of time in having repairs made, the cost of repairs, and the danger of breaking down at critical times, are serious matters, and the careful man will take them into consideration before making his selection.

We do not know an artificial leg with an ankle joint that is now made, that has ever been made, or, perhaps, ever will be made, that will not cost from five to twenty-five dollars a year to keep in repair. The delicacy with which an ankle joint must be constructed in order to be light and small enough for its narrow limits, and the immense strain that it must resist at times, are conditions incompatible with durable mechanism.

The fact that persons walk, run, and perform all kinds of labor on artificial legs with rubber feet without ankle motion is evidence that the ankle mechanism is unnecessary. Men, women, and children with rubber feet run, walk, skate, and dance. Work, regarded not many years ago as impossible, is now being daily performed with facility. The farmer follows his plow on a rubber foot, the blacksmith works at his forge, the sailor climbs his rigging, the builder erects houses, and persons of every vocation attend to their affairs with as little concern and hindrance, operating on one or a pair of our rubber feet, accomplishing as much as their associates who are in possession of all their natural limbs.

How Long Will a Leg Last?—The question is frequently asked, "How long will an artificial leg last?" There is but one reply: it depends upon the care the leg receives. We have patrons who are still wearing artificial legs that were made for them twenty-five years ago, and the legs still appear to be in fair condition. These are exceptional cases and should not be referred to, any more than should the experiences of those who, through abuse and carelessness, destroy their artificial limbs in an unexpectedly short time. An average made of the frequency with which our patrons renew their substitutes, fixes the period at about eight years. This does not imply that a leg will not last longer. Necessity by no means occasions all renewals; wearers want new legs much the same as they want new coats, before the old ones are completely gone. Wearers become as proud of their artificial limbs as they do of articles of apparel; those financially able frequently supply themselves with several, so as to have a reserve for emergencies. Accidents are as likely to occur to the substitute as to the real ones. Men have been run over by vehicles and have had their artificial legs crushed instead of their natural ones. When accidents of this kind occur, the limbs must be sent to the manufacturer for repairs. The wearer who is fortunate enough to have a duplicate which he can put on is at a great advantage. Taking all these facts into consideration, and fixing the average life of an artificial leg at eight years is certainly estimating on a fair basis.

Shoes and Stockings.—All artificial feet should be dressed with stockings and shoes, as are natural ones. The wear and tear on shoes and stockings, when the feet articulate at the ankles, are enormous and have been a source of complaint. This annoyance is removed by the use of rubber feet, for shoes on rubber feet look and wear like those worn on the natural, as the wrinkling at the toes and other parts is nearly identical in both. We have heard patrons say that in five years their rubber feet have saved them in the cost of stockings and shoes enough to buy a new leg.

How Soon after Amputation Should an Artificial Leg be Applied?—As soon as the stump is thoroughly healed and the patient has regained sufficient strength to go about on crutches, it is time for him to consider the matter of procuring an artificial leg. Before procuring one some attention should be given to the preparation of the stump.

Treatment of Stumps.—Tight bandages should be worn from

the moment the stump is healed until the artificial leg is applied. Bandages are inexpensive and can be frequently renewed. The stump corset suggested by some is made as follows. A block of wood is carved to the shape and dimensions of the stump; a piece of substantial leather is moulded upon this form, the edges running down the front are permitted to remain apart about two inches, eyelets are put on each edge to admit of lacing, straps to hold it in place are attached as shown in the cuts. A shoemaker or saddler within the reach of the wearer can usually be found who will make the corset at little expense. No matter how soft and pliable the corset is made, it has not the adjustability of ordinary bandages, therefore its use is not encouraged.

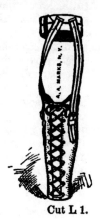

Cut L 1.

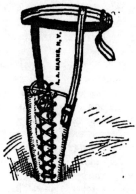

Cut L 2.

Cut L 1 represents one with suitable straps for leg amputation and Cut L 2 represents one for a thigh stump.

The knee and hip joints should be moved very frequently, and the stump rubbed vigorously in order to maintain mobility.

No matter what means are employed to reduce a stump before an artificial leg is applied, it is doubtful if all the changes can be brought about. As a rule stumps become smaller from wearing artificial legs. The pressure received from the socket has a tendency to force absorption and solidify the tissues. The extent of this emaciation cannot be conjectured. Some stumps do not change even when artificial legs are worn for years. On the other hand, we know many cases where the stumps have grown larger. The matter is governed by the disposition of the wearer, his occupation and his activities.

If a stump reduces after an artificial leg is worn, some compensative adjustment must be employed, lining the socket with thick material as leather, felt, or cloth, or by wearing a number of socks on the stump, one drawn over the other is the most convenient way, but in case of great shrinkage, so much so that such fillings are objectionable, it will be necessary to remove the socket from the leg and substitute a new and smaller one. We do this work for our customers at small expense, but new measurements and diagrams are required and the entire leg must be sent to us.

If the stump is one that will yield to pressure it will not only become smaller under the influence of the bandage or corset, but must grow still less by the use of the artificial leg. Under such circumstances, it is an important economical question to determine whether it may not be wiser to immediately apply a leg and change the socket, should it become necessary, than waste time in bandages or shrinking corsets.

THE GAIN IN APPLYING A LEG IMMEDIATELY.—The immediate use of an artificial leg enables the wearer to dispense with crutches at the earliest possible moment, to gain the freedom of his arms, attend to his vocation, and take healthy and vigorous exercise. The cost of a new socket to fit a reduced stump is insignificant when the advantages of wearing an artificial leg during the interval the stump is changing are taken into account.

Walking on crutches is dangerous, a slip or fall may seriously injure a stump. An artificial leg is the best protective device for the stump.

The single exception to the wisdom of early applications is in amputations which result from malignant diseases.

DANGERS IN DELAY.—If a stump is permitted to go for six months without performing its share of work, it will become weak, nervous, and disordered, and circulation will become sluggish. It is much more difficult to use an artificial leg on a stump that has been permitted to get into this condition than if applied immediately after it has healed.

We have applied artificial legs within a month after amputation with good results, although this time is exceptionally brief. It is impossible to indicate the exact length of time that should elapse between the amputation and the application; it is safe, however, to say that a limb can be judiciously applied as soon as the wound is healed, even if there be tenderness on the amputated surface. It is well to remember, in this connection, that with rare exceptions the end of the stump bears no pressure whatever.

It is a common error to assume that a stump will become hard and tough in time. Nothing can harden or toughen it except use, and there is no better way to toughen a stump than to use a leg. The hands of a laborer are strong and hard because he uses them in performing his work. Those of a person not accustomed to manual labor are soft, tender, and delicate, and become easily blistered because they have not been disciplined. Exactly the same principle is applicable to stumps.

Surgeons are at variance in their views on this topic. Some advise an early application, others insist on their patients waiting an unreasonable length of time. The surgeon who has studied the subject in all its bearings invariably agrees with the advice given above.

CORK LEGS.—The term " cork leg " has long and frequently been used to designate an artificial leg. The prevailing impression is that there is or has been an artificial leg made principally of cork. This is an error and should be corrected. Cork is known to every mechanic as a very friable substance, on account of which it has not strength enough to form any part of the supporting structure of an artificial leg.

The origin of the term "cork leg" is not known. It has, however, been said by credible authority, that the term originated from the fact that years ago very good artificial legs were made in Cork, Ireland, which were called Cork legs, the same as legs made in London are called London legs, those made in New York are called New York legs, etc.

There have been many doggerels written in which the word cork is used to designate an artificial leg.

Thomas Hood, in his Golden Legend, "Miss Kilmansegg and Her Precious Leg," speaks of cork and wooden legs, neither of which was good enough for the fastidious Countess:

> "She couldn't, she shouldn't, she wouldn't have wood,
>   Nor a leg of cork if she never stood!
>   And she swore an oath, or something as good,
>   The proxy leg should be golden!"

It is evident that at the time the above was written, many years ago, the term "cork leg" was misunderstood the same as it is now.

CHAPTER XIII

ARTIFICIAL LEGS FOR THE AGED

To be deprived of a natural leg after having passed the allotted span of life is indeed a calamity, and the thought of wearing an artificial one is entertained with forebodings. Will not the infirmities of age come fast and heavy? Has not the shock sapped the vital reserve so that early decline will make the purchase an unprofitable one? Is the prospect of living a few years promising enough to justify the attempt? These are questions of gravity that come with force especially to those in moderate circumstances.

As is shown in another part of this book, the loss of a leg, no matter how old or enfeebled the patient may be, instead of hastening the fatal day, has a tendency to give a new lease of life. The removal of a diseased leg serves as a tonic to the entire system. If the finger of death has been laid upon the foot, as in senile gangrene, remove the foot and the decay will cease.

Like cutting the dying limbs from an old tree, the vital forces will be more generously distributed among the remaining parts and the tree will take on new life.

It is no greater task to learn to walk on an artificial leg than to learn to use crutches, and as a matter of fact an artificial leg is much safer. To put an aged person in a rolling chair and deprive him of the health-giving walks is to invite disaster. The aged as well as young will rust out sooner than they will wear out.

Age must not be taken into consideration; as soon as the stump is healed an artificial leg should be obtained; in a very brief time the wearer will be able to get about without depending upon others. Walks in the open air and healthful exercise will be indulged in, and gratifying results will follow.

A few cases bearing on this matter may be cited:

The Rev. Edward Beecher, of Brooklyn, N. Y., brother of the famous Henry Ward Beecher, lost a leg by accident in his eighty-fourth year. For several years prior to that time there were evidences of senility, and when he met with his accident it was not supposed he had vitality enough to survive it. Amputation, however, was proceeded with. Mr. Beecher recovered from the shock, and in a very short time was convalescent. He was soon able to take short walks on crutches, but the fear of falling made the task difficult and exhausting.

The writer well remembers when he was summoned to this distinguished clergyman's house. He was seated in a chair, looking very tired. He had just returned from a walk on crutches. "I am a very old man," he said, "and I do not think I have long to live. The idea of buying an artificial leg appears to me a piece of folly; but my friend, Mr. Sage, is insistent that I should get one and try it. Whether I succeed or not, it will make no difference to you, but considerable with me. If I ever learn to walk on the leg I know I shall feel better, and I am going to try."

The leg was made and applied, and in a very brief time he acquired the art of walking on an artificial leg. He moved cautiously at first, but soon got so that he could put entire confidence in the limb. He took long walks daily, and attended to his church and parish work with renewed vigor. The leg was much easier for him to walk on than crutches, and gave him a feeling of security. He wore it for eight years, when he died at the age of ninety-two. Is it reasonable to assume that, if Mr. Beecher had not applied an artificial leg, but had resigned himself to the cot or rolling chair, he would have lived to that ripe age? Did not the walking that he was able to do, and the open air exercise, contribute to his health, and add to his life? The denial of an artificial leg would certainly have been a severe punishment to this good man for having lost his leg in old age.

Charles Van Brunt, of Long Branch, N. J., had his foot amputated on account of senile gangrene when he was seventy years old. An artificial leg was applied as soon after the amputation as prudence admitted, and he lived for fifteen years and wore the leg constantly. He died at the age of eighty-six. During much of the time he performed the duties of school janitor.

George Hinman, New Haven, Conn., had his leg amputated when he was eighty years old. He obtained an artificial one and wore it continuously for four years, during which he was active on his feet and walked long distances.

Mrs. Susanna Brown had her leg amputated above the knee when she was seventy-three years of age, a result of an accident. An artificial leg was applied four months after the amputation. She wore it three years and was active in domestic work. Dr. A. L. Britten, of Athens, Ill., writes about this case as follows:

"Mrs. Susanna Brown, of Cantrall, Ill., for whom you manufactured an artificial leg after she had passed her seventy-third birthday, found it eminently satisfactory. She was helpless in no sense. She could, and did, ascend and descend stairs without assistance, and without fear of falling."

David Penfield lost his leg on account of gangrene when he was seventy-two years of age. Dr. White, of Franklin, N. Y., in one of the letters says of the case: "The facts in regard to David Penfield are briefly told as follows: He was in the seventies when I first saw him, and had had two attacks of cerebral apoplexy, which left one arm and one leg paralyzed to such an extent as to make walking and use of arm impossible. Gangrene presented itself and I amputated the foot of the affected leg. He recovered, and I obtained an artificial leg from you for him. He very soon learned to use it, and was able to walk about fully as well as before his trouble. He lived a considerable time after he obtained the leg, and found it a source of great comfort. His family and I regard the wearing of the limb as having added to his comfort and health."

Nelson Stevenson, Salem, Ind., had his leg amputated above the knee when sixty-seven years of age. An artificial leg was applied a few months later, which he wore for over three years.

Frederick Triebold, St. Paul, Minn., had his leg amputated above the knee when seventy-four years of age (in 1894). An artificial leg was applied eight months after the amputation which he is still wearing (1905). Dr. A. H. Steen, in writing of the case, says, "Frederick Triebold considers the artificial leg made for him indispensable, his health is good, and he wears the leg at all times."

Russell Perkins lost his leg in 1894, when he was sixty-nine years of age. An artificial leg was applied within eight months. Dr. William R. Lough, of Edmeston, N. Y., says, "Mr. Perkins gets along well with his artificial leg. He does his chores around the farm, and frequently comes to town. He does not use a cane and gets along very well."

James R. Bugbee lost a leg when he was seventy-six years of age on account of a fall. He had an artificial leg applied, which he is still wearing with great comfort. In one of his letters he says, "I am now seventy-nine years old. I am able to do my work around the house and garden, which I positively could not do with crutches."

William P. Hiller, of Nantucket, Mass., lost a leg in the Civil War. He is still living, and has worn an artificial leg continuously since. He is now eighty-two years of age.

Mr. Bradford Beal had his leg amputated in 1894 at the age of eighty-three. The leg was applied the following February, and he wore it with comfort and relief for over five years. We quote from a letter: "I am wearing the artificial leg constantly. I go about the house without cane or crutch. I have walked a mile from home and back a number of times without fatigue."

Equally encouraging reports can be given of hundreds of similar cases.

CHAPTER XIV

ARTIFICIAL LEGS FOR INFANTS AND CHILDREN

THE PROBLEM CONSIDERED.—It is a serious problem that confronts the parents of a child who has had one or both legs amputated. The parent, in happy possession of all his limbs, realizes more keenly than the child the misfortune that has happened. An artificial leg is, no doubt, the immediate and only remedy that can be suggested, but even this presents thoughts of expense for remodeling, and the question is often asked if the benefits will justify the costs incurred, and whether it may not be better to wait until the child has obtained his growth, before equipping him with the needed limbs.

A child, however young, is as greatly disabled by the loss of a leg as an adult. If one leg is lost he becomes dependent on crutches; if both legs are lost, he has to be carried in the arms or pushed about in a rolling chair, or is obliged to hitch himself about on his haunches as best he may. Such methods are at once unnatural and objectionable; they have a hurtful effect on the physique of a growing child, as well as harming the limbs, stumps, and joints. Walking on a pair of crutches for any length of time pushes the shoulders forward, settles the neck in the chest, and the spine fails to develop the sustaining strength demanded in later life.

Walking on one crutch, as most children do, cants the body sidewise, elevates one shoulder above the other, tilts the pelvis, and produces an over-development of one side of the body at the expense of the other. If the use of crutches is continued throughout the growing period, the disproportions resulting from unequal development will bring troubles that will last through life and imperil health. The stump, being pendent from the body and performing no functions, will become poorly adapted to the use of an artificial leg. The muscles will become atrophied, the joints enervated, and the range of motion lessened. It will be troublesome to wear an artificial leg under these conditions, and the task of disciplining the stump will be more difficult. It is doubtful if the harm thus done can ever be righted.

We can cite many cases where the neglect to apply an artifical leg to a growing child has been the cause of physical weaknesses that have been impossible to correct. Contracted hips and knees, weakened spines, deflected and rotated stumps, are a few of the many ills that have been traced to this neglect.

Failure to apply artificial legs in double amputations is

attended with more serious consequences. The stumps are held in flexed positions and subjected to such unnatural influences that the wearing of a pair of artificial legs, when undertaken later on, is greatly hampered. The art of balancing is forgotten and has to be learned again. The hip joints, having been in flexed positions during the greater part of the development period, have become more or less set, and extension is difficult and pain-ful when the erect position is attempted.

SUPPORT FROM THE PELVIS MORE NATURAL.—An artificial leg applied to a child, no matter how young, supplies a support to the amputated side that is the nearest approach to nature. It gives freedom to the arms, the joints and muscles are kept in ac-tivity. Being propped from the pelvis instead of from the shoul-ders, the spine, chest, and shoulders are not distorted, but are as free to perform their functions as if the child had never lost a limb. All the parts of the body maintain their proper relations and develop symmetrically.

The child invariably becomes expert in the use of one or a pair of artificial limbs, if applied soon after amputation; he mingles with other children, and engages in the same sports and exercises, the variety, which makes him strong mentally and physically, keeps him healthy, and prepares the foundation for the vigorous manhood and active life before him.

ALTERATIONS FOR GROWTH.—A child will outgrow his artificial leg, but this does not entail a serious loss; the leg can be altered in length and size to accommodate his growth and devel-opment. The expense attending such changes is not large, no greater than that of changing or renewing crutches, or repairing rolling chairs.

The only growth of the child that affects the length of the arti-ficial leg is that which takes place in the sound leg from the knee to the floor. A child may, in the course of two years, grow four inches in his entire height, but the growth in the sound leg, from the knee to the floor, will be less than an inch. It is, therefore, evident that a child growing four inches in height will not require his artificial leg to be lengthened over an inch.

FREQUENCY OF ALTERATIONS.—The frequency with which an artificial leg worn by a child is lengthened, is about once in two years, oftener if the growth is more than usually rapid, and the expense attending each lengthening is not over $5.00. In fam-ilies where economy has to be exercised to an extreme degree, the lengthening of the leg can be deferred, if necessary, by in-creasing the thickness of the sole and the heel on the shoe worn on the artificial foot as soon as growth requires. The size of the leg can be increased, and the foot can be enlarged, and in this way the leg can be made to last from five to ten years. It will thus be seen that in extreme cases a child can be supplied with an artificial leg, and the leg can be kept in proper length, at an expense of about $2.50 a year. We can hardly conceive of a parent who is so poor that he cannot meet this expense, or who socket was made to fit the stump snugly, the joints were placed on the sides to harmonize with the natural knee joint; a thigh piece incased the thigh. The leg would swing when the child was carried, and forced the stump to move at the knee.

In a few months the child began to creep. The mother was surprised one morning to find her standing by the chair, putting some of her weight on the leg. It was not long before she began to walk, then to run and play. The leg was lengthened quite frequently, and enlarged several times. During her childhood she ran and romped about as other children, went to school, and was as happy as any of her companions; she is now a young lady of twenty-two. Although her parents were in moderate circumstances, they always felt that their daughter's health and perfect development were important, and they denied themselves many things, but considered themselves amply compensated for the care they had given to the needs of their daughter.

Carrie K., when seven years of age, was run over by a carriage and lost her left leg. An artificial one was applied as soon as the stump had healed. The distinguished Dr. James Knight, the founder of the Children's Hospital in New York City, took the case in hand, and realizing the importance of putting the child on a leg instead of keeping her on crutches, interceded in her behalf. A leg was applied and she grew up with it; she developed gracefully and now is a woman of forty-three years. Cut M 6 represents her as she appeared when brought to us in 1869. Cut M 7 represents her with artificial leg applied, and Cut M. 8 gives her as she appears to-day, a thankful wife and a happy mother.

Thomas Kehr, when eight years of age, was run over by the cars, both of his legs were crushed, the right was amputated four inches below the body, and the left two inches below the knee. As soon as the child recovered from the operation Dr. Samuel J. Brady, of Brooklyn, advised that he be provided with a pair of artificial legs with rubber feet. They were obtained and applied, and the manner in which the young man got along is clearly stated in Dr. Brady's letter of 1876, from which we make the following extract: "I have thoroughly examined the case of the boy Thomas Kehr, who has been wearing a pair of artificial legs for six months. About a year and a half ago he was run over and both of his lower limbs were so crushed that I amputated them, the one well above the knee, the other an inch and a half below. At the time of the operation many expressed the wish that death would occur, as the lad being very poor, it was thought that his future would not only be a burden to himself, but that his support, should he reach man's estate, would depend upon the charity of the public, as it was considered an impossibility for him to serviceably use artificial limbs.

"I am thankful that I can say that Marks' artificial legs have made his future worth the living.

"I saw him two weeks after he had put the legs on for the

first time, and it astonished me greatly to see the remarkable use he had so soon acquired; since then I have seen him many times, and quite recently I saw him walking without the use of canes. He has, much to my astonishment, been fully and absolutely restored.

"I attribute the wonderful success in this boy's case mainly to the superior results achieved by your inventions, and to the

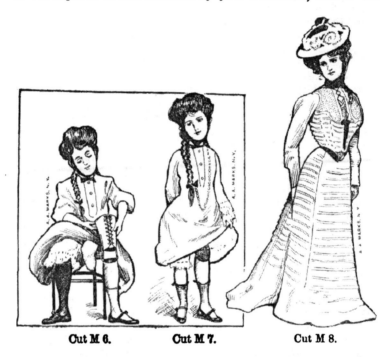

Cut M 6.   Cut M 7.   Cut M 8.

fact that the legs were put on so soon after the amputations that the stumps had not had a chance to forget their functions."

Mr. Kehr is now a man of forty years. He is an active, capable, energetic workman, in perfect health, earning his livelihood and maintaining a family. If this man had been neglected in his childhood, he would be to-day a helpless object of pity, instead of a self-supporting member of the community,

Annie L. Beckwith lost her leg below the knee in 1887, when she was seven years of age. An artificial leg was immediately applied. It has been lengthened several times since. She is now a woman of good proportions, strong and healthy. Cuts M 9 and M 10 represents her as she appears without and with her artificial leg.

Manuel Parraga, of San Salvador, Central America, had his leg amputated above the knee in 1876, when eleven years of age. An artificial leg was applied immediately. His weight at the time was seventy-five pounds. The lad has developed into a full-

George W. Sheridan, son of General George A. Sheridan, was thrown from a carriage by a runaway horse, when he was ten years old. One leg was crushed and had to be amputated below the knee. Nine months later his mother, becoming solicitous about the child's development, insisted on an artificial leg being obtained, this in opposition to the advice of her husband and family medical adviser. The mother gained her point, and a leg was applied, and the child used it immediately, and the effect upon his health was surprising. We quote from the General's letter: " My son is now fifteen years of age. He has worn a leg of your make for the last five years, always with comfort and satisfaction. When visiting him at his school a while since, I found he was out for a day's fishing. When he returned and stated where he had been, the teacher remarked that he had walked at least ten miles. George skates on steel or roller skates, rides a bicycle, and in short enjoys to the full the usual sports of boys of his own age. I now realize that it would have been a mistake, almost a crime, to have made the boy wait until he had stopped growing before supplying him with your artificial leg."

Hattie L. Moore had her leg amputated at the age of thirteen. Six months after the operation an artificial foot was applied. She wore it five years without lengthening. The growth of the natural foot, from the ankle down, was not great enough to require any alteration in the artificial foot. We quote from her letter: " My foot was amputated when but a child of thirteen, and as soon as the stump had healed, I had one of your admirable rubber feet supplied, made and fitted from measurements. It fitted me as if I had gone to New York and had had the foot fitted by your own hand. I have used the foot four years now, to the untold satisfaction of myself, and the utmost gratification of my friends, who often tell me that they would never notice anything peculiar about my walk. I have lived with people nine months without their discovering that I was lame.

" I am at present doing a daughter's part of housework, standing on my feet the greater part of the time."

William E. Shaw, leg amputated for injury to the knee. An artificial one was applied when nine years of age. To quote from his father's letter: " My boy has had great success with the artificial leg that you made for him. He can walk and get about excellently. He would not be without it for anything. It is unquestionably the best thing for a child, when he has lost one of his legs, to get an artificial one without delay."

John Kershaw, leg amputated above the knee, railroad accident. Artificial leg applied when ten years of age, immediately after the healing of his stump.

Dr. A. C. Dedrick writes: " I passed John Kershaw in the street three months ago. From the success in his case I certainly advise the application of an artificial leg to a young and growing lad as soon as the stump has healed. John Kershaw has been able, thanks to the artificial leg, to enjoy his early life equally with others not so unfortunate. He plays football, baseball, and all other sports. I think he would have lost all power of stump if the leg had not been employed. The stump is only about six inches long, and would in all probability have become flexed if he had grown older without a leg to keep the hip joint in condition."

Flossie Lee, leg amputated below the knee. Artificial leg applied when four years of age. Dr. G. A. Harris, of Chepachet, R. I., writes, "Flossie Lee has worn an artificial leg, which you fitted her five years ago, continuously since that time, except when sent to you for lengthening. It is needless to say that her health, in both mind and body, is different from what it would have been had she been confined to the house all these years. She has been to school, and runs about like other children, which means everything to a growing child. No change has been made in the leg all these years, except the increase in length."

Thomas McAleer, leg amputated above the knee on account of accident. Artificial leg applied when seven years of age. Dr. D. K. Dickinson writes: "McAleer, whom you so nicely fitted with an artificial limb for amputation above the knee joint, has received great satisfaction. I recommend the application of a limb by all means in similar cases."

Ettie Stangl, leg amputated below the knee in 1889. David Jones, of Richardson County, Neb., writes in regard to the case: "Ettie Stangl, to whom you applied an artificial leg when she was very young, has worn it continually. She does not appear like a cripple, she moves about so naturally. I can say that the artificial leg was a source of comfort to her, and I think providing her with the limb when she was so young was the best thing that could be done for her health and comfort."

Mary Wiley, both feet amputated in 1891; cause, railroad accident. Artificial feet were applied several months later. She was then eight years of age. This little girl is a forcible example of the wisdom of applying artificial limbs to children, especially when both are amputated.

Clarence Wintersgill, both legs amputated; right, six inches below, and left, three inches above the knee; cause, railroad accident. Artificial legs applied within a few months. Age, seven. Dr. R. F. Wintersgill writes as follows: "In regard to my son's case, the application of a pair of artificial limbs has been a wonderful success. He was but seven years of age when you made his limbs, but learned rapidly how to use them. He now skates, rides a horse, goes to school, and walks several miles without resting. I was advised not to get Clarence any limbs until he had ceased growing and had almost made up my mind to wait, but to look at my little child sitting out in the yard helplessly, and to think that he must do so until he had finished growing, made me almost frantic. In the meantime, one of my neighbors provided me with one of your books, and I studied it day and night until I came to the conclusion to try a pair of your legs, with the results mentioned above.

"You will remember, Clarence's left leg is off above the knee and the right below the knee. He was wearing his artificial limbs one year after amputation, and if I had to do it over again he would wear them in one month."

John E. Palmer, leg amputated below the knee. Artificial leg applied within six months; age, nine years. His father, Bradford Palmer, writes: "I am glad to let you know what success my boy has had in using his artificial leg. He was only nine years old when he commenced wearing it. I can say that it has afforded him the greatest satisfaction, and he could in no way be induced to do without it. He is growing fast and has the best of health."

Anton Gaub, leg amputated in 1884. Artificial leg applied within a few months after amputation; age, four. Gaub is now (1905) twenty-five years of age, full grown and well developed. He has always used the leg and never cared for crutches. He is strong, in good health, and walks great distances without becoming fatigued. He is actively engaged in business. His parents refer with pride to their decision in putting him on an artificial leg when he was so young.

Roscoe E. Bosworth, leg amputated below the knee in 1890; age, nine years. His father, Levi Bosworth, of Worcester County, Mass., writes: "I consider that it was a very wise thing on my part to have supplied my boy with an artificial leg when he was so young. He now has full use of his knee and hip joints, which I think would have become greatly impaired if he had not used the leg. He is now in good health, well developed. Crutches, which he used for a short time, always made him sick.

"Roscoe has skated, ridden a bicycle, and done almost everything other boys do. If I had a child only two years of age and he needed an artificial leg I would put one on immediately."

Roy V. Bryant, leg amputated above the knee when seven years of age; artificial leg applied immediately. His father writes as follows: "My son has worn his artificial leg constantly, with the exception of times when it has been at your factory for lengthening. He is now twenty years of age. He has grown straight, strong, muscular, well developed. I am thoroughly convinced, from the experience in my own son's case, that an artificial leg cannot be applied when a child is too young."

Carl T. W. Banks, leg amputated above the knee; railroad accident; artificial leg applied within six months after amputation. His mother writes: "The question of applying an artificial leg to a young child was one of great thought to me. Many of my friends thought it unwise to do so, but I could not bear to see my son Carl going on crutches, so I got a leg and had it put on when he was only seven years old. He has been wearing it since, and he is now well developed, strong and healthy. During his childhood days he played with other boys, in all kinds of weather and at all kinds of games."

Emma Zern, leg amputated above the knee. Dr. J. William Trabert, of Annville, Pa., writes: "Emma Zern's leg was amputated in the lower third of the thigh in 1890, when nine years of age. She received an artificial leg from you within six months. She has been wearing the same constantly. In the following spring she grew 2½ inches. The leg had to be lengthened, but it did not cost very much to do it.

"At first I was doubtful that a child of her age should have an artificial limb, but am now convinced that a child cannot be too young, as this case has shown."

Nellie Cartwright, at the age of eleven, met with an injury to her leg that necessitated an amputation below the knee. Six months after an artificial limb was applied. Her father writes: "I purchased an artificial leg from you for my daughter in 1893. She was then eleven years old. She has used the leg constantly. I am delighted with the results and prepared to say that I recommend the use of artificial limbs to children of any age, and the sooner the child has a leg applied after losing a natural one the better it will be for that child. There are two reasons that should induce a parent to act promptly: First, an artificial leg enables a child to walk naturally, promoting good health and symmetrical growth. Second, a child becomes accustomed to the use of the limb while young and active and will ever afterwards use it with better results than it could if the use was delayed until maturity."

Clara Giere, leg amputated below the knee; age, eight. An artificial leg was applied immediately. Dr. E. Alonzo Giere, of Hayfield, Minn., writes: "The artificial leg which I obtained for Clara has given good satisfaction. The child has grown and the leg has had to be lengthened. She is still using it with comfort."

Dr. A. R. Eaton, of Elizabeth, N. J., under date of March 31, 1904, writes: "The facts of my case are as follows: In March, 1891, I had my left leg so badly crushed as to require a supracondylar thigh amputation (Gritti-Stokes type). In May of the same year I applied one of your artificial legs and wore it for a considerable length of time. Since I have attained my growth I have had another one made. The leg was a blessing to me from the start. As a matter of fact, I would have been lost without it at any time. I walk easily long distances, sometimes ride a bicycle, other times ride a horse; I play tennis, golf, etc. In fact, do with ease and facility almost all ordinary things.

"My observation leads me to believe that this excellence of locomotion is only possible with the Marks leg, for I see cases similar to my own using ankle-joint legs who are able to enjoy only ordinary usefulness.

"In regard to the application of artificial legs to young and growing children, I can say that my own case is an example. The artificial leg was applied when I was thirteen years old. I am now fully grown and am a physician engaged in active practice. My professional knowledge tells me that it is a most advisable procedure, for the use of a leg strengthens the stump, prevents atrophy of joint structures and soft parts, and trains a child in the use of a leg, and when he reaches adult life he will have perfect control over it, and he will become strong and healthy."

Charlie Moore, at the age of eight, had his leg crushed by a wagon. Amputation was above the knee. His mother writes: "My little son, Charlie Moore, when eight years of age, met with an accident that resulted in the amputation of his right leg. He went on crutches two years. He was pale and sickly and grew but little. The doctor said he was sure that the constant use of crutches would induce spinal disease or lung trouble. I therefore resolved to get an artificial leg for him. I did so, and as a result he now has good health, is well grown and thoroughly developed. I advise buying your make of artificial limbs for young and growing children. They are light and strong in construction and easily lengthened."

CHAPTER XV

HOME MEASUREMENTS

Our system, devised and inaugurated years ago, by which measurements and diagrams for artificial limbs can be taken at home by the family physician or the subject himself, assisted by some member of his family, and our method of fitting and constructing artificial limbs from such data, have proved so satisfactory that we encourage those desirous of saving long, tedious, and expensive journeys to have their limbs made from measurements while they remain at home.

This feature has placed our facilities and skill within reach of those who are in need of artificial limbs, no matter how distant they may reside from us; it affords an opportunity to obtain the best at the least possible expense and trouble.

So successful have been the results obtained from this method that expressions of gratitude and commendation have come from the most distant parts of the world. Men of prominence, as well as those not so frequently in public mind, have benefited by the plan.

We have customers living within a few miles of New York City who are so actively engaged that they prefer to have their limbs fitted from measurements under the guarantees we give, rather than absent themselves from their homes.

To encourage persons to have their limbs made in this way, we agree to make all changes or reconstructions without charge, whether such are required on account of errors in measurements or changes in stumps, or any other cause whatever.

If anyone desires to be present at the fitting, we will not dissuade him from his intentions, and will give him immediate attention on his arrival.

As soon as measurements and diagrams are received, we subject them to the closest scrutiny, and if errors or omissions are discovered, they are returned for corrections, and if there are any indications that successful fittings from measurements are doubtful we do not hesitate in notifying the party to that effect. As soon as we accept the data we assume all risks, we make the leg accordingly and forward it to the client with full instructions for its application. Should it fail to fit properly, it can be returned with particulars, and we will alter or reconstruct it without charge.

INSTRUCTIONS WHEN ONE LEG IS AMPUTATED

DIAGRAMS.—First, make a diagram of both the sound and amputated legs. This is done by removing the clothing and sitting

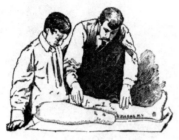

Cut N 1.

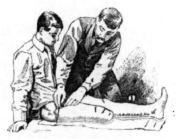

Cut N 2.

on a large sheet of paper, with both the sound leg and the stump extended and slightly spread apart, the foot pointed directly

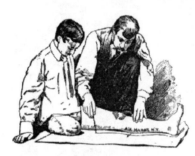

Cut N 3.

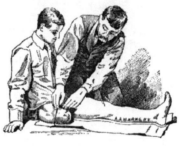

Cut N 4.

upward. Beginning at the body, draw a pencil down the outside of the sound leg from the hip, around the heel and up the inner

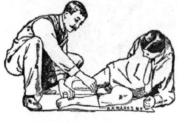

Cut N 5.

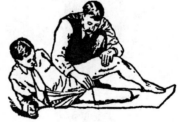

Cut N 6.

side to the body. Then carry the pencil down the inner surface of the stump and around the outer side to the hip. Cuts N 1 and N 2 show the manner in which this is done if the amputation is below the knee; Cuts N 3 and N 4 show the same if the amputation is in or above the knee. For side diagrams, it is necessary for the patient to lie on one side with the knee bent at right angles and then pass the pencil around the leg, as shown in Cut

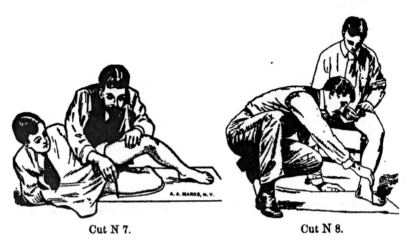

Cut N 7.   Cut N 8.

N 5. If the amputation is below the knee, turn on the amputated side, resting the exterior surface of the stump and thigh on the paper, and mark around it, as shown in Cut N 6. Then, without changing the position of the body, flex the knee to about right angles, and mark around the thigh and stump, as illustrated in

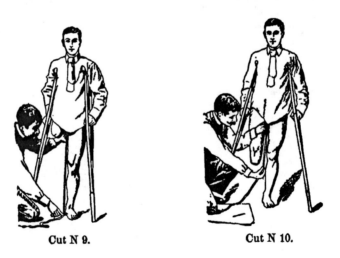

Cut N 9.   Cut N 10.

Cut N 7. These diagrams will show the amputated leg in two positions, one with the stump fully extended, and the other flexed at right angles. If there is a limited motion in the knee joint, special care must be taken that the limits of extension and flexion are shown in the diagrams. Then place the foot on the paper and draw a line around it, as shown in Cut N 8.

MEASUREMENTS.—After the diagrams come dimensions. Measuring should be done in the morning when the stump is not

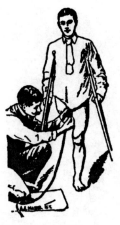
Cut N 11.

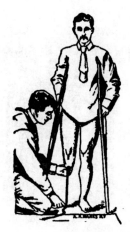
Cut N 12.

swollen; a tape line should be used. Begin with measuring the distance from the crotch, or perineum, to the floor—the end of the tape line must be put close to the body between the legs and carried vertically down to the floor (see Cut N 9); in the same

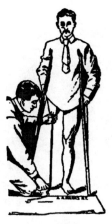
Cut N 13.

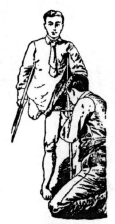
Cut N 14.

way measure the distance from the crotch to the end of the stump (see Cuts N 10 and N 11). Measure from the end of the stump to the floor, as shown in Cut N 12 or Cut N 13.

While still standing take the circumferences of the sound thigh, beginning close to the body, as shown in Cut N 14, repeat at points two inches apart, until the knee is reached, then take the circumference of the knee around the knee-cap, then the following

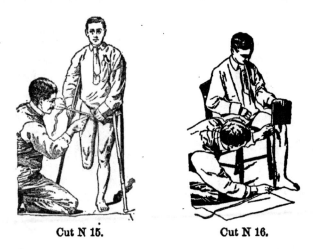

Cut N 15.   Cut N 16.

circumferences; the leg immediately below the knee-cap, the calf, smallest part of the ankle, just above the joint, the heel and instep, the instep, the foot at the base of the toes; then measure the length of the foot.

If the amputation is below the knee, take the circumference of the thigh close to the body (see Cut N 15) and repeat these cir-

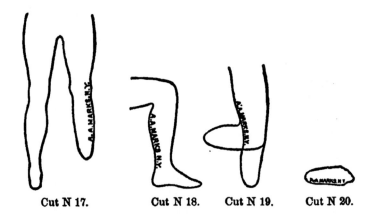

Cut N 17.   Cut N 18.   Cut N 19.   Cut N 20.

cumferences at points two inches apart until the entire thigh is measured; then take the circumference of the knee around the knee-cap; then take the circumferences of the stump, beginning immediately below the knee-cap, and repeating at points two inches apart until the entire stump is measured. If the amputation is in or above the knee, take the circumference close to the body and repeat at points two inches apart until the entire stump is measured.

After the circumferences have been taken, measure the distance

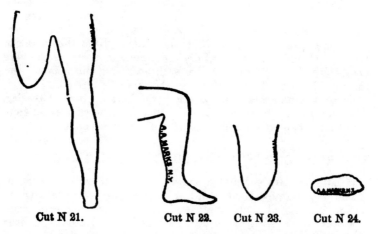

Cut N 21.   Cut N 22.   Cut N 23.   Cut N 24.

from the top of the knee of the sound leg to the floor when seated in a chair, with the leg bent at right angles (see Cut N 16).

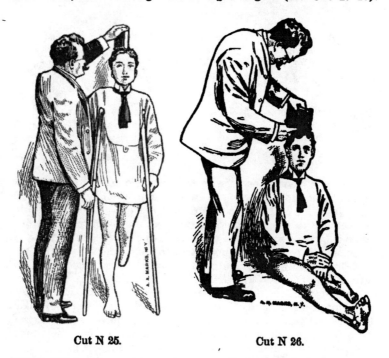

Cut N 25.   Cut N 26.

Write all these lengths and circumferences on the diagrams in their respective places.

If correctly made, the diagrams of an amputation below the knee will resemble those figured in Cuts N 17 to N 20; for amputation in or above the knee they will resemble Cuts N 21 to N 24.

Other required measurements include the height of the person when standing erect on the sound leg. This can be taken by standing against a wall and the height marked by a book or carpenter's square (see Cut N 25); the distance from that point to the floor should then be carefully measured; then sit on the bare floor, with the back against the wall, and note the height from the top of the head to the floor, as shown in Cut N 26.

These heights are wanted to verify the length given of the leg. The height from the head to the floor when sitting subtracted from the height when standing is equal to the length of the leg.

INSTRUCTIONS WHEN BOTH LEGS ARE AMPUTATED

If both legs are amputated, either above or below the knees, or if one is amputated below and the other above, it is necessary to make diagrams of each stump and thigh, presenting both front and side views, with knee joint extended and flexed to as near right angles as possible. These can be taken by disrobing and

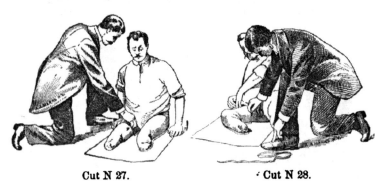

Cut N 27.   Cut N 28.

sitting on a piece of paper with the stumps extended and marking around them from body to the ends with a pencil held perpendicularly (see Cut N 27). Then turn to one side so that the exterior surface of the thigh and stump will rest on the paper; the stump extended, mark around the thigh and stump, then bend the knee to about right angles and mark around thigh and stump (see Cut N 28). A similar diagram must be made of the other thigh and stump (see Cut N 29). After these diagrams have been made, circumferences should be taken by passing a tape line around each thigh, close to the body, and repeating at points of about two inches apart until the thighs and stumps have been measured. Care should be given to take the measurements when the stumps are not swollen and to draw the tape line moderately tight, as shown in Cuts N 30 and N 31. Write all the measurements in plain figures in their respective places on the diagrams. Sit on the floor, with back against the wall, and mark, by book or square, the distance from the top of the head to the floor, as illustrated in Cut N 32. Send this measurement, together with former height,

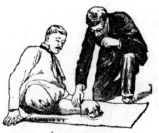

Cut N 29.

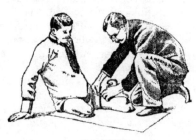

Cut N 80.

that is, the height before amputation. If the full former height is to be restored that fact should be noted.

Stumps that reach to the ankle joints or knee joints should be reproduced in plaster.

The following questions should be answered in every case: Name of patient? Post-office address? Occupation? Age?

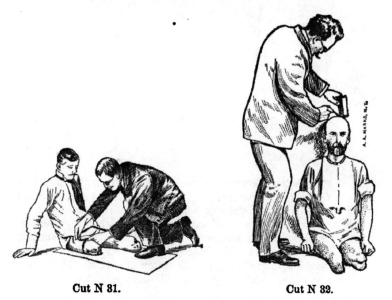

Cut N 31.   Cut N 32.

Weight? Cause of amputation? When was the amputation performed? Which leg amputated? Has an artificial leg been worn? For how long? Name of the party ordering the leg? His address? Is the leg to be made and fitted from measurements in the absence of the patient?

If it is proposed to take weight on the end of the stump, that fact should be noted.

If the amputation is in the ankle joint or in the foot, the diagrams and measurements are the same as are required in amputations above the ankles.

PLASTER CASTS.—Plaster casts are only required of stumps that reach to the articulations (knee or ankle joints) or in the feet, and of deformed limbs, and of amputations that have resulted from deformities.

The method of making a plaster cast depends upon the condition of the stump. For tapering stumps, the following is the simplest: Remove the clothing, shave all hair from the stump or fasten it down with paste, or thick soap, as otherwise it will

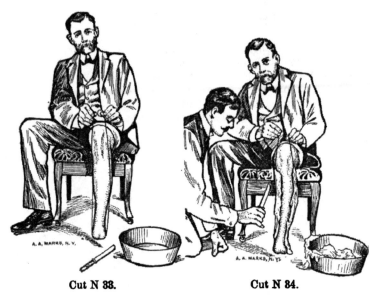

Cut N 33.   Cut N 34.

cling to the plaster. Then take two quarts of thick, quick-drying plaster of Paris, such as used by dentists, put a quart of water in a bowl and sprinkle the dry plaster in it, mix thoroughly. It should be made about as stiff as "pancake dough;" then spread it over all sides of the stump to the thickness of at least half an inch. The stump must be held perfectly still until the plaster has become hard, which will be about ten minutes. Then draw it from the stump and the inside will be a counterpart of the stump.

If the stump is larger at the end than immediately above, as in the case of partial foot, ankle-joint, or knee-joint amputations, the plaster must be broken off in large pieces and put together after the stump is removed, or the string method can be used, as follows: A piece of strong, thin cord is passed loosely up each side of the limb (see Cut N 33), to which it is made to adhere by thick plaster (see Cut N 34). Work quickly, using about four quarts of slacked plaster and cover the entire limb to a thickness of not less than half an inch. As the leg must be held vertically,

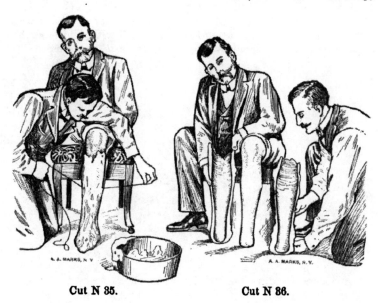

Cut N 35.   Cut N 36.

the plaster must be quite thick, otherwise it will flow down. Every part, the back, sides, front, and end, must be liberally covered. As soon as the plaster has become a little set, the string can be

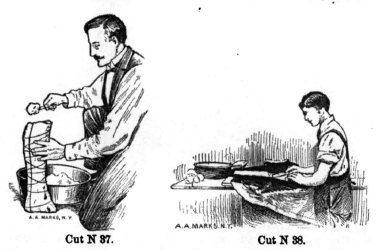

Cut N 37.   Cut N 38.

pulled gently downward (see Cut N 35), cutting the mold into longitudinal parts. It must now be left alone, so as to thoroughly harden, which will take about ten minutes; the mold can then be

separated on the line cut by the string and the two parts
removed (see Cut N 36). These parts can then be greased or
oiled on the inside and put together and bound with a string; the
inside can then be filled with thin plaster of Paris (see Cut N 37).
When the mold is filled, it should be laid aside for several hours,
when it will have become so hard that the shell will yield to slight
pressure and break off, uncovering a facsimile of the stump.

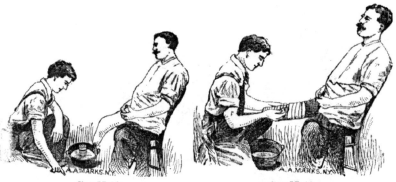

Cut N 39.   Cut N 40.

The plaster bandage method is an excellent way of taking a
cast of a flabby and tapering stump. A sheet of old muslin or
cheesecloth is cut into strips about two inches wide and sewed
into lengths of about twelve feet long. Three such strips are
usually needed. Dry plaster should be spread on the strips which
are then rolled up very tightly (see Cut N 38). No more plaster

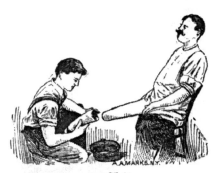

Cut N 41.

should be put on than will fill the meshes. The stump should be
prepared by removing the hair or fastening it down with paste or
thick soap. The plaster bandage roll must be immersed in water
and allowed to remain until the bubbles cease to come to the
surface (see Cut N 39). It is then taken from the water and
wrapped around the stump while being unrolled, beginning at
the end of the stump and continuing to a little above the knee

(see Cut N 40), then work down and up again, covering the stump with three or more layers or until all the bandages have been used. Allow the bandage to remain on the stump until it becomes hard, when the stump can be withdrawn (see Cut N 41). The plaster bandage will form a mold of the stump, which can be sent to us as it is, or it can be greased and filled with slacked plaster, and a true cast made, as previously described.

Casts and molds should be sent packed in sawdust to prevent breakage. If shells are sent, they must be filled with sawdust, to prevent collapse in transit.

CHAPTER XVI.

PRICES—ACCESSORIES—TERMS OF PAYMENT—
GUARANTEE

Artificial Feet for Partial Feet Amputations, described on pages 27 to 36	Cut C 2	each	$ 30.00
	Cut C 5	"	50.00
	Cut C 18	"	60.00
	Cut C 25	"	60.00
	Cut C 27	"	60.00
	Cut C 28	"	100.00
Artificial Feet for Ankle-Joint Amputations, described on pages 37 to 44	Cut D 7	"	60.00
	Cut D 12	"	60.00
	Cut D 14	"	60.00
	Cut D 16	"	60.00
	Cut D 21	"	100.00
	Cut D 23	"	100 00
Artificial Legs for Below-Knee Amputations, described on pages 45 to 69	Cut E 2	"	100.00
	Cut E 7	"	100.00
	Cut E 17	"	100.00
	Cut E 28	"	65.00
	Cut E 40	"	100.00
	Cut E 44	"	100.00
	Cut E 46	"	100.00
	Cut E 50	"	100,00
	Cut E 51	"	100.00
Peg Legs for Below-Knee Amputations, described on pages 67 to 71	Cut E 54	"	15.00
	Cut E 55	"	30.00
	Cut E 56	"	75.00
Ferrules and Rubber Tips for Peg Legs, described on pages 71 and 72	Cut E 57	complete	2.00
	Cut E 58	each	1.25
	Cut E 59	"	.75
Suspenders, described on pages 71 and 72 .	Cut E 60	set	2.00
	Cut E 61	"	3.00
	Cut E 62	"	4.00
Straps attached to corsets	Cut E 63	"	1.50
Or, $0.75 for each strap, corsets to be furnished by wearer.			
Artificial Legs for Knee-Bearing Stumps, described on pages 73 to 77	Cut F 5	each	100.00
	Cut F 9	"	100.00
Peg Legs for Knee-Bearing Stumps, described on pages 77 and 78	Cut F 11	"	15.00
	Cut F 12	"	75.00
	Cut F 13	"	50.00
Artificial Legs for Disarticulated Knee Stumps, described on pages 79 to 83 .	Cut G 7	"	100.00
	Cut G 8	"	100.00
Artificial Legs for Thigh or Femoral Stumps, described on pages 84 to 93 . . .	Cut H 5	"	100.00
	Cut H 15	"	100.00
	Cut H 25	"	75.00

Peg Legs for Thigh Stumps	Cut H 26	each	$50.00
	Cut H 27	"	75.00
Suspenders, described on pages 94 to 97 .	Cut H 28	set	4.00
	Cut H 34	"	8.00
	Cut H 35	"	5.00
Straps attached to Vests	Cut H 36	"	8.00
Or, $0.75 for each strap, Vest to be furnished by wearer.			
	Cut H 37	"	6.00
Straps attached to Corsets	Cut H 38	"	8.00
Or, $0.75 for each strap, Corset to be furnished by wearer.			
Artificial Legs for Hip-Joint Amputations, described on pages 98 to 100 . . .	Cut I 5	each	100 00
	Cut I 7	"	150.00
Artificial Feet and Legs for Deformities, etc.,	Cut K 3	"	30.00
	Cut K 7	"	60.00
	Cut K 11	"	60.00
	Cut K 16	"	60.00
	Cut K 17	"	100.00
	Cut K 20	"	60.00
	Cut K 22	"	100.00
	Cut K 25	"	60.00
	Cut K 27	"	60.00
	Cut K 29	"	100.00
	Cut K 21	"	100.00
	Cut K 33	"	100.00
	Cut K 35	"	100.00
	Cut K 36	"	125 00
	Cut K 38	"	100.00
	Cut K 41	"	100.00
	Cut K 42	"	100.00
	Cut K 46	both	150 00
	Cut K 51	each	100.00
	Cut K 54	"	100.00
	Cut K 57	both	200.00
	Cut K 59	"	200.00
	Cut K 61	each	60.00
	Cut K 63	"	125.00
	Cut K 66	"	125.00
	Cut K 69	"	60.00
	Cut K 71	"	75.00
	Cut K 72	"	75.00

ACCESSORIES.—Needful supplies, as indicated below, are furnished without extra charge.

Artificial Foot for partial foot and ankle-joint amputation. A suitable sock for the stump, an extra lacing.

Artificial Leg for below-knee amputation. A suitable suspender, one long and one short stump sock, pocket oil can, screwdriver, and extra lacing.

Artificial Leg for all other amputations. A suitable suspender one sock for stump, lubricant for the knee-joint, screwdriver, extra spring, etc.

TERMS OF PAYMENT.—Payment is required in advance with every order. If preferred, one-half can be advanced and the balance paid on delivery. This is the plan on which payments are reasonably and properly required on all articles that are made to order.

GUARANTEES.—A guarantee for a period of five years covering material and construction is given with each leg.

CHAPTER XVII

HANDS AND ARMS, NATURAL COMPARED WITH ARTIFICIAL

HISTORY.—Artificial hand and arm construction has advanced with that of artificial legs. The modern arm is calculated for general purposes, the ancient had only one object in its design. M. Sergius (167 B. C.), referred to by Pliny, wore an artificial arm, with which he held his shield while in battle, and released Cremona from siege. The artificial arm made for a celebrated tenor of the sixteenth century was used successfully in his histrionic gesticulations; the arm of the celebrated Surgeon Pare, as well as the productions of Lorrain, Sebastian, Bailiff, Verduin, Serre, Wilson, and De Graef, and all the early makers, had but few functions to perform.

There is a strong inclination to the belief that artificial arm construction has retrograded, and that those of modern times are not as useful as those of the early masters. Visitors to European museums, where many of the archaic substitutes are exhibited, are impressed by the profuse and extravagant labels and catalogues, ascribing to the wearers miraculous deeds of valor, performed in battle.

We are in position to state that historic substitutes were useless beyond the specific purposes for which they were designed, and were greatly inferior to those of modern construction. The ancient arm weighed from twenty to thirty pounds, was made of steel, copper and leather, and could be worn only on a long and powerful stump. The modern arm weighs from one to two and a half pounds, is made of rubber, wood, rawhide, leather, and metal, and can be worn on short, enervated, and nervous stumps to advantage. They have a range of utility infinitely greater than those used by warriors centuries ago.

The need for artificial arms has never been as great as now. The incentive to invent and improve is always responsive to demand. Want begets supply, and competition is the stimulus that carries improvements close to the goal of perfection.

THE DEMAND GREATER.—The demand has increased in direct proportion to the utilization of machinery in the industries and to the expansion of methods for rapid transportation. As the mileage of railroads increases, the mutilation of the human body is more frequent. The electric trolley has maimed more than the horse-cars of a decade ago. The mowing machine and the reaper have cut off more limbs than the scythe or cradle, dynamite has mutilated the human body more than the black powder of former days. These agencies, necessary for quick results, are dreadful implements of death and mutilation.

SIMPLICITY.—In recent years the tendency of the arm manufacturer has been to simplify construction; the earlier devices were complicated, burdensome to carry, expensive to maintain, and unreliable. No one will now tolerate a clumsy, heavy, noisy, complicated, and unwieldly arm; neat adaptation to the stump, lightness and naturalness of appearance, durability and utility, are the only essentials that will satisfy.

WHAT AN ARTIFICIAL ARM MUST DO.—The artificial arm must conceal the loss, protect the stump, restore a natural appearance to the dismembered side, provide a medium that will force the stump into healthful activity, and, in the way of utility, it must assist the opposite hand, carry articles of moderate weight, and, if the stump is powerful, the hand must be capable of cutting food on the plate and carrying the morsels to the mouth. The modern arm is capable of all this, and still more. A pen can be placed between the finger and thumb, and, after a little practice, the wearer will learn to write quickly and legibly. Implements capable of specific functions can be held in the hand or in the socket. A ring will help the farmer in guiding the handles of his farming tools; it will assist the blacksmith in wielding the sledge. A pair of pincers is capable of holding the work of a jeweler, a claw hook, a clevis, a hand vise; in fact, a great variety of implements have their distinct uses. While these attachments are capable of a large range of adaptation, there is a limit beyond which art and science cannot go. These operations of the natural hand that depend on the brain for their functions cannot possibly be performed by mechanical devices.

THE NATURAL HAND A MARVEL.—The intelligence with which the natural arm is endowed is the result of the system by which mental force is carried from the brain to the distant fingers. The human hand and arm are marvels of mechanism, their combinations of motions are almost limitless, their functions vast, their capabilities beyond comprehension. The motion of the shoulder is circumrotary; those of the elbow, flexion and extension; those of the wrist, rotary, circumrotary, flexion, and extension, and the fingers are capable of a range of accommodation almost limitless. Every joint is connected by powerful sinews, tendons, muscles, nerves, and blood vessels, which perform their work in conveying the commands of the mind to the most distant parts, and in compelling an instantaneous obedience. The hand that is capable of placing the delicate works of a watch is capable of placing the stones of a cathedral. And yet the human arm is but a machine, useless by itself.

THE BRAIN.—The brain is the vis-viva that renders it capable of its wonderful work. If the medium that conveys the wishes of the mind to the arm be destroyed, if the co-ordination be impaired, the natural arm ceases to be any more valuable than an artificial one of the crudest type.

An artificial arm, no matter how ingeniously it may be constructed, pales into insignificance when its functions are compared with those of the healthy arm nature has given us. Nevertheless, it is far more useful than the natural arm that has become palsied.

SELF-REPAIRING.—The natural arm has other endowments, aside from its responsiveness to the will. The power of repairing itself is one of its mysterious attributes. The bearing surfaces of the bones would grind away, the tendons would stretch and become inert if this process were not in constant operation. If a muscle becomes lacerated, or a tendon detached, or a bone broken, the work of reparation soon restores the injured part to its normal relations. Every drop of blood that flows through the arteries carries new material to replace the waste, and every drop of blood that flows through the veins carries away the particles that have become diseased and detached. In old age, when the human repair shop becomes disorganized, the entire physical mechanism breaks down, and the end soon follows.

SENSE OF TOUCH.—Another great and important endowment of the natural hand is the sense of touch. This sense is susceptible of cultivation. The contact of the fingers will convey the information that the substance is soft or hard, liquid or solid, dry or wet. The blind man is capable of reading by the tips of his fingers. When we place our hands in our pockets, we know by this sense whether we take hold of a key or a jackknife, a handkerchief or a lead pencil. The moment we touch the object we know what motions the fingers are to make and the strength required to put that object within our grasp.

An artificial hand is absolutely devoid of sensation. When we call to mind the fact that an artificial arm, made with joints, springs, and cords cannot be endowed with mental sympathy or with the power of repairing itself, or with the sensation of touch, we must become reconciled to the fact that it is necessarily of limited capacity.

STORIES MISLEADING.—We are frequently amused by reading newspaper articles on artificial arms, made by forgotten mechanics, "that are fully as good as natural arms." We frequently have to listen to the narration of some magical performances of men who wear artificial arms. We recall an article that appeared in a Canadian newspaper, of a woman who had a pair of arms adjusted to her person, supplementary to her natural ones. She became so dexterous in manipulating them that when in a public conveyance she would hold a book in her artificial hands, and, while apparently reading, would, with her natural hands, pick the pockets of those who sat next to her.

We have also read the story of a politician who lost his arm in the Civil War, and who had an ingenious artificial one applied that enabled him to shuffle a deck of cards, pick up a glass of beer and carry it in his mouth; and, on one occasion, when in a barroom brawl, he liberated a spring, and the arm immediately began its pugilistic movements, with more vigor and more deadly results than possible for the natural arm. Quite recently a New York paper gave a page to the description of an artificial arm, made by a German prothesist, that incases the undeveloped arm of the Emperor of Germany; the description of the arm and the functions it was capable of performing were extremely absurd and amusing to those acquainted with prothesis, but to laymen unacquainted with the subject, there was a strain of plausibility that must have made some persons believe that at last a mechanic is on the earth who is as skillful as Divinity Himself.

CHAPTER XVIII

IS IT PROFITABLE TO BUY AN ARTIFICIAL ARM?

If I procure an artificial arm, will I make any practical use of it? If I do not, can it in any way contribute to my physical or mental comfort? Is the risk worth taking?

These are the questions that have to be answered. They weigh heavily upon the minds of those who find it necessary to exercise economy in their purchases.

Whether male or female, rich or poor, the feasibility of substituting a member that has been lost must be thoughtfully considered.

Let us first take up the question of ornamentation.

ORNAMENTATION.—That a person will make a better appearance with an artificial arm properly dressed than with an empty sleeve,

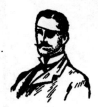

is obvious. To conceal any physical defect is a natural aim. There is nothing so distressing, especially to a sensitive person, as the exhibition of any imperfection in his anatomy.

The glass eye is worn for no other purpose than ornament. It fills a sightless socket and conveys the impression that the natural eye is there; it does not restore vision nor fulfill the optical functions, yet thousands of them are worn with a feeling that they are indispensable. They certainly look well, and are to be preferred to the cloth patch frequently seen. The man with a hunched back pays his tailor very dearly for the skillful adjustment of pads in his coat, so as to minimize the visibility of his deformity.

Any deficiency of the body that becomes conspicuous will attract attention and invite comment and sympathy. No person who maintains his self-respect, no matter what his disability may be, cares to be constantly reminded of it, and the commiseration of others, above all things, is the most abhorrent. To be frequently asked: "How did it happen?" "Did you lose your arm in the war?" "Were you in a railroad collision?" or to have such utterances as: "Poor, unfortunate man!" "How he must have suffered!" "What a terrible loss!" whispered within your hearing, may, for a while, be accepted in good part, but their repetition soon becomes annoying and odious.

An artificial arm will conceal the loss, restore a natural appearance to the person, avoid observation and comment, and after it has been worn a short time will become companionable and necessary to the wearer's mental comfort.

The Russian prince, Galitzin, obtained an artificial arm of us to cover a deformed and undeveloped member, the conspicuousness of which had given him much solicitude. He was elated over the results and pronounced the purchase a most satisfactory one, fully paying him for his long journey from Moscow to New York.

Miss Julia Shay Lindsay, of Polk County, Minn., struggled with this subject for some time, and finally ordered an artificial

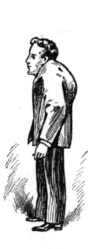 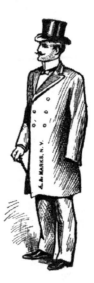

hand. The results that followed are clearly set forth in a letter recently addressed to us: "It is over five months since I received the artificial hand which my doctor ordered for me. I am very much pleased with it. No one can tell the artificial hand from the natural one. In this, it is a source of great comfort."

A. T. Basden, of Hamilton, Bermuda, who had both of his arms amputated between the elbows and wrists, wrote recently, as follows: "The artificial arms you sent me fit acceptably. They meet with my expectations. I find them helpful and especially valuable, as they hide my misfortune. Prior to the application of the arms, I suffered considerably with my stumps, but since wearing them the pain has entirely ceased."

HYGIENE.—This part of the subject, considering the importance it bears to the general health and welfare of the individual, has not been sufficiently emphasized. With much pleasure we quote

from Dr. Schenck, of Cincinnati, Ohio: " Pain is the cry of a
hungry nerve for food.

" When a part of the body becomes inactive, as is the case with
the stump of an amputated arm, the inability to receive the
necessary activity on account of the abbreviation of its length,
permits the stump and muscles to fall into a quiescent condition;
in consequence there occurs a stagnation in the venous system,
which depends entirely upon muscular activity for the return of
the venous blood to the lungs for aëration, from whence it is again
pumped by the heart to the different parts of the body, in order to
carry nourishment and oxygen to the tissues so that the normal
metabolism can occur, and thus produce the physiological tone
required for a healthy individual.

" As such, an abbreviated member, unassisted, cannot contribute
the necessary energy for its welfare; because of the above-ex-
plained pathological condition, it must suffer and lose its normal
tone and indirectly, as in diseased organs of the body, affect the
general economy in a more or less degree, depending upon the
temperament of the individual.

" So that, from the hygienic view, an artificial arm will cause
the defective part to functionate, causing activity of the remaining muscles, and thus stimulate its circulation, giving to the
part the required nourishment and preventing the accumulation
of effete material and dismissing a conspicuous deformity, which,
no matter how indifferent the unfortunate assumes to be, has
some influence upon his nervous system, all of which, being
improved, is conducive to promote a healthy tone to the whole
body."

It is not an infrequent occurrence for a person to complain of
peculiar, dull aches, or nerve twitchings, or sharp, stinging darts
of pain in his stump. Investigation will disclose the fact that
these are nervous disturbances, due to muscular inactivity, and, as
soon as stumps are forced to do something, the distress will almost
invariably disappear.

Dr. Cook, United States Examining Surgeon, puts this phase
of the subject in an interesting and unique light:

" When a limb has been amputated, the stump, or remaining
portion, takes on queer antics and assumes conditions that are
in accordance with well-known physiological and psychological
laws.

" For instance, it is no uncommon occurrence for a man who
has lost a part of his leg by amputation to have a severe pain in
the heel, foot, or toe of the lost member, or for those who have
lost parts of their arms to have excruciating pains in the wrists,
hands, or fingers of the amputated parts. To those unaccustomed
to these nerve complications this may appear absurd, but they
are facts well known to neurologists.

" It would seem that the stump, or part remaining after amputation, either resented the indignity that it had been subjected to,
or else made its sorrow for its loss manifested by these means.

"The man who allows an amputated arm to hang indolently by his side makes a mistake. The muscles above the stump shrink and waste away for a lack of nourishment, and the nerves become irritable and neuralgic. An undisputed physiological law is that 'action increases strength,' and the reverse is just as true, that inaction produces weakness.

"Place an artificial arm on the idle stump and it at once begins to get a better circulation of the blood, the muscles begin to develop, and the nerves have something to think about besides their terminals."

Dr. L. G. Armstrong, of Boscobel, Wis., in emphasizing the importance to persons who have had legs or arms amputated, to procure artificial ones, presents in a forcible way the penalty that must be paid if a stump is permitted to become indolent:

"Artificial limbs have added much to afflicted humanity in the way of happiness and comfort.

"Physiology teaches plainly that the want of use of any part begets weakness. Atrophy of the muscles is sure to follow, which is the legitimate consequence of the neglect. To prevent this, begin using the stump as soon as it is thoroughly healed, when the adhesions are perfect, save atrophy, and put the muscles to their new use. Neuralgia of the stump is always sure to follow, or it may even antedate the withering away of the muscles for the want of proper use. Get a well-made, perfectly fitting limb, and you have at once removed the cause of nervous disturbances and the mental shock. You have added much to the person's ability to earn a livelihood. My experience is that artificial limbs are soon accepted, and soon used to advantage, and so much so that money would not induce the wearers to do without them. My advice is to get an artificial limb at the first practical moment, after the stump is perfectly healed."

Dr. T. P. Smith, of Tacoma, Wash., says: "During the last fourteen years you have fitted a great number of my patients with artificial limbs, and they have all given entire satisfaction. The proposition that a limb, whether a stump or whole, needs and is benefited by motion, is so self-evident as not to call for discussion; a stump becomes useless without it.

"I am in the habit of using motion in all cases of fracture, as well as in all cases of amputation, to prevent atrophy of the muscles, and stiffening of the joints, and as soon as a stump, after amputation, is healed, I insist on applying an artificial limb. Until the limb comes, I insist on the patient doing the best he can toward exercising and using his stump. After the limb is adjusted he will naturally use it, and that will prevent the stump from becoming flabby and fat.

"In conclusion, I will say that I know of no way to retain the use of a leg or arm, except it be early fitted with an artificial limb, and the sooner it is done the better. In spite of bandaging, and such motion and exercise as patients can give their stumps, they become large and flabby."

Dr. Geo. E. Powell, La Crosse, Wis., writes: " We have had your artificial limbs for twenty years and consider them the best made. We have never applied one that did not give satisfaction. Many arm stumps that were soft and doughy to the feel, became strikingly firm and vigorous with the use of artificial arms."

Dr. Chas. F. Noe, of Amana, Ia., states: " I wish to say that in my experience a well-fitting artificial arm exercises a beneficial influence on the stump, due to the stimulus given to circulation and nutrition, and thus preventing stagnation from disuse."

Dr. J. H. Sieling, of York, Pa., says: " The arm that you sent me recently has done more work than my fondest hopes expected; it has not only had a helping influence on my patient's stump, but adds greatly to his appearance. He is able to execute some very helpful acts with the elegant equipment; he eats, by its help, very artistically indeed. I am only too glad to add a word of commendation whenever opportunity offers."

Carl M. Person, of Webster County, Neb., states: " I will write to you and let you know that my arm is all right. I have worn it every day since I got it, and have never been chafed or experienced any inconvenience. The arm is useful as well as ornamental. I find that the exercise my stump receives from it prevents those dull pains that I suffered from for so long a time, and I value it for this reason far more than the money it cost."

William F. Starner, of Carroll County, Md., writes: " I have been wearing one of your artificial arms for about three years, and am well pleased with it. I can do most any kind of work. The arm exercises my stump, and keeps it in a more pleasant condition."

The utility to be derived from an artificial arm depends very largely upon the length of the stump, the strength of the muscles, and the aptitude of the wearer. The stump must be long in order to provide a lever with which to control the hand and forearm in lifting such articles as may be placed in the hand. Although the artificial arm is very light, the power to elevate it must come from the muscles in the arm and shoulder, and when the stump is very short, and the muscles weak, the utility of an artificial arm is lessened. But, notwithstanding these conditions, the artificial arm should be worn on the shortest of stumps. There are persons who have more aptitude than others, and perform feats under adverse conditions that are marvelous; some with short stumps do more than others with long ones. It is safe to say, however, that any person, no matter how short a stump he may have, may, with patience and application, learn to operate an artificial arm, and derive a reasonable compensation from it. Ambition, application, and thoughtful effort will overcome many difficulties. If one person can learn to write quickly and legibly with an artificial hand, why should not another? If one person can handle a farming implement, such as a hoe, rake, ax, or wheelbarrow, or a carpenter can drive his plane, hold a nail or carry tools, there is no reason why others should fail.

CHAPTER XIX

WOODEN HANDS. RUBBER HANDS

OLD METHODS.—During the first decade of our prothetical career (from 1853 to 1863), we manufactured mechanical hands, they were carved from wood with fingers jointed at the knuckles, controlled by straps operated by the shoulder. By a forward motion of the opposite arm, the strap would apply a pulling force to the artificial hand and force it to open. By relaxing, the strain on the strap would be released and the hand would close. It would seem as though a hand of this character would be useful and valuable, but when the invariableness of the spring tension, the oppressive harness to be worn, and the exertion required to operate the straps were considered, it was doubtful that the results obtained justified the means employed.

NEW METHODS.—In 1863 our attention was attracted to the utilization of rubber, the resilient nature of which appealed to us as being better adapted to the purposes of an artificial hand than harsh, unyielding wood or metal. The rubber hand was thereupon invented. It was cast in a mold made from the model of a natural hand, and it was attached to the end of the artificial forearm by means of a spindle. The fingers were flexible and would yield under pressure, having sufficient elasticity and adhesion to hold light articles. It presented a natural appearance and was pleasant to the touch. It was far more durable than the wooden hand. It might fall or strike a hard object and would not break. It could be slipped from the socket and a hook, knife, fork, brush, ring or other implement put in its place. For a number of years this hand found many purchasers, and was

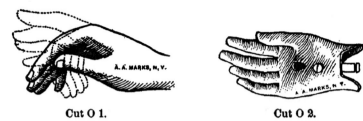

Cut O 1.   Cut O 2.

greatly admired. Improvements were suggested from time to time.

DUCTILE FINGERS.—A fortunate thought was that of changing the fingers from flexibility to ductility. Flexible fingers would move under pressure, but as soon as that pressure was released they would return to the positions in which they were cast. The ductile fingers admit of change of position. The wearer can, by the opposite hand, or by pressing the fingers against some resistant object, change their positions from full extension to clinched. The hand with fingers partly closed is sufficiently firm to carry a valise or package. Cut O 1 represents the rubber hand partly closed. The dotted lines indicate the positions of extension and flexion in which the fingers can be bent.

PALM LOCKS.—A lock embedded in the palm, shown in Cut O 2, receives and holds implements with firmness. A hand brush, a knife and fork (as shown in Cut O 3) can be thus placed and have the appearance of being grasped by the fingers. When it is required to carry articles of considerable weight for a great length of time a steel hook is slipped in the palm socket, and, concealed by the hand, it is held with sufficient strength to carry an article of one hundred pounds in weight. A knife or fork can be put in the same socket; the latter will hold a piece of meat while it is being cut with the opposite hand, and will convey food to the mouth. A brush placed in the palm lock can be used in washing the opposite hand. When it is desired to remove an implement a little pressure is applied to the button and the implement is released, and can easily be taken from the socket.

WRIST CONNECTIONS.—Rubber hands are attached to forearms by various methods.

Cut O 3 represents the spindle method. A steel spindle is attached to the base of the hand, and made to fit a locking plate secured to the base of the forearm socket. The hand when so placed will rotate at the wrist if the wearer wishes. When it is

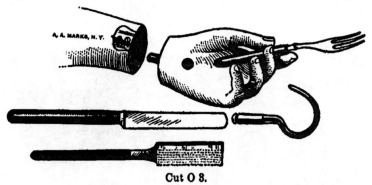

Cut O 3.

desired to remove the hand a little pressure applied to a button will release the hold, it can then be taken from its place. When it is desired to prevent the hand from rotating a set screw is turned inwardly, and the hand is clamped firmly in one position. A variety of implements are illustrated in the cuts O 4 to O 7, each can be placed in the forearm substituting the hand.

CLAMPS.—Cut O 8 represents a new device for a wrist-joint connection, it is intended for a person who works at the bench. The

end of the forearm is made of aluminum, and provided with a
sliding jaw operating as a vise. A cold chisel can be held firmly
at any convenient angle, shown in Cut O 9; a saw-file can be used
to advantage, as shown in Cut O 10. A jeweler's hammer, or in
fact any implement with a handle not greater than ⅝ of an inch
in diameter can thus be held in a thoroughly practical way.

FLEXION.—The mortise and tenon wrist connection is preferable

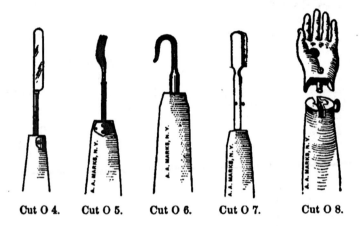

Cut O 4.   Cut O 5.   Cut O 6.   Cut O 7.   Cut O 8.

to any wrist mechanism that admits of flexion and extension.
Cut O 11 represents this method. The mechanism consists of
a series of interlaying strips, held together by a bolt, which forms
the axis of motion. Rotation of the arm is obtained, when de-

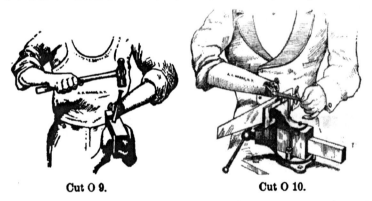

Cut O 9.   Cut O 10.

sired, by means of a bolt connection introduced immediately
above the wrist joint.

Cut O 12 represents the mortise and tenon connection, the hand
flexed holding hook. Cut O 13 shows the hand extended, with
fork held by the palm lock, the knife and other implements are
held in the same way.

For laborers who wish to obtain the greatest variety of practical uses from artificial arms, the spindle connection at the wrist (Cut O 3) is preferable. This device admits of greater strength and enables the wearer to press the artificial hand against any object desired to be held in place. The mortise and tenon wrist

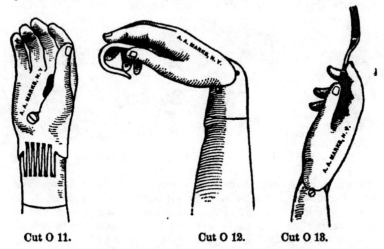

Cut O 11.   Cut O 12.   Cut O 13.

connection, illustrated in Cut O 11, is chosen by persons seeking ornament more than utility.

When lightness is a paramount consideration it is advisable to have the hand permanently attached at the wrist.

This method obviates any metal connection, and thereby lessens the weight.

SPRING THUMB.—We have a mechanical device by which the thumb can be made to move at its base, away from or toward the fingers. Cuts O 14 and O 15 represent the hand with the thumb ab-

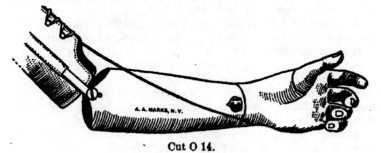

Cut O 14.

ducted; this is effected by tension applied to a cord passing from the under side of the base of the hand upwardly to the elbow. Cut O 16 represents the hand with thumb pressed against the finger. As soon as the tension of the abductor cord is released, the thumb will be forced by a strong spring to press against the index and middle fingers. When the abductor cord is connected with the artificial arm above the elbow, the thumb will press against the forefinger when the elbow is flexed, and will draw away from it when the elbow is extended, as shown in Cut O 16. The abductor cord may be carried up the arm, over the back, around the opposite shoulder, by which it will be controlled. When thus

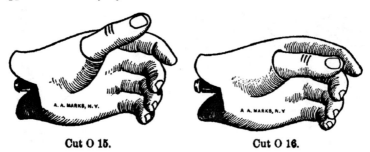

Cut O 15.   Cut O 16.

connected. it is independent of elbow motion and is operated by a movement of the shoulder or contraction of the chest.

As considerable mechanism is required in the spring thumb, the construction is more or less complicated, and we do not advise its selection except in special cases. In double amputations, when all dependence must be placed upon artificial means, spring thumbs are advantageous; but in single amputations they prove to be quite useless; the remaining natural hand becomes so adept that it performs about all the work that prior to the amputation was performed by both hands.

GLOVES ALWAYS TO BE WORN.—Artificial hands and parts of hands must be gloved at all times. This is necessary in order to conceal the fact that they are not real. Artificial hands, whether made of wood, rubber, or other material, may be modeled to the shape of nature, and have all the graceful lines, creases, and folds that are found in the natural hand..

They may be painted and tinted with artistic nicety, yet it is not possible to impart to them the characteristics which distinguish nature from art. The natural hand has a different tint in the forenoon than it has in the afternoon; when the fingers are extended there are more creases in the skin than when they are flexed; when the hand is at labor it is broader and the muscles and blood vessels show with more prominence than when at repose. An artificial hand, no matter of what material it may be constructed, cannot possess this metamorphic power. It, therefore, must be concealed by a glove, otherwise it will be conspicuous.

CHOICE OF MATERIAL FOR SOCKETS.—Sockets for artificial arms may be made of wood, leather, or aluminum, to suit the wishes of the purchaser. Makers of experience are united on this point, and advocate the use of tough, light wood. Wood is capable of being worked into convenient shapes, which it will retain indefinitely. It is lighter than any other material that can be used.

and when strengthened with rawhide is sufficiently strong for most purposes. It is also a non-conductor of heat, and when varnished does not absorb perspiration. The objection to leather is its flexibleness. While this may appear to be desirable, it is actually the cause of trouble. A socket that is flexible cannot be comfortable to wear, as it does not place the pressure at points of toleration; instead, it distributes it uniformly over the entire surface, causing pressure to come as much on sensitive parts as elsewhere. Leather absorbs perspiration, becomes foul and offensive, and unless extraordinary methods are used to keep it clean it will become hard and dead, it will crack and fall to pieces.

Leather sockets are sometimes unavoidable; they will be spoken of in due course.

Metal sockets are objectionable on account of their weight, liability to corrode from perspiration, and their disposition to hold heat. When arms are to be made for persons who work in water, such as dyers, laundrymen, fishermen, oystermen, etc., it will be necessary to use metal, such as aluminum, which receives no injury from exposure to moisture free from salt.

A rubber hand permanently attached to an aluminum socket will provide a useful, resistant, and durable arm, and when frequently cleaned and coated on the inside with sweat-proof enamel or paint, will last a great many years.

CHAPTER XX

PARTIAL HAND AMPUTATIONS

The loss of a finger may be lamentable, but it cannot be considered a serious impairment. The remaining fingers as a rule are competent to perform all the labors that are usually demanded of the complete hand. Yet there are times when the substitution

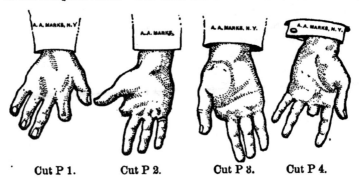

Cut P 1.　　　Cut P 2.　　　Cut P 3.　　　Cut P 4.

of a lost finger is essential, either for cosmetic effect or to equip the hand for some special purpose; for example, playing the piano, or other musical instrument.

THE LOSS OF ONE FINGER.—Cuts P 1 to P 6 represent hands from which one finger has been removed. An artificial finger

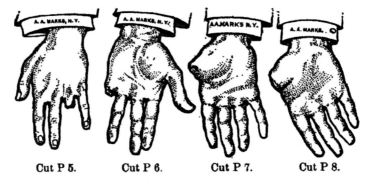

Cut P 5.　　　Cut P 6.　　　Cut P 7.　　　Cut P 8.

similar in appearance to that illustrated in Cut P 9 meets the needs of each case. The loss of the thumb, far more than of a finger, impairs the usefulness of the hand. It is, therefore, more important to substitute that loss. Cuts P 7 and P 8 represent hands from which the thumb has been removed. An artificial thumb similar to that shown in Cut P 10 is suitable for such cases.

MATERIALS.—Artificial fingers and thumbs are made of rubber,

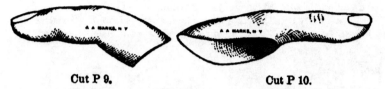

Cut P 9.   Cut P 10.

or silver. Rubber is desirable, if flexibility is an object; silver has the greater durability, is neater, lighter, and

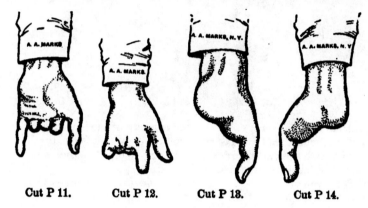

Cut P 11.   Cut P 12.   Cut P 13.   Cut P 14.

more practical. The price is the same for each. When ordering send a plaster cast of both the mutilated and opposite

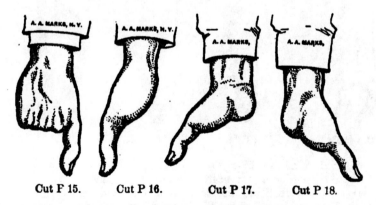

Cut F 15.   Cut P 16.   Cut P 17.   Cut P 18.

hand, one is required for fitting, and the other as a guide in shaping the outside to correspond with its mate on the opposite hand. If the stump, either finger or thumb, is very short, it will be necessary to hold the substitute in place by straps passing around the base of the hand, or by a glove. If the stump is long, the substitute will remain in place without additional support.

It is important that the artificial part should be covered at all times by a glove, as it is not possible to give it the characteristics of nature closely enough to defy detection.

THE LOSS OF TWO OR MORE FINGERS.—Cuts P 11 to P 22 represent hands from which two or more fingers have been removed.

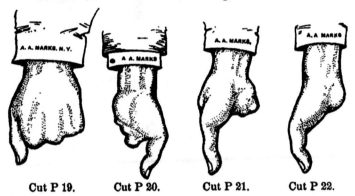

Cut P 19.   Cut P 20.   Cut P 21.   Cut P 22.

An artificial part for any of these cases consists of rubber fingers attached to a socket that incases the remaining part of the natural hand. This is essential in order to hold the fingers together and provide means for securing them to the stump.

Cut P 23 represents an artificial hand devised to supply the amputation of index and small fingers. Cut P 24 represents

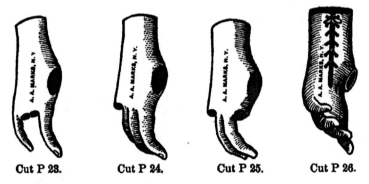

Cut P 23.   Cut P 24.   Cut P 25.   Cut P 26.

an artificial hand suitable for use when the index, middle, and small fingers are amputated. Cut P 25 shows an artificial part to substitute the loss of middle and ring fingers. Cut P 26 represents an artificial hand, suitable for a palm amputation, in which the natural thumb remains. The fingers in all the above hands are made ductile, rigid, or flexible, according to the choice of the wearer. For those who do little work and wish to combine ornament with utility, the ductile fingers should be chosen. For a laboring person, who wishes to lift heavy weights and do hard work, the rigid fingers are better. And for those who wear artificial fingers and parts of hands for ornamental purposes only, the flexible fingers give the greatest satisfaction.

INDIVIDUAL FINGERS.—Where the amputation of one or more fingers has been made at the first or second joint, it will not be

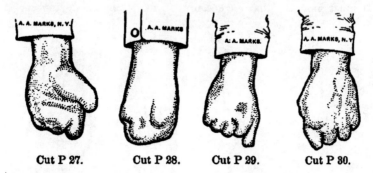

Cut P 27.   Cut P 28.   Cut P 29.   Cut P 30.

necessary to have the artificial fingers connected at their base; separate fingers, as represented in Cut P 9, can be used.

Amputations that have been made in the palms of hands are capable of prothetic treatment, giving natural appearances to the mutilated members as closely as conditions will admit. If the remaining part of the hand provides a stump that will control the artificial part, a considerable amount of utility can be looked

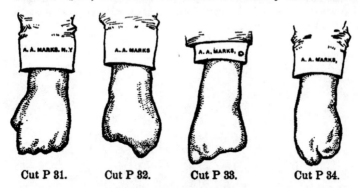

Cut P 31.   Cut P 32.   Cut P 33.   Cut P 34.

for; but if the stump is of such a character as to offer little or no leverage by which the artificial parts can be controlled, scarcely anything beyond ornament can be assured.

CONSTRUCTION.—The hand below the fingers is made of rubber, combined with canvas and leather, providing a socket for the remaining part of the amputated member; this is laced on line with the palm. If the remaining thumb is greatly abducted, as shown in Cuts P 19 and P 20, caused by the weakening of the flexor muscles, it will be difficult to apply an artificial part that will possess more than an approximate approach to nature in appearance. It will, nevertheless, materially improve the hand and add to its utility.

When amputations remove the thumb, as well as the fingers, as shown in Cuts P 27 to P 37, the artificial hand required will resemble that shown in Cut P 38. This hand is similar in construction to that previously described.

It must be noted that on account of the stump occupying the

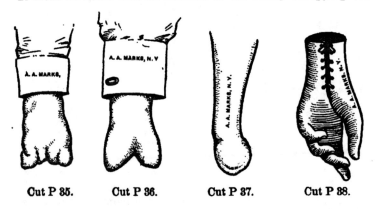

Cut P 35.   Cut P 36.   Cut P 37.   Cut P 38.

interior of the artificial palm, there can be no mechanism in the hand. When it is desired to have an appliance connected with the artificial part that will hold implements of utility, rings passing over the fingers, or plates riveted to the palms, must be used. These are only furnished when they are especially requested at the time the order is placed.

CHAPTER XXI

WRIST-JOINT AMPUTATIONS

When a hand is amputated at the wrist articulation, the ulnar

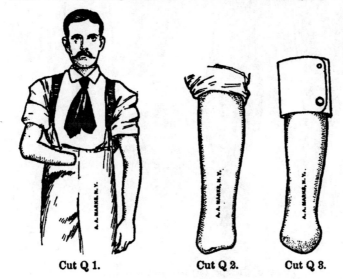

Cut Q 1.   Cut Q 2.   Cut Q 3.

and radial (or styloid) processes are sometimes trimmed off, and

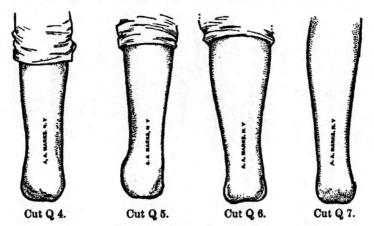

Cut Q 4.   Cut Q 5.   Cut Q 6.   Cut Q 7.

sometimes left as they are, as these prominences form means by
which the artificial part can be held firmly to the stump.

FLAT ENDS.—Cuts Q 1 to Q 7 represent amputations in the wrist, in which the styloid prominences of the ulna and radius

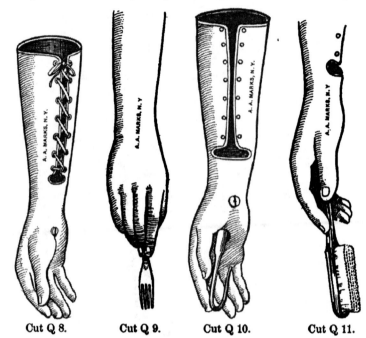

Cut Q 8. Cut Q 9. Cut Q 10. Cut Q 11.

are present. These stumps require artificial arms constructed on the plan shown in Cut Q 8. The hand is of rubber, with ductile fingers, a locking arrangement is imbedded in the palm, as

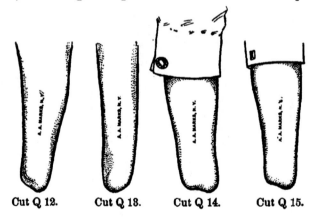

Cut Q 12. Cut Q 13. Cut Q 14. Cut Q 15.

described. The hand is permanently secured to a leather socket, which is formed on a cast of the stump. The arm thus constructed is then placed on the stump and laced down the frontal line. Implements for the table, working, and for washing, etc., can be placed in the palm, where they will be held firmly. Cuts Q 9, Q 10, and Q 11 show the various implements in place.

TAPERING ENDS.—When the styloid prominences have been removed and the stump becomes a tapering one, as shown in Cuts Q 12 to Q 15, an artificial arm constructed on the plan of that

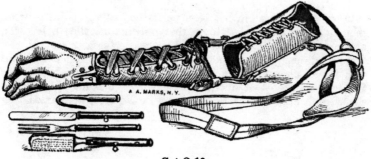

Cut Q 16.

represented in Cut Q 16 must be used. This arm is practically the same as that shown in Cut Q 8, with the exception that it is supplied with attachments that go above the elbow and connect with suspenders resting on the shoulders and passing around the body. These are essential to keep the arm from slipping off the tapering stump. Useful implements can be held in the hand, as shown in Cuts Q 9, Q 10, Q 11.

CHAPTER XXII

FOREARM AMPUTATIONS

When an amputation has been performed at any point between the elbow and wrist, the stump that remains is called a forearm, or radial stump. Cuts R 1 to R 6 represent forearm stumps of a variety of lengths and conditions. The most suitable artificial arm for an amputation of any of the above is illustrated in Cut R 7. The socket is of wood, leather, or metal, as may be selected, shaped interiorly to receive the stump in the most accommodating

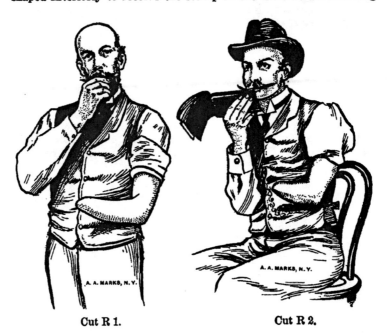

Cut R 1.   Cut R 2.

way. The outside is given the contours of the natural arm as closely as conditions will admit, it is then covered with rawhide and enameled a natural tint.

LEATHER ELBOW JOINTS.—The arm being intended for a long radial stump, the connection with the upper arm piece (incasing the muscle part) is of flexible leather, so as to permit a great range of motion; being adjustable, it can be tightened or loosened, as required; it is absolutely noiseless and very strong; being flexible, it admits of rotation of the forearm. The hand is of

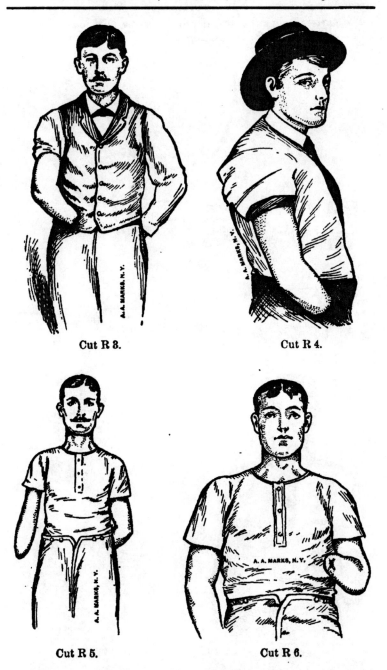

Cut R 3.

Cut R 4.

Cut R 5.

Cut R 6.

rubber, with ductile fingers, as heretofore described. The connection at the wrist is by the spindle or the mortise and tenon method, or the hand can be permanently attached.

The part incasing the arm above the elbow is made of leather, with suitable straps for regulating pressure.   Shoulder straps and

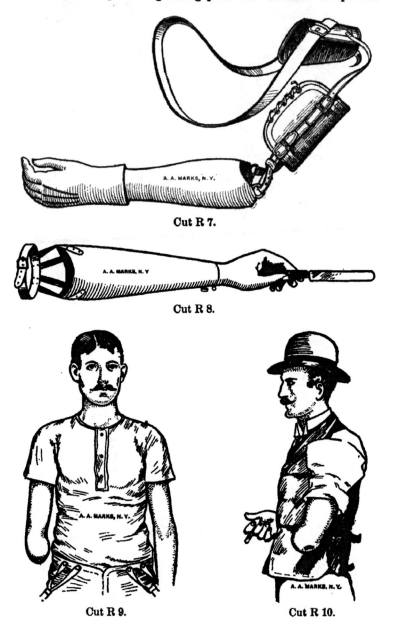

Cut R 7.

Cut R 8.

Cut R 9.

Cut R 10.

suspenders are attached to the upper part of this section.

Arms of this construction are thoroughly available for stumps below the elbow five or more inches in length.

It is sometimes desirable in long radial stumps to secure the arms by a narrow strap above the elbow instead of by the long

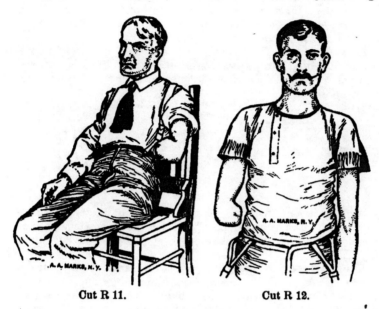

Cut R 11.   Cut R 12.

leather muscle part. Cut R 8 represents an arm of this character. This method of attachment is adequate when the artificial arm is

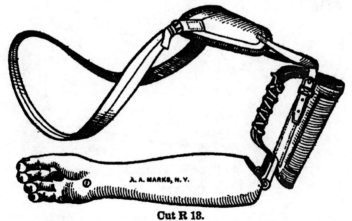

Cut R 13.

not used for carrying heavy articles or in performing laborious work.

STEEL ELBOW JOINTS.—Radial stumps that are shorter than five inches, as shown in Cuts R 9 to R 12, require a firmer method of securing the stump socket to the upper-arm part than the leather joint above described. Cut R 13 represents an artificial arm constructed practically the same as R 7, differing in the elbow joint. Steel hinge joints are used instead of leather. While there is less freedom in the elbow movement, the steel joints place the arm under firmer control of the stump.

SHORT STUMPS.—This arm is, as a rule, made with hand permanently attached, in order to minimize weight. When an amputation below the elbow leaves a stump so short that when flexed the

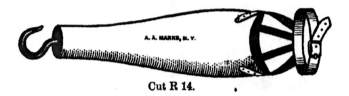

Cut R 14.

projection beyond the line of the upper arm is insufficient to control the movements of the elbow, it must be treated the same as an amputation in the elbow joint, as described in the following chapter.

ARMS WITHOUT HANDS.—Peg arms for radial stumps are of several kinds, made of wood, leather, or aluminum; they are practically artificial arms without hands. Cut R 14 represents a peg arm without long muscle part or suspenders. Cut R 15 shows a peg arm with long muscle part and suspenders; both the

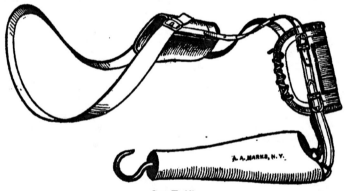

Cut R 15.

above peg arms are constructed in the same manner as those heretofore described, the absence of the hand is the only difference. Farming, shop, and other implements can be devised for specific purposes and held in the ends of the forearms.

SUSPENDERS.—Cut R 16 represents a suspender suitable for an arm for a radial amputation. Suspenders must be renewed occasionally, according to the demands that are made upon them by the wearer. If the arm is used by a laboring person and he perspires very freely, a new suspender will be required more frequently than if less destructive conditions prevail. The suspender can be procured independent of other parts. It consists of a

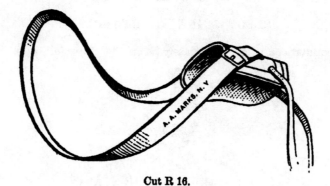

Cut R 16.

plate of leather shaped to rest on top of the shoulder and fit close to the neck. A webbing strap passes around the body under the opposite arm and buckles to the suspender in front.

CHAPTER XXIII

ELBOW-JOINT AMPUTATIONS

Amputations in or immediately below the elbow joints, leaving

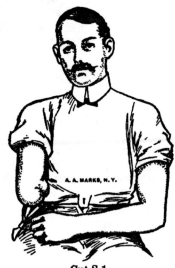

Cut S 1.

stumps so short they cannot be availed of in controlling the arti-

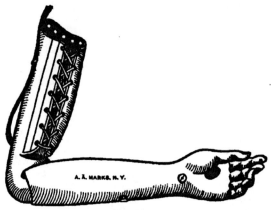

Cut S 2.

ficial elbow joint, require artificial arms of special construction.

206

The presence of the condyles, or bony prominences, affords an opportunity for fitting that will secure firmness without employing shoulder straps, or, if not dispensing with them entirely, simplifying them very materially.

SHORT RADIAL STUMPS.—Cut S 1 represents an amputation a little below the elbow joint, but very close to it, leaving a stump so short that it cannot be utilized. A suitable arm is illustrated in Cuts S 2 and S 3. This arm is especially designed for an amputation through the elbow joint.

CONSTRUCTION.—The forearm is made of wood, shaped to the contours and dimensions of the natural arm, excavated to receive

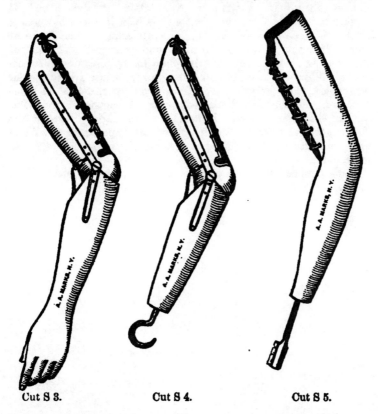

Cut S 3.   Cut S 4.   Cut S 5.

the stump properly and to reduce weight, covered with rawhide to obtain strength, and finished in enamel. The hand is of rubber, attached to the forearm by either of the methods heretofore described. The palm is provided with a locking arrangement that will hold implements of utility. The elbow joint is of the ginglymoid pattern and is operated by a flexion strap under control of the opposite shoulder. The elbow joint is provided with a locking arrangement that will hold the arm in flexed position when desired. The socket receives the stump, which, on account of its enlarged extremity, is inserted from the front and held by lacing. Cut S 3 represents an artificial arm practically the same as an S 2, except that the stump is placed in the socket from the rear instead of the front. Cut S 4 represents the same with the hand slipped off and a hook inserted in the end of the forearm. This can only be done when the arm is so constructed that the hand is connected with the forearm by the spindle attachment. In style S 3 the upper section is made entirely of leather, formed on a cast of the stump, modified as the conditions require.

ARMS WITHOUT HANDS.—Peg arms for elbow-joint amputations are found useful for laboring purposes. Cut S 5 gives the simplest form. It is without articulation at the elbow. It receives the stump from the front and is held in place by lacing; it may be made of wood, leather, or aluminum. When made of wood it is strengthened with rawhide and enameled. The end of the socket is provided with a wrist plate for holding useful implements. When the conditions of the stump require, a suspender is provided which rests on top of the shoulder and held in place by a strap passing around the body under the opposite arm. The arm, as shown in the cut, is usually made slightly bent at the elbow and approximately the length of the opposite arm. When elbow-joint motion is required it becomes the same as S 4, without a hand.

Suspenders are the same as those used on arms for above-elbow stumps.

CHAPTER XXIV

ABOVE-ELBOW AMPUTATIONS

An amputation at any point between the shoulder and elbow produces what is known by surgeons as a humeral stump. Cuts T 1 and T 2 are fair examples.

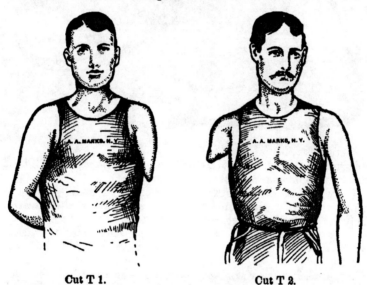

Cut T 1.   Cut T 2.

Artificial arms suitable for humeral stumps are usually provided with artificial elbow articulations, which are flexed and extended by a swing of the body or by the contraction of the shoulders.

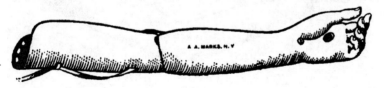

Cut T 3.

Cut T 3 represents such an arm extended at the elbow, and Cut T 4 represents it with the elbow joint flexed.

This arm is usually constructed of wood, shaped to the contours and dimensions of the opposite arm, excavated to reduce weight, covered with rawhide to add strength, and enameled a flesh-like tint. The hand is of rubber, attached to the forearm by either of the methods heretofore described. The palm is provided with a locking arrangement for holding laboring, eating, and other useful implements. The joints at the elbow are of a

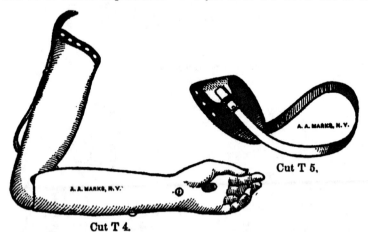

Cut T 5.

Cut T 4.

substantial character, combined with an attachment that will hold the forearm at one or more desired angles.

Elbow Lock.—The locking arrangement is released by pressure applied to button protruding from the under side of the forearm. Suitable suspender is represented in Cut T 5. This can be renewed, as occasion may require. By an ingenious attachment rotation of the elbow is obtained when length of stump will permit.

Peg arms for upper-arm amputations are of several kinds. Cut T 6 represents the least expensive. It is usually made of wood, excavated to receive the stump properly and to reduce weight, and

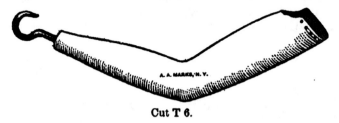

Cut T 6.

shaped on the outside to have the form and dimensions of the opposite arm. The end of the socket is provided with a catch that will hold implements of utility. This arm is partly flexed and immovable at the elbow, as it is found to be more convenient that way. If a peg arm with elbow-joint motion is wanted, it becomes the same as T 4 without a hand.

pad that runs well above the top and over the shoulder, resting on the shoulder close to the neck. The stump is held in position by a strap passing around the body under the opposite arm. The elbow joint admits of flexion and extension, and is provided with

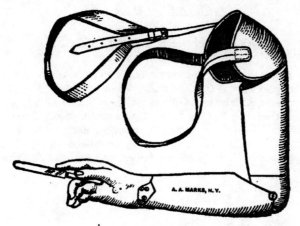

Cut U 6.

a locking arrangement that will hold it at right angles. The attachment can be released by pressure applied to a press-button immediately under the forearm. Cuts U 6 and U 7 represent the arm flexed at right and oblique angles.

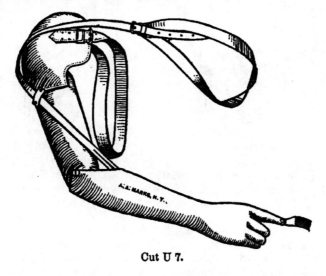

Cut U 7.

Peg arms for shoulder-joint amputations are practically the same as those for above-elbow amputations, and are described in previous chapter.

CHAPTER XXVI

DOUBLE ARM AMPUTATIONS

The amputation of both arms is a deplorable loss and presents the strongest appeal to the artificial limb maker. The subject is absolutely dependent upon others unless artificial arms are applied. He is neither able to feed himself, prepare his food, dress himself, or perform labor of any kind. Something must be done to better his unfortunate condition. If not, he is obliged to remain dependent upon some kindly disposed friend or relative. Anything that

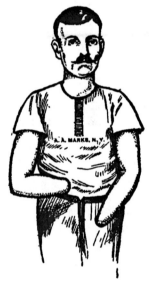 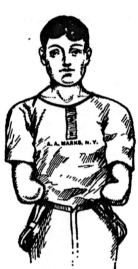

Cut V 1.   Cut V 2.

will help him in his condition, no matter how little, will be a benefit and will materially lessen the burden on others.

Cut V 1 represents the amputation of both forearms, leaving stumps that are long and powerful. Cut V 2 represents double forearm amputations, stumps short. Cut V 3 shows artificial arms applied. Artificial arms, under control of long and powerful stumps, will enable the wearer to prepare his food at the table, convey it to his mouth, perform labor of a great variety, carry articles of considerable weight, write a legible hand, open and close a door, and attend to the adjustment of his own attire

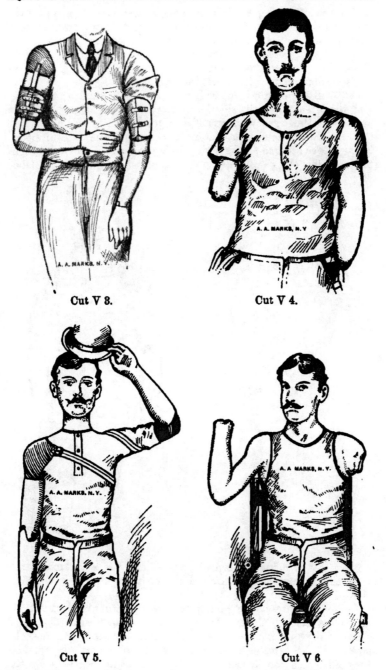

Cut V 3.

Cut V 4.

Cut V 5.

Cut V 6.

to a reasonable degree. When the stumps are short, the range of utility is correspondingly lessened.

The use of spring thumbs is always desirable in double arm amputations, and unless otherwise instructed, we assume that they are wanted and construct the hands accordingly.

Cut V 4 represents double arm amputations, one immediately above the wrist, and the other above the elbow. Cut V 5 represents similar cases, with artificial arms applied.

Cut V 6 represents amputations of the right hand at the wrist and the left arm at the shoulder. A pair of artificial arms were applied to this case with gratifying results.

The right artificial arm was under control of the natural elbow. The left was secured to the stump by straps with a locking attachment at the elbow and clamp at the wrist. Considerable labor

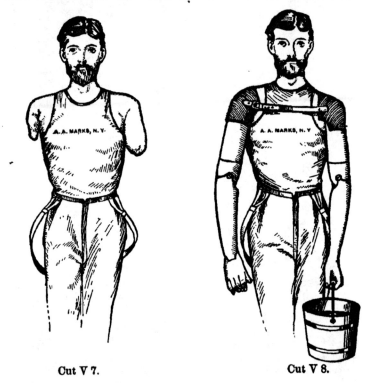

Cut V 7.   Cut V 8.

was capable of being performed by the right, the left arm depending upon a strap passing around the body for flexion and extension of the elbow.

Cut V 7 represents a young man with both arms amputated above the elbows, the result of a railroad accident. Cut V 8 shows him with a pair of artificial arms applied. As may be surmised, the arms were of very limited use, but, nevertheless, they mitigated his affliction to a compensating degree. By the working of his right shoulder, he was able to bring the artificial forearm to right angles. In this position it would remain, providing a means by which articles could be laid on the forearm and carried. His left arm could be flexed by means of the stump, which was long and powerful. When at extension, a pail, basket, or valise could be carried, and other services performed. The arms rescued him from a life of absolute idleness.

Cut V 9 represents a man who, while attending his duties on a railroad, was overtaken by a severe storm, and before he could reach shelter, both feet and hands were frozen. It was necessary to amputate the right hand between the thumb and wrist and the left at the base of the fingers and thumb. The great toe was removed from the right foot, and left leg amputated a little above

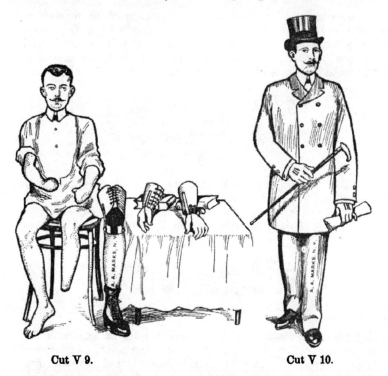

Cut V 9.   Cut V 10.

the ankle. The same cut shows a pair of artificial hands and an artificial left leg suitable for the case. Cut V 10 represents the limbs applied. Each hand had moving thumbs, which were connected with levers, operated by the forearm. When the stumps were flexed the levers would force the thumbs against the index and middle fingers. When the stumps were extended this pressure was released, and the thumb was permitted to withdraw. An artificial leg was applied to the left side. By these appliances this person was rendered capable of earning his livelihood.

CHAPTER XXVII

APPLIANCES FOR DEFORMITIES, EXCISIONS, WEAKENED JOINTS, ETC.

In cases of ununited fractures of either bone of the forearm or of the elbow joint or upper arm, it is necessary to apply a brace constructed upon durable lines and capable of being removed and readjusted as conditions require. Cut W 1 shows an apparatus for an ununited fracture. The forearm and muscle parts are con-

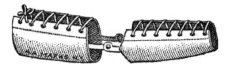

Cut W 1.

structed of material sufficiently firm to serve the purpose. They are connected by articulating joints that work in harmony with the elbow, or supply the elbow motion; the parts are adjustable by lacing, they hold the bones in place and give strength and firmness

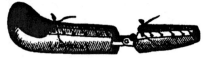

Cut W 2.

to the fractured member. Cut W 2 represents an apparatus for elbow-joint resection or for dislocated shoulder joint. The forearm and muscle parts are made of suitable material and are connected by steel joints. The muscle part is provided with a hood, which

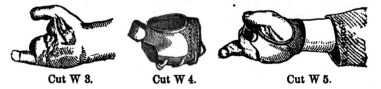

Cut W 3.   Cut W 4.   Cut W 5.

rests comfortably upon the shoulder. When necessary, a strap connected with the hood is passed around the body, holding the appliance firmly in place.

Cut W 3 represents a hand mutilation, the subject being a sailor, requiring an appliance that would enable him to hold a rope, tie a knot, climb the shrouds, and carry articles about a vessel. Cut W 4 represents a socket composed of canvas, rubber,

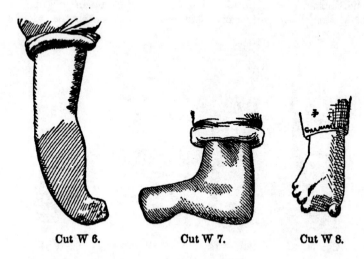

Cut W 6.   Cut W 7.   Cut W 8.

and leather, formed to fit the mutilated hand, with apertures to admit the passage of the remaining fingers; a steel, flattened hook was riveted between the apertures. Cut W 5 represents the apparatus applied, which proved to be useful and satisfactory.

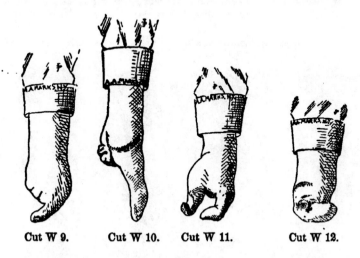

Cut W 9.   Cut W 10.   Cut W 11.   Cut W 12.

There are many cases of deformities, resections, etc., of the upper extremities that can be treated practically the same as amputations. They require artificial parts that incase the weakened members and strengthen them.

Hands and parts of hands are attached to malformed members so as to correct the deformity and supply the want to a degree sufficient to make the remaining parts useful. Cut W 6 represents a deformity of the forearm, the elbow joint possessing normal conditions. This deformity case was treated as an amputation below the elbow, adjustments to meet the peculiarities of the

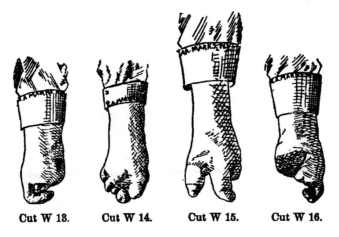

Cut W 13.   Cut W 14.   Cut W 15.   Cut W 16.

stump. Cut W 7 represents a deformity of elbow joint and forearm, a very slight movement remaining in the elbow, the forearm terminating in an enlargement. An artificial arm, constructed similar to one for wrist-joint amputation, was made and applied.

Cuts W 8 to W 20 represent congenital deformities of the hands.

In these cases, the conditions being somewhat similar to ampu-

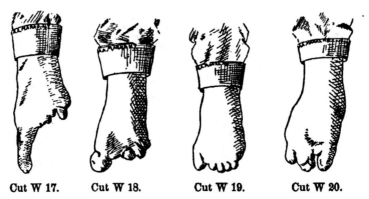

Cut W 17.   Cut W 18.   Cut W 19.   Cut W 20.

tations, artificial hands for partial hand amputations, as illustrated and described in Chapter XX., were applied.

Cut W 21 represents a European prince of distinguished lineage. When an infant, he fell from his nurse's arms, paralysis of the right arm followed. As he grew to manhood, the affected member grew in length, but failed to develop in size. It was limp and useless. In 1893 he came to us, and, upon examination, we found that the entire right side of the thorax was undeveloped, and that an artificial arm could be applied without producing noticeable disproportion. The case was treated the same as a shoulder-joint amputation, and an arm constructed accordingly was attached outside the withered member. The supporting part covered a great area of the shoulder, chest, and back; this held

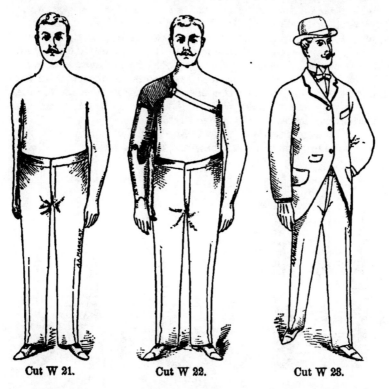

Cut W 21.   Cut W 22.   Cut W 23.

the artificial arm in place, as shown in Cut W 22. In dressing, the withered arm was (as had always been the custom) permitted to rest close to the body, the clothing was placed between the artificial and the withered arm, and, when dressed, the prince presented an appearance that was beyond criticism, as shown in Cut W 23.

CHAPTER XXVIII

ARM IMPLEMENTS

Implements for artificial arms are of endless variety: hooks, knives, forks, clevises, claw-hooks, pincers, clamp rings, are a few of the many devices that have been made for persons whose occupations demand something aside from the usual line. Each arm we make is supplied with a hook, knife, fork, and brush. These are included in the cost. Additional implements are furnished when desired, and if a customer desires one made to order for any special purpose, we will gladly make it for him. Our charges for the same will be moderate.

Cut X 1 represents a table knife, Cut X 2 a table fork, Cut X 3 a hand or nail brush; these are fitted to slip in the palm of

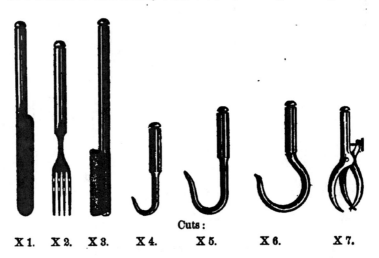

Cuts:

X 1. X 2. X 3. X 4. X 5. X 6. X 7.

hand or in the end of the forearm. They are of great assistance at the table and in washing the opposite hand.

Cuts X 4 and X 5 are hooks to be carried in the palm of the hand or in the end of the forearm. They are made with straight shanks, so that they can be received in the palm, are of two sizes, large and small, as shown in the illustrations.

Cut X 6 is a round hook, to be used in the end of the forearm. The curved back prevents it being placed in the palm of the hand. Cut X 7 is a claw hook, to be used in the end of the forearm. One part is made with two prongs and the other with one; it can be opened, closed, and set. This device enables a mechanic to clasp a tool with firmness.

Cuts X 8 and X 9 show rings which can be placed in the end of the forearm. One is immovably attached to the shank, and the other is loose; either is serviceable for mechanics and farmers. Through the ring the handle of a tool, or farm implement, can slide, while the tool is directed by the opposite hand.

Cut X 10 shows a clevis to be used for holding shop or farming implements. A quarter-inch hole must first be bored through the handle of the tool to be held, then the pivot pin unscrewed and the clevis placed over the handle, the pivot pin passed through one tine of the clevis, through the hole in the handle, and then

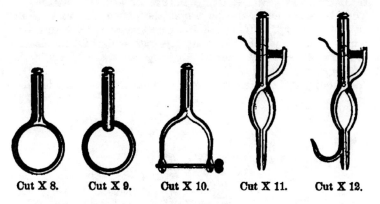

Cut X 8.   Cut X 9.   Cut X 10.   Cut X 11.   Cut X 12.

screwed into the other tine. This will hold the tool in an accommodating way, and permit it to swivel.

Cuts X 11 and X 12 show implements for light laboring purposes. X 13 and X 14 show the improved utility hook which can be used for more general purposes. The jaws are opened by a leather strap running up the arm connecting with the muscle section. When the artificial arm is extended the strap is pulled upon and the jaws of the pinchers open. When the arm is flexed the strap is released and the spring of the pinchers forces the jaws together, holding whatever may be placed between them.

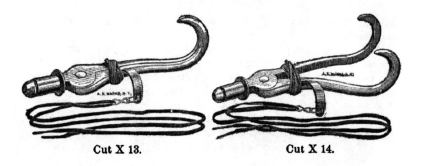

Cut X 13.   Cut X 14.

CHAPTER XXIX

UTILITY

Although claim is not made that an artificial arm possesses functions comparable to those of the natural, it is contended that a reasonable and a compensating amount of utility is assured.

The wholesome effect an arm has on the stump, that of keeping it in a healthy and vigorous condition, protecting it from injuries, forcing it into healthful activity, together with its ornamental aspect, are sufficient reasons for wearing one, even if utility is totally ignored.

As before stated, there are persons who have more aptitude than

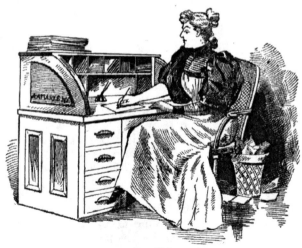

Cut Y 1.

others. Some with very short stumps do more than others with long ones.

Notwithstanding how short a stump may be, there is always a possibility of its controlling an artificial arm to advantage. If one person can use an arm on a short and difficult stump, there is hope that every person can do likewise, no matter what length or kind of stump he may have.

A few cases are presented, to give some idea of the scope of the value of artificial arms from the utility point of view.

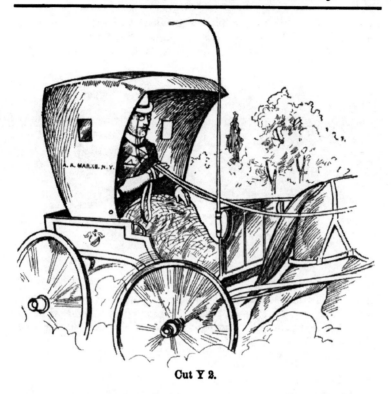

Cut Y 2.

One of our lady patrons is an amanuensis. While she is holding and guiding a pen with her rubber hand, she is keeping the paper from sliding on the desk with her natural hand. She writes

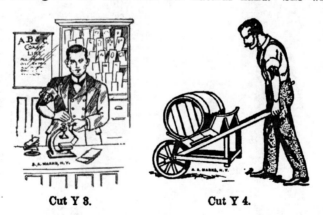

Cut Y 3.   Cut Y 4.

quickly and legibly and earns her livelihood by that employment. Cut Y 1 represents her at the desk.

One of our patrons, a physician, who is engaged in general country practice, wearing an artificial arm for amputation below

the elbow, finds his rubber hand convenient and valuable in holding the reins of his horse while driving. (See Cut Y 2.)

Mr. Woolley, of Ohio, is a ticket agent at a railroad station.

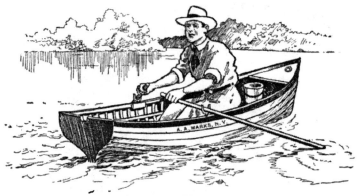

Cut Y 5.

He has held the position for a number of years to the satisfaction
of the company. He holds tickets in his natural hand while he
operates the stamp and dating machine with the rubber one.
(See Cut Y 3.)

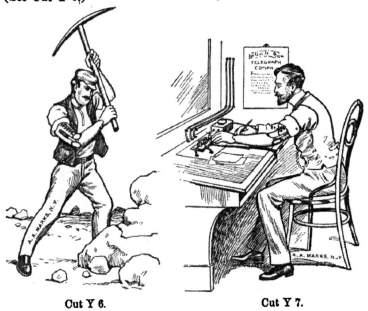

Cut Y 6.   Cut Y 7.

W. G. Bray, of Dunklin County, Mo., lost his arm below the
elbow some years ago. He has worn an artificial one since. He
is a clerk in a store and has to handle all kinds of heavy mer-

chandise. He handles a wheelbarrow to advantage. (See Cut Y 4.)

Cut Y 5 represents a customer who uses his rubber hand in rowing a boat; he is a farmer, located on the banks of a river, and finds it necessary to cross the stream frequently.

Mr. Ely, of Windham County, Conn., has no difficulty in working with other laborers and earning laborer's wages, although he has to do a great amount of work with the pickax. His right arm is artificial. (See Cut Y 6.)

A physician in Michigan writes that his patient, for whom he bought an artificial arm, has learned to operate the key of his

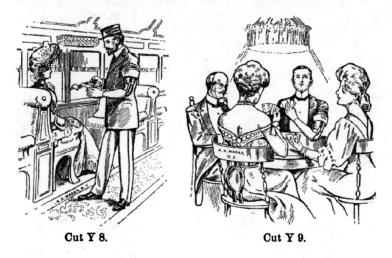

Cut Y 8.   Cut Y 9.

telegraph apparatus very skillfully with his rubber hand. (See Cut Y 7.)

The accompanying Cut Y 8 portrays a railroad conductor who wears an artificial arm and holds the ticket in his rubber hand while he operates the punch with the other.

A patron, residing in Providence, wears an artificial arm on a short shoulder stump; he could not be induced to do without it; it exercises his shoulder, improves his appearance. He finds the rubber hand a great convenience in holding cards while playing whist, a game he is greatly attached to. (See Cut Y 9.)

CHAPTER XXX

DIRECTIONS FOR TAKING MEASUREMENTS FOR ONE OR A PAIR OF ARTIFICIAL ARMS

Place a sheet of paper (about twenty or thirty inches) on a smooth table, remove all clothing from the upper part of the body, and place both arm and stump on this paper at full length. Be sure that the edge of the paper presses closely against the chest. Pass a long pencil down the inside of the arm (Cut Z 1), around the fingers, and up the outside to the shoulder. Then pass the pencil around the amputated side, from body around end of stump, and up to the shoulder (Cut Z 2). Bend the elbow of the sound arm to about right angles, mark from the shoulder around the elbow, down the forearm, around the hand, up the inside

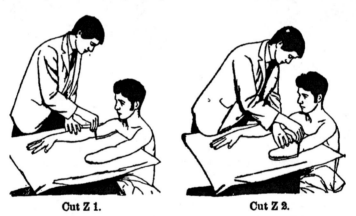

Cut Z 1.   Cut Z 2.

to the shoulder (Cut Z 3). Bend the elbow of the amputated arm to right angles and mark around it, from the shoulder to the end of the stump (Cut Z 4). If these diagrams are correctly made, they will resemble Cuts Z 5, Z 6, Z 7, and Z 8.

With a tape line measure the distance from the point of shoulder to the point of elbow of the sound arm, also the distance from the armpit to the bend of elbow (indicated by dotted lines in Cut Z 7). Measure the distance from the point of the shoulder to the point of the elbow of amputated arm, also the distance from the armpit to the bend of elbow. Give the circumference of each arm at points two inches apart, beginning close to the body. These circumferences are represented by dotted lines A, B, C, D,

E, and F of sound arm, and the dotted lines A, B, C, D, E, F, G, and H in the diagram of the stump (Cut Z 5). Then give the circumference of the hand at the base of the thumb, the circumference of the palm at the base of the fingers, the circumference

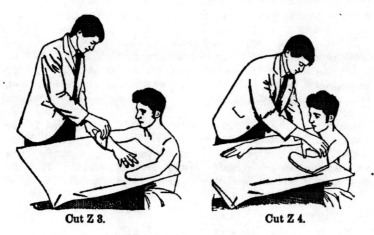

Cut Z 3.   Cut Z 4.

of the thumb at the first joint, represented by dotted lines G, H, and I (Cut Z 5).

If one arm is amputated in or above the elbow, the diagrams

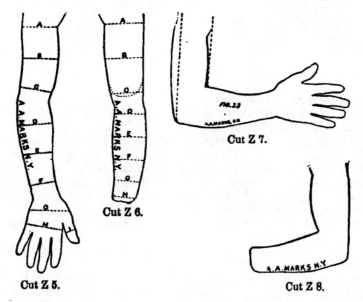

Cut Z 6.

Cut Z 7.

Cut Z 5.   Cut Z 8.

and measurements of the sound arm called for by Cuts Z 5 and Z 6 are required, and only one diagram of the stump, together with circumferences at places two inches apart, the distance from point of the shoulder to the point of the stump and from arm-pit to the point of the stump are also required.

If both arms are amputated above the elbow, diagrams of each stump, and the distances from the point of each shoulder to the point of each stump, and from armpit to the point of each stump are required, also the circumferences of each taken at points two inches apart.

If both arms are amputated below the elbows, the diagrams and measurements may be taken as suggested by Cuts Z 6 and Z 8.

All amputations in the shoulders, elbows, or wrists, or in the hands, leave extremities that are bony, more or less sensitive, requiring very exact fitting. Such stumps should be reproduced in plaster.

Answers to the following questions should be attached to the blank and forwarded with every order: Name of patient? Post-office address? Occupation? Age? Cause of amputation? When was amputation performed? Which arm amputated? Has the patient worn an artificial arm? If so, whose make? Name of

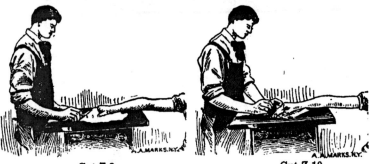

Cut Z 9.   Cut Z 10.

party ordering? His address? Is the arm to be made and fitted from measurements in the absence of the wearer? To what address shall it be shipped?

Plaster casts of arm stumps are only required in amputations in the wrists, elbows, shoulders, and in the hands, and in other cases when there are peculiarities that cannot be clearly indicated by the diagrams. A dentist, wax flower maker, or plaster statuette maker is familiar with the manipulation of plaster, and if one is available he should be employed for the purpose. The operation, however, of taking a plaster cast is not difficult, and can be done by almost any person.

The simplest method is as follows: Remove all clothing, shave away all hair, or stick it down with glue, paste, thick plaster, or thick soap. Then place about two quarts of plaster of Paris in a basin containing one quart of water, stir it up thoroughly, so that the plaster will become pasty. Then spread it upon the stump, until it is entirely covered with at least one-half an inch in thickness. The stump should be kept very quiet until the plaster has become hard, at which time it can be withdrawn, and the plaster will form a mold of the stump. This can be sent to us, or, if preferred, the inside can be greased and filled up with slaked plaster of Paris, which, when hard, can be taken from the mold.

If the end of the stump is large, or if there are prominences on the stump, it will be necessary to make the mold in two parts, so that they can be separated when hard, and the stump removed. The simplest way is to spread a little slaked plaster on the table, lay the stump upon it, pressing it down until it sinks half way into the plaster (see Cut Z 9). Then lay pieces of thin, wet paper all over the exposed surfaces of the plaster. Then pour and

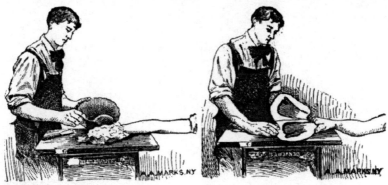

Cut Z 11.   Cut Z 12.

spread plaster on the top of the stump (Cut Z 10). Let the plaster run down the sides on the paper. The stump should be covered with at least one-half inch in thickness. When it has become thoroughly hard, the piece of paper will permit the plaster to separate and the stump can be withdrawn. The mold thus produced can be sent to us, or, if preferred, a plaster facsimile of stump can be made from it, by first speading oil or grease in the mold, then placing the two parts together, tying them by a string; then mix plaster of Paris to about the thickness of cream and pour it inside the mold. When this has become hard, the mold can be separated and the cast withdrawn.

ARMS FITTED FROM MEASUREMENTS

Artificial arms can, as a rule, be fitted from measurements and diagrams, while the wearers remain at home. The same reasons that are given for fitting artificial legs from measurements apply to arms. The guarantees that we give protect the ordering party in the strongest possible way. Should an arm fail to fit acceptably, when made from measurements, it may be assumed that the stump has changed, or that there are peculiarities about the stump which have not been made known. No matter what conditions may be responsible for such misfit, the arm can be returned, with particulars, and all the needed alterations or reconstructions will be made by us without charge, or, if the wearer desires, he can at that time call upon us and have the arm refitted and readjusted directly to his stump. It will thus be seen that the conditions under which fittings are made from measurements are entirely in the interest of the wearer. As a rule, fitting from measurements results in saving the party expense, annoyance, and loss of time in traveling.

CHAPTER XXXI

PRICES, ACCESSORIES

Artificial Fingers for Partial Hand Amputations, described on pages 194 to 197	Cut P 9	each	$30.00
	Cut P 10	"	30.00
	Cut P 23	"	50 00
	Cut P 24	"	50 00
	Cut P 25	"	50.00
	Cut P 26	"	50.00
Artificial Hands for Partial Hand Amputations, described on pages 197 to 198	Cut P 38	"	50.00
Artificial Arms for Wrist-Joint Amputations, described on pages 199 to 201	Cut Q 8	"	35.00
	Cut Q 9	"	35.00
	Cut Q 10	"	35.00
	Cut Q 11	"	35.00
	Cut Q 16	"	50 00
Artificial Arms for Forearm Amputations, described on pages 202 to 206	Cut R 7	"	50.00
	Cut R 8	"	40.00
	Cut R 13	"	50.00
Peg Arms for Forearm Amputations	Cut R 14	"	30.00
	Cut R 15	"	40.00
Suspenders for Forearm Amputations	Cut R 16	"	2.00
Artificial Arms for Elbow-Joint Amputations, described on pages 208 to 210	Cut S 2	"	75.00
	Cut S 3	"	75 00
Peg Arms for Elbow-Joint Amputations	Cut S 4	"	65.00
	Cut S 5	"	50.00
Artificial Arms for Above-Elbow Amputations, described on pages 211 and 212	Cut T 3	"	75.00
	Cut T 4	"	75 00
Suspenders for Above-Elbow Amputations	Cut T 5	"	2.00
Peg Arms for Above Elbow Amputations	Cut T 6	"	50.00
Artificial Arms for Shoulder-Joint Amputations, described on pages 213 to 215	Cut U 5	"	75.00
	Cut U 6	"	75.00
	Cut U 7	"	75.00
Appliances for Deformities, Excisions, Weakened Joints, etc., described on pages 220 to 223	Cut W 1	"	50.00
	Cut W 2	"	50.00
	Cut W 4	"	25.00
	Cut W 22	"	75.00
Arm Implements	Cut X 1	"	.75
	Cut X 2	"	.75
	Cut X 3	"	1.25
	Cut X 4	"	1.25
	Cut X 5	"	1.25
	Cut X 6	"	1.25
	Cut X 7	"	5.00
	Cut X 8	"	2.00
	Cut X 9	"	2.50
	Cut X 10	"	3.00
	Cut X 13	"	3.00

Cut X 11	"	8.00
Cut X 12	"	9.00

ACCESSORIES.—Artificial arms for wrist-joint, forearm, elbow-joint, above-elbow and shoulder-joint amputations will be accompanied, free of charge, with necessary suspenders, sock for the stump, knife, fork, hook, brush, pair of kid gloves, etc.

Peg arms for the above amputations will be accompanied with all the above-mentioned articles except gloves.

CHAPTER XXXII

TERMS OF PAYMENT, INSTALLMENT PAYMENTS, GUARANTEE

ADVANCE PAYMENT AVOIDS DELAY.—An article so important as an artificial leg or arm, which has to be made expressly to order for the person who is to wear it, should be paid for in advance. Time and expense are saved by doing so. If, however, objection is made to paying the full amount in advance, one-half the value can be forwarded with the order and the balance paid on delivery.

HOW TO MAKE PAYMENTS.—Remittances can be made by bank draft on New York, by postal money order, by express money order, or by money package by express. All drafts should be made payable to the order of A. A. Marks.

OUR RELIABILITY.—Every assurance is given that the interests and the welfare of the wearer will be subserved in every detail. Our reliability and business and financial standing can be ascertained by consulting any mercantile agency.

SUCCESS MOST IMPORTANT TO US.—It is of the greatest importance to us that every client shall be satisfied, not only with the fitting and construction of his artificial limb, but that he shall become clever, skillful, and dexterous in its use. He must do this in order to reflect credit on our skill. We take as much pride in the successful results of our work as do our clients.

As manufacturers, we cannot afford to neglect, or hastily dismiss a case, or show a lack of interest, or the least hesitancy in doing everything that is possible for the relief and comfort of our patrons. Wisdom compels the strictest integrity in the discharge of every obligation. Trouble and expense are not to be considered when disappointment and displeasure can be averted. No establishment can exist long that becomes careless, or allows its conduct to be criticised or impugned.

ADVANCED PAYMENTS ARE IN THE INTEREST OF THE WEARERS.—Payments in advance may be looked upon by some as arbitrary and unreasonable, but by the man of business they are viewed in the proper light, and not objected to. As a matter of fact, the best and most skillful services are always paid for in advance. If you wish to send a letter, you must attach a stamp to the envelope, and the stamp must be paid for when purchased, before the letter is delivered. This may appear to be a small matter, but to publishers and business men who have large correspondence, it amounts to hundreds of dollars every day. If you wish to send a telegram, you must pay for it in advance. If you want a telephone in your house, you must pay a month's fee in advance. If you wish to travel by land or sea, you must buy your ticket before you start; not after you have finished your journey. If you want a Lorenz to perform a surgical operation, you must pay him before he leaves his home. If you want a Makart to paint your portrait, you must pay him before he will entertain your order. And so it goes, the world over. The best talent and the most skillful services are only obtainable by paying in advance for them. The richest men—the most reputable merchants—have always to yield to these terms when they seek the best.

The same can be said of artificial limbs. The best can only be obtained by meeting the maker's terms. The poorest, those made by the inexperiencd, can be obtained upon any terms that the purchaser may wish to make.

The question then resolves itself into whether the applicant prefers to get the best limb, and pay for it in advance, or whether he is willing to put up with the product of an unskilled maker, merely to have his notion indulged regarding payment.

ARTIFICIAL LIMBS ON TRIAL, PREJUDICIAL TO SUCCESS.—It has been said that "things that are not paid for are good for nothing," and, as a matter of fact, articles that are constructed and sold under the consideration that they can be accepted or rejected, are, as a rule, rejected. It is safe to estimate that at least seventy-five per cent. of the artificial limbs that are made and delivered by small, inexperienced, and eager manufacturers, with the understanding that they can be tried for a reasonable length of time, and if not satisfactory, can be returned, are thrown back on the hands of the maker, and as these terms are only allowed by the maker of small means, he cannot afford to lose the time and material expended in the rejected limb. He, therefore, makes some slight alterations in the limb, and passes it to the next victim. There is, therefore, a strong probability, when placing an order with a manufacturer who permits his work to be returned, of getting a limb that was originally made for some other person.

WHY CORRECTLY MADE LIMBS ARE NOT ALWAYS PLEASANT AT THE START.—An artificial limb, no matter how scientifically it may be made and correctly fitted, is not a very comfortable article to wear during the period required to get accustomed to it. During this time there are many moments of discouragement. The stump, being weak, soon tires and fails to control the limb, and because of this weakness, the wearer gets discouraged and either concludes that the limb has not been properly made and fitted, or that his stump is of a character that will never control one. If the leg is not paid for, it will in all probability be rejected and returned to the maker during one of these periods when the wearer is in a discouraged frame of mind.

PATIENT ENDEAVOR BRINGS ITS REWARD.—If, on the other hand, the limb is paid for, the effort to wear it will be repeated again and again, until finally the task is accomplished, and the services derived will prove to be valuable beyond calculation. Viewing the subject in this aspect, it will be seen that the fact that the limb is paid for has a stimulating effect on the wearer, impelling him to put forth further effort.

MONEY DEPOSITED IN BANKS NOT ACCEPTABLE.—The proposition to place money for the payment of the limb on deposit with some bank, to be paid to us as soon as the limb is received and found satisfactory, is often made. We invariably decline to accept such terms, as money deposited is subject to such conditions that the feature of security is removed. The money cannot be drawn, unless the party ordering the limb gives his consent. If he declines to accept the limb from caprice, or hasty judgment, he can demand his money, and we have no redress.

INSTALLMENT PAYMENTS.—We are willing to accept payments on the installment plan to accommodate those in indigent circumstances, provided such obligations are imposed as will make the payments absolutely sure from the legal point of view. On an order for an artificial leg the first payment must be at least one-third its value, and for an artificial arm, one-half its value; and this amount must accompany the order. The balance can be paid in large or small amounts—weekly, monthly, or at other periods—as may be desired. Deferred payments must be secured by the indorsement of a reliable business person who has an acceptable mercantile rating.

DEFERRED PAYMENTS MUST BE GUARANTEED.—The deferred payments can be made by promissory notes, one note for each payment, signed by the party ordering the limb, and also by the party offering himself as security, or they can be secured by a letter written by the party guaranteeing the payments. The following is an example that will be acceptable:

Place.....................Date...........

A. A. MARKS, New York:

Dear Sir—Mr. .... desires to procure from you an artificial leg, and wishes to pay for the same in the following manner: .... dollars will be advanced with the order and .... dollars will be paid at the rate of ten dollars per month, beginning one month after the delivery of the leg.

In case of failure to meet the payments as agreed, or in case of default due to any cause whatsoever, you may hold me responsible, and upon demand I will pay the same to you.

Signed ....

Post-office address, ... Occupation, ...

ACCEPTABLE GUARANTORS.—We know no mercantile agency that quotes the financial standing or business liability of professional men, such as ministers, lawyers, doctors, farmers, retired men, employees, or agents. Mercantile agencies only give the standing of credit of those who are actually engaged in commercial or manufacturing industries. For this reason, we require the signature of a person engaged in business.

We believe there are but few dishonest persons; those whose motives and impulses are entirely void of integrity. Promises are made in good faith, but because of inability to keep them, they frequently go by default. A man without means, and being in need of an artificial leg, will assume almost any obligation, in order to procure one. He has the promise of a situation as soon as he can go without crutches. The future is promising and bright. He will go to his minister, or to his doctor, or his legal adviser, and as a rule, he will receive his favor. The clergyman or the doctor will promise to go security for him. The limb is obtained; the man wears it; he gets the situation, and earns fair wages; he becomes a little careless in his expenditures, or some relative or friend becomes afflicted and requires some financial help from him. The time arrives for payment to be made, and the young man has no money. The minister, or the doctor, who has guaranteed the payments, feels that it is unjust to be called upon to make payments. He writes a pitiful letter, and time is extended. This is repeated until patience becomes exhausted, and drastic measures have to be resorted to. It suddenly dawns upon the manufacturer that it would be poor policy to force payment out of the minister, or to make enemies with the doctor, and the matter is dropped, the manufacturer suffering the loss.

This is an old, old story, so often enacted in life that the manufacturer has been forced to accept no guarantors, except men engaged in business who have acceptable mercantile standings, and are prepared to meet losses, should the party default.

OUR GUARANTEE.—Every artificial leg or arm delivered by us is accompanied by a guarantee giving the assurance to the wearer that the artificial limb is constructed of the best material, and in a thoroughly workmanlike manner, and if any defects present themselves, we obligate ourselves to remove them without charge, provided the limb is delivered to us as soon as the defects have become known, and before the limb has become further damaged on account of being worn when out of order. The guarantee covers a period of five years from date of delivery.

CHAPTER XXXIII

PENSIONERS OF THE UNITED STATES ARMY AND NAVY FURNISHED WITH ARTIFICIAL LIMBS AT GOVERNMENT EXPENSE

THE ORIGINAL LAW.—It has been the purpose of the United States Government, since the early part of the Civil War (1862), to furnish artificial limbs to those who lost their natural ones from injuries received while in service. The first law, passed in 1862, gave one limb for each amputation, and to soldiers and sailors only. It was soon amended so as to include officers.

THE AMENDED LAW.—In 1870, a new law was passed, which increased the number of those entitled to artificial limbs, and repeated the issue every five years. This law was in force for twenty years.

THE NEW LAW NOW IN FORCE.—In the early part of 1891 Congress enacted additional pension laws, and added to the list hundreds of thousands of soldiers who had never before received pensions, and who had never dreamed of receiving any. The same Congress adopted measures by which additional benefits were given to the beneficiaries of the artificial limb laws. The old law was amended so that the issue was changed from five to three years. This was done not because soldiers required new limbs so frequently, but as an additional gratuity to the maimed. The law, as amended, reads as follows:

"Every officer, enlisted or hired man, who has lost a limb or the use of a limb in the military or naval service of the United States is entitled to receive, once every three years, an artificial limb or apparatus. The period of three years is reckoned from the last maturity subsequent to March 3, 1888."

Those whose maturity under the old law occurred between March 3, 1886, and March 3, 1888, were given a new date: namely, March 3, 1891 (the day the bill became a law).

TRANSPORTATION FREE.—Necessary transportation to the manufacturer is only issued when the order calls for an artificial limb to be made by the government manufacturer who is located the nearest to the applicant; if the limb chosen is to be made by a manufacturer more distant, transportation will not be given, but the order will be issued just the same, provided the applicant is willing to have the limb constructed from measurements or will pay his own traveling expenses.

THE BOND.—As manufacturers to the United States Government, we have met the requirements of furnishing bonds with two sureties, of five thousand dollars each, for the faithful performance of our work.

A blank application for an artificial limb and transportation will be sent upon request. The same can be filled out, signed, and mailed to us. As soon as we receive it, we will ascertain the date that the applicant will be entitled to a new limb, and at the proper time will pass the application to the proper officials.

Those who reside at a great distance, and do not care to travel, can remain at home and have their limbs constructed and fitted from measurements. We extend to them every protection, every assurance, every guarantee, and assume every risk, exactly as we do to civilians.

We have on file the measurements, diagrams, records, and dimensions of all the artificial limbs made by us since the founding of our house, and can duplicate any limb at any time.

If a soldier wishes to have a limb duplicated, he will not be required to send any additional measurements.

We advise pensioners to procure artificial limbs under the laws, and apply for them promptly upon the maturity of their claims, and lose no time.

When Congress makes changes in any law, the law in force up to that time becomes null and void. No one can predict what Congress will do, any more than he can predict what public sentiment will be on any issue. Should a party clamoring for extreme economy in the administration of public affairs become dominant, there is no telling what would be done in cutting down allowances.

ADVANTAGES IN REGISTERING WITH US.—As pensioners seldom keep records concerning themselves, we make it a point to notify them a little prior to the date of their maturity. Any change, or threatened change, in the law affecting the issue of artificial limbs is watched by us and communicated immediately to those on our records whom the law may affect. It is, therefore, to the advantage of the pensioner to keep within touch of us; to inform us of his change of address, and to see that our records are complete, so far as rank, company, regiment, number of pension certificate, etc., are concerned.

CHAPTER XXXIV

CHEAP ARTIFICIAL LIMBS

From the International Journal of Surgery

CHEAPLY MADE LIMBS NOT SAFE.—From time to time the newspapers chronicle severe accidents happening to the wearers of artificial limbs as the result of faulty construction. Here is an instance taken from the Cincinnati *Enquirer* of December 19, 1901:

"Fred Rentz was severely injured last evening, about five o'clock, by falling on the street at Central Avenue and Liberty Street. His fall was due to a cork leg breaking. The unfortunate man was taken to a hospital by Patrol No. 5."

INVITING DISASTER.—There is material in this brief item for profound thought on the part of every man who has occasion to require an artificial leg. There is material, too for a sermon on the iniquity of dealers who sell artificial limbs of inferior or defective workmanship. That there are many persons who commit the folly of risking their bodies, and possibly their lives, upon poorly made limbs for the sake of the few dollars saved thereby, and that there are dealers who are willing to encourage them in this folly, may be proved to the satisfaction of anyone who will read the daily papers carefully. Every few days cases are reported similar to the above, and in almost every case the disaster may be traced to the same cause—poor material or inefficient workmanship.

Mr. Rentz undoubtedly wore a cheap leg—cheap in construction, but very costly in the price he ultimately paid for it in money, suffering, and lost time. Some weakness in the wood or leather or steel (there is no cork in any artificial limb) was revealed by an accidental slip which brought an unusual strain upon it, and caused it to give way just when he had most need to rely upon it. The saying that "no chain is stronger than its weakest link" applies with the fullest possible force to an artificial leg. Every part may be perfect except one, and yet that one is certain to precipitate a fall of serious if not fatal results.

The adage that "the best is the cheapest" applies to almost everything that one may require. It applies without exception to the purchase of artificial limbs. The steeplejack will not make use of a cable unless he knows that it has been tested and proved to be capable of sustaining the weight that he will bring to bear upon it. The caisson worker will not descend below the bed of a river unless he is assured that the air-pumps are in perfect working order. No more should the wearer of an artificial limb trust himself upon it unless proved material, skill, and honesty have entered into its construction.

CONFIDENCE NECESSARY TO SUCCESS.—The essence of success in walking with an artificial leg is confidence. To learn to manipulate the limb is a very simple matter, but unless the wearer knows that he can rely upon it as thoroughly as he would upon his natural legs he will never be able to walk well or to move about with a sense of perfect freedom. There are thousands of persons walking about to-day on Marks' artificial legs whose intimate friends are not aware that they have lost any of their natural members. They do not limp or hobble, and they do not find the slightest difficulty in moving about as freely as their most active neighbors—all because they have confidence; they know that every bit of material that enters into the leg is carefully tested and proved before it is used, and that, therefore, it cannot possibly give way under ordinary use or at some critical moment when they most need its support.

A vast amount of care and trained ability enters into the construction of a thoroughly reliable artificial leg, foot, or arm. It will not be sufficient to use ordinary material, or even the best material that can be bought through the ordinary channels of trade.

SELECTION OF MATERIAL.—As the first step in the manufacture of the artificial leg, an expert visits the woods and selects the tree from which the material is to be cut. To do this is no easy matter, and requires long experience. The tree must be neither too young nor too old. It must be free from knots and must have a firm, even grain that it will be equally strong in every part.

When the tree has been felled it must be cut into lengths and carefully split into sections, use being made only of the main body of the tree trunk in which the grain is firm and even. Only a small portion of the ordinary tree is available for this purpose.

When the wood has been thus carefully selected, it is by no means ready for use. It must then be kiln-dried, so as to be thoroughly shrunk before it can be utilized. About four years is required in this process before the stick of timber can be manufactured into an artificial leg.

It is not the wood alone that is selected with such careful attention to its strength and wearing qualities. The steel which goes to form the braces and joints of the leg is first carefully tested to detect the existence of any flaws or defects and to prove that it is capable of carrying a larger weight than it will be called upon to support.

The leather for the jacket which forms the upper part of the leg is selected with equal care. Only the strongest and most valuable parts can be used; the rest must be thrown away or used for some other purpose. The buckskin lacings are also a matter of solicitude, and are subjected to thorough tests to determine the weight they will sustain.

Even a more delicate matter is the proper vulcanizing of the rubber foot which plays an important part in every successful artificial leg. The elasticity of the foot depends upon the exact degree of heat applied to the rubber. Thus, at every step in the selection of material, the greatest care and judgment must be exercised.

The need of practical experience and expert judgment does not end with the selection of materials. Equal skill is needed to assemble them properly. An artificial leg, to be a source of comfort and usefulness to its wearer, must fit perfectly, and no two persons can be fitted by exactly similar legs. The highest skill of the artisan is required to meet and make allowances for all the little peculiarities of each individual wearer. It is ridiculous to assume that it is possible to fit all comers with artificial legs simply by carrying a few sizes in stock.

The worst mistake that the prospective purchaser of an artificial limb can make is to patronize one of the cheap establishments which are continually being started by disgruntled apprentices or discharged workmen. It seems incredible that a man who will not permit his horse to be shod by an incapable blacksmith, or his beard to be trimmed by a man of no experience as a barber, will nevertheless trust the delicate and vital task of supplying an artificial limb for himself or a member of his family to a crude bungler or a cheap mechanic. Yet such cases come to notice frequently. Too late, when permanent injury has been done to some delicate blood vessel or tender nerve center, or when a bad fall and broken bones have taught the lesson that better counsel might have imparted in the beginning, he turns to the firm that has a long-established reputation for efficiency, reliability, and honest dealing.

How much better—yes, how much cheaper—it would be to intrust one's self in the beginning to a firm the members of which have gained a thorough knowledge of the subject through a business experience of years, which spares no expense to secure the most perfect materials for its artificial limbs, which employs the most carefully trained and thorough workmen, which owns the most important and successful patents for artificial limb appliances, and the name of which is a guarantee of good faith, good workmanship, and satisfaction to its customers!

CHAPTER XXXV

DO THE MAIMED DIE YOUNG?

A FALSE BELIEF.—There appears to be a belief, shared by the medical profession as well as the laity, that the amputation of one or more of the limbs from the human body necessarily curtails the allotted years of man, that there is a law that establishes a ratio between the length of the life of the normally equipped man and that of the dismembered one. That the ratio is according to the extent of the dismemberment. If a man is born to live three score and ten years, provided he retains all his limbs, the loss of one limb will take, say, ten years from that allotment; and if he loses two limbs the lopping off of a few more years will be the consequence.

WHAT OUR RECORDS DISCLOSE.—During our career as prothetications we have had opportunities to investigate. An examination of our records, which comprise the histories of many thousands of maimed persons, has led us to the conclusion that the dismembering of the human body plays no part whatever in shortening life. Our records date back to 1853, and it is a fact that, of the entire number of our patrons, less than twenty-five per cent. have died, and most of those have died from old age or accident, and in no case can we learn of a death that can be directly ascribed to the loss of a limb. We know of very few persons wearing artificial limbs who have suffered or died from pulmonary or cardiac diseases, and those who have fallen under those diseases were affected before their limbs were amputated. It is not an uncommon occurrence for octogenarians who have been our patrons for years to order new limbs, expecting to live long enough to wear them out.

AMPUTATIONS REVITALIZE THE SYSTEM.—As we investigate this subject more thoroughly we are persuaded that amputations revitalize the entire person, and render it not only possible but probable, that, on account of amputations, the lives of the subjects will be prolonged, comparatively immune to disease.

It is obvious that diseased and mangled limbs that cannot be cured will cause death if they are not removed; but this is not the phase of the question we are discussing. Will the length of life of the person who has had his limb removed on account of disease or injury be less than it would had his limb never been diseased, injured, and amputated? While it is absolutely impossible to give a direct reply to this question we believe, and we say it with all sincerity, that the compensation for the loss of a limb lies in assured good health and prolonged life. Numerous instances support this belief and many of them are of national reputation.

ILLUSTRATIONS.—Rev. Edward Beecher reached the age of eighty-four. Evidences of senility were apparent. By making a false step he fell from a railroad train and had one of his legs so badly crushed that it had to be amputated. He recovered from the operation and had an artificial leg applied. He lived for eight years and enjoyed excellent health and remarkable physical strength and mental energy. It was his custom to take long walks every day, to preach sermons on Sundays, lead prayer meeting during the week, and in fact, perform all the duties expected of a clergyman. From the moment he recovered from the accident that deprived him of his leg, new life and renewed energy came to him. He was a stronger, healthier, and more sprightly man after the accident than he had been for a number of years prior to it.

Governor Wade Hampton lived to be an octogenarian. He had a leg amputated a number of years before and wore an artificial one up to the time of his death. He was up to the last moment mentally and physically strong.

John Pearson lived to be eighty-five years of age. He lost a leg when seventy, recovered quickly, obtained an artificial leg, enjoyed vigorous health, giving his time to his railroad interests almost up to the moment of his death. General Butler, General Wager Swayne, and scores of others have more than fulfilled the biblical allotment and enjoyed many years of active life after having been deprived of one of their limbs.

It is a remarkable fact that there are very few maimed persons in insane asylums. Records of suicides are almost free of the crippled. The mental as well as the vital forces appear to become stimulated by the dismemberment.

ATHLETES.—Dare, Melrose, Conway, Leland, and Fitzpatrick are one-legged acrobats whose muscular developments are the envy of the world. Few possessed of natural limbs can vie with them in athletic activities.

It is a noticeable fact that persons who lose their legs become powerful in their arms, large in chest and girth, and persons who lose their arms become powerful in their legs and large in girth. The loss of one part of the body stimulates the growth of the remaining parts.

COMPENSATION.—A reasonable explanation may be found in the hypothesis that the removal of a part of the body lessens the demand on the vital forces and permits the supplying reservoirs to contribute more abundantly to the remaining members. If it overtaxes the heart to force the blood through all the avenues of the body, will not its labors be lessened if some are cut off? And will not the remaining avenues receive a larger share of the life-giving essences? If the nervous system is taxed to its limit, will not the tax be lessened if a part of the nerve organization be removed? If a tree is permitted to grow unpruned, it will sap itself by many choking branches and the trimming up of the limbs always gives vigor. The tree will grow larger, stronger, and will live longer.

It has been said that a maimed person takes care of himself, does not expose himself to the elements, or to the dangers that beset other human beings; that on account of being crippled, he is compelled to be more cautious than others; he cannot indulge in the riotous, inebriate course which wrecks so many lives. In this connection we will say, and we speak from knowledge, that a person who is deprived of one or more of his limbs is not necessarily a convert to a life of virtue. He is not always the sober man, the epitome of morality that some persons think he is. He goes through life in the same careless manner as other healthy mortals, doing what he ought to do, and many times what he ought not to do. He sometimes observes propriety, but oftentimes is as reckless as his companions. There are, however, many maimed persons who are sober, industrious, thoughtful, and prudent. The same habits, indulgences, and discretions that are found among those in possession of their natural limbs are found in about the same proportion among those who have been amputated.

GRATITUDE.—It is also an error to suppose that the loss of a limb induces despondency. There will not be found a class of people who are less lugubrious and who lament their losses as little as that class of humanity having abbreviated extremities. We recall the visit of a man some years ago who had both of his legs and one arm amputated. After reciting a harrowing tale of a railroad collision and fire, weeks of suffering at the hospital, and his recovery to health with only one of his four limbs remaining, he closed his narrative with the ejaculation: "Thank God, it was no worse!" This illustrates fairly well a crippled man's disposition. He is more thankful that he has not lost more, than he is regretful for having lost so much. He is constantly meeting with persons who, in his mind, have met with greater hardships than himself. It is an ordinary occurrence for a one-legged man to meet a one-armed man, and for each to say to the other, "I prefer to be as I am rather than as you are."

A cripple is neither a cynic nor a pessimist. His misfortunes have driven from him whatever there may have been of the choleric. Being always in good health, he is a happier and a more contented man than the dyspeptic, the rheumatic, or the gouty man, who is in possession of all his limbs. It is a common occurrence for a man wearing two rubber feet to take consolation from the fact that he can never be troubled with corns, gout, or suffer the torture of having some ponderous lout tread on his feet.

Nature, with her usual generosity, compensates for every misfortune. We look about us and see conditions that are appalling, and are impelled to pour out our commiseration; but we little think how useless, how unsolicited, and often uncharitable it is for us to do so. Those that are the most afflicted need our commiseration the least. Their minds and dispositions have already been prepared by Nature to bear their misfortunes, and they dislike to have others notice or mention them, much less to shed tears over that which they so little regret themselves.

CHAPTER XXXVI

AWARDS

1858. The first Exposition at which A. A. Marks exhibited artificial limbs was at the Crystal Palace at New York in 1858. As that exhibition was destroyed by fire no awards were given.

1859. AMERICAN INSTITUTE, NEW YORK CITY.—The silver medal was awarded to A. A. Marks for his superior artificial limbs.

1865. AMERICAN INSTITUTE, NEW YORK.—After a careful and extended examination, and practical tests of the various kinds of artificial limbs, the First Premium Gold Medal was awarded to A. A. Marks.

1867. AMERICAN INSTITUTE, NEW YORK, FIRST PREMIUM.—Marks' Patent Artificial Limbs have frequently been before the Institute and continue to sustain their former reputation. The First Premium awarded.

1869. AMERICAN INSTITUTE, NEW YORK.—A. A. Marks Best. This limb is constructed with an india-rubber foot, which from its elasticity does away with the necessity of motion at the ankle, and also obviates entirely that heavy, thumping sound when the foot strikes the ground in walking. The control which the wearer has over it and its movements, so closely resembling those of the natural limb, entitles it to the highest commendation. First Premium awarded.

1870. AMERICAN INSTITUTE, NEW YORK.—The especial point of excellence appears to be the rubber foot, by the use of which all complications in the construction of an ankle joint are avoided. First Premium awarded.

1871. AMERICAN INSTITUTE, NEW YORK.—The artificial limbs with rubber feet and rubber hands are especially recommended for their simplicity, durability, and easy movements. First Premium awarded.

1872. AMERICAN INSTITUTE, NEW YORK.—The artificial limbs manufactured by A. A. Marks continue to merit approval, and are entitled to all the confidence the public have reposed in them. First Premium awarded.

1873. AMERICAN INSTITUTE, NEW YORK.—After full and impartial examination of the articles above described, the undersigned Judges make report that they find the artificial limbs on exhibition by A. A. Marks worthy of the confidence heretofore reposed in them. We cheerfully indorse all that has been said of them by former examiners, *their simple construction, easy movements, durability, etc.* First Premium awarded.

1874. AMERICAN INSTITUTE, NEW YORK.—We consider the artificial limbs of A. A. Marks of great value. A great improvement

—better than any known to us; and entitled to the highest award. First Premium awarded.

1875. AMERICAN INSTITUTE, NEW YORK.—We regard the artificial limbs presented by Mr. Marks superior to all others in practical efficiency and simplicity. First Premium awarded.

1876. CENTENNIAL EXHIBITION, PHILADELPHIA, PA.—The Judges having examined Marks' artificial limbs respectfully recommend the same to the United States Centennial Commission for the highest award, for the following reasons, viz: Utility, Workmanship, and Adaptation to Purposes Intended.   Highest award given.

1876. AMERICAN INSTITUTE, NEW YORK.—The judges consider the limbs made by A. A. Marks remarkable for simplicity of construction, durability, efficiency, and comfort to the wearers. Special Gold Medal awarded.

1877. AMERICAN INSTITUTE, NEW YORK.—After a full and impartial examination of Marks' artificial limbs, the Judges report that they consider the exhibit of great value and entitled to highest award. Medal for Superiority awarded.

1878. AMERICAN INSTITUTE, NEW YORK.—Having received the Medal of Superiority in 1877, The Diploma for Maintained Superiority is awarded at the Exhibition of 1878.

1881. INTERNATIONAL COTTON EXPOSITION, ATLANTA, GA.—First Premium, Gold Medal, awarded for the following reasons:

First. Simplicity in the mechanism of the knee joint and its excellent movement. Second. Durability. Third. Rubber Foot, possessing many excellent qualities and compensating for the absence of the motion in the ankle joint. The highest award was declared in favor of A. A. Marks.

1885. THE WORLD'S INDUSTRIAL AND COTTON CENTENNIAL EXHIBITION, NEW ORLEANS, LA.—The Jurors having carefully examined the exhibits of artificial limbs concur in recommending the award of the First Class Medal to A. A. Marks, New York. Gold Medal awarded.

1889. THE JOHN SCOTT LEGACY PREMIUM AND MEDAL.—John Scott, late of Edinburgh, by his will made in the year 1816, bequeathed a sum of money to the Corporation of the City of Philadelphia, directing that the interest and dividends received therefrom shall be laid out in premiums, to be distributed among ingenious men and women who make useful inventions, and that therewith shall be given a medal with this inscription:

"TO THE MOST DESERVING."

The great improvements in artificial limb construction consist in the substitution of rubber for wood in both the foot and hand.

The rubber foot consists of a wooden block rigidly secured or formed with the leg and extending downwardly to within about two-fifths of the distance from the ankle to the sole, and forward to nearly the first articulation of the metatarsus and toes; this block is covered with india-rubber.

The action of such an artificial foot is that of an elastic segment of a wheel. The shock of placing the weight upon the heel at each step is avoided by the elastic cushion of rubber forming the heel, and as the weight is progressively transmitted to the forward part of the foot, by the combined effect of muscular exertion in the remaining part of the natural limb, and the momentum previously acquired, an easy flexure of the toes takes place, which, reacting elastically as the weight is transferred to the other limb, giving an easy and naturally appearing movement. Such artificial feet are, upon trial, found to be easier to use, lighter, and more comfortable.

The desire to adapt the india-rubber hands to changes of flexure, for purposes of better and more natural appearance and to grasp light objects, led Mr. Marks to improve them by making a light wooden core in the palm or metacarpal portion of the hand and inserting ductile metallic wires in such core, which extended centrally through the fingers. By bending the fingers they retain the form in which they are set.

The latest improvement in artificial limbs consists in forming the leg and foot part of a single piece of wood, having the grain curved naturally in its growth, such pieces being procured from the parts of the trunk contiguous to the roots and branches of trees; limbs made in this way are stronger with the same amount of wood remaining in them than when made of parts glued together, and are made waterproof, which is a valuable feature when the occupation of the wearer exposes it to constant dampness, or to water itself, as in fishing, mining, dredging, etc.

The above report was presented to the committee appointed by the City of Philadelphia, under the auspices of the Franklin Institute, and it was unanimously decided that the John Scott Legacy Medal and Premium be awarded to A. A. Marks.

1891. AUGUSTA EXPOSITION, AUGUSTA, GA.—Seven Gold Medals and Awards for distinct and separate features of excellence.

First. For Improved Artificial Legs with Rubber Feet.

Second. For Improved Artificial Arms with Rubber Hands.

Third. For Superior Methods of Suspenders for Artificial Legs and Arms.

Fourth. For Superior Crutches and other Auxiliaries for Cripples.

Fifth. For a Combined Knife and Fork for the use of one-armed men.

Sixth. For Improved Waterproof Artificial Legs, carved from natural crook timber.

Seventh. For Improved Artificial Legs and Arms with Aluminum Sockets.

1893. THE ELLIOTT CRESSONS GOLD MEDAL, awarded to A. A. Marks for aluminum socket artificial legs and arms, as stated in the following report:

At the stated meeting of the committee on Science and the Arts of the Franklin Institute, held February 1, 1893, the following report was adopted and ordered to be issued:

This invention consists of an improved method of making artificial limbs, adapted to amputations in the ankle, or below, in the tarsus or metatarsus, in which the former modes of construction, with articulated ankle joints of wood as the material, were impracticable and unsatisfactory. The new method of construction involves the use of aluminum as the material to form the shell socket or sustaining frame, as it might be called, the aluminum shell supporting the body, and forming the attachment for the elastic rubber foot, which acts as a rolling elastic segment simulating the functions of the natural foot in walking, and acting as an elastic cushion in relieving the wearer from the jar or shock of resting the weight upon the limb.

Your committee has examined the limbs in the course of manufacture, and as completed and as in use by wearers. When clothed, they give no indication in walking that they are not natural feet.

It is clearly apparent that the invention is one affording much-needed relief to persons heretofore greatly embarrassed, and further that the surgeons may save much more of the patient's body from mutilation than heretofore, and yet render comfortable and satisfactory artificial limbs practicable.

In view of these points of excellence and well-attested evidence thereof the committee awards the Elliott Cresson Medal to Mr. Marks, of New York.

1893. WORLD'S COLUMBIAN EXPOSITION, CHICAGO.—The judges appointed to investigate artificial limbs decided in favor of Marks' artificial limbs and recommended to highest award on the following points of excellence.

First. RUBBER FOOT. (*a*) Its close approximation to the motions and actions of the natural foot.

(*b*) Its durability and lightness; the yielding and elastic qualities of rubber supply requisite motion without necessitating mechanism.

(*c*) Phalangeal assistance. The methods of construction and connection with the body of the leg in each case are such as to provide assistance in walking from the anterior portion of the foot, at the same time maintaining the height of the wearer when walking, same as is obtained from the natural foot; the feature of phalangeal assistance avoids limping, and removes the fear of toppling forward when standing.

(*d*) The elasticity of rubber affords a yielding medium to alight upon, thus avoiding jars and concussions to the stumps.

Second.—KNEE JOINTS. (*a*) The construction of knee joints is such as to render them capable of adjustment, thus obviating the noise that follows attrition.

(*b*) The disposition of the knee spring, which assists extension of the lower leg, is such as to become neutralized when the leg is flexed to a given angle; this avoids " kicking out " of the lower leg when the wearer is sitting and unguarded.

(*c*) Safety lock. This attachment is combined with the knee mechanism, and provides against treacherous flexing of the knee, thus avoiding dangerous falls.

Third. The production of waterproof legs from natural crook timber with rubber feet attached.

Fourth. Aluminum sockets, especially designed for stumps that extend to the ankle and in the body of foot.

The advantages obtained by the utilization of this metal are as follows:

(*a*) The production of a socket that can be closely fitted to the stump, without touching or allowing painful contact with any of the tender spots on the stump, at the same time possessing sufficient strength to properly support the wearer.

(*b*) The construction of a socket that will possess the requisite strength without conspicuously enlarging the ankle.

Fifth. Roller Suspenders. The object of this method of suspending an artificial leg to the wearer is to avoid the moving and rubbing of the shoulder straps on the shoulders.

First. THE RUBBER HAND. (*a*) Being composed of rubber, is pleasant and natural to the touch and durable in construction.

(*b*) The fingers, being ductile, can be placed into accommodating positions.

(*c*) The palm of the hand, being provided with a locking socket, is capable of holding implements of utility with firmness.

Second. The ability to detach the hand at the wrist for laboring purposes.

Third. Rotation of hand at wrist.

Fourth. The elbow joint, with lock for holding the arm in a flexed position.

Fifth. Fingers and parts of hands made of rubber.

Sixth. Rotation of upper arm socket.

In conformity with the Judges' report, the highest award (medal and diploma) was declared in favor of A. A. Marks, New York City.

Two additional diplomas were awarded by the Board of Lady Managers, one for DESIGN, and the other for INVENTION.

1895. COTTON STATES AND INTERNATIONAL EXPOSITION, ATLANTA, GA.—This certifies that the appropriate jury has awarded to A. A. Marks of New York City the Gold Medal "For the most complete exhibition of ingenious mechanics for the relief of physical defects and deformities, namely: Artificial Legs, Rubber Feet, Artificial Knee Joints, Self-Adjusting Suspenders, Artificial Arms, Rubber Hands, Duplex Elbow Joints, and Aluminum Socket Legs; also for Imitating the Movements of Knee, Elbow, Wrist, and Finger Joints."

1896. AMERICAN INSTITUTE, NEW YORK.—After a full and impartial examination the Judges made report:

That the exhibit of A. A. Marks of artificial limbs, deserves the highest award for the following reasons.

First. To the rubber foot with imbedded metallic mattress spring.

Second. To the flexible fingers on artificial hand, and their great adaptability to everyday use.

Third. The use of aluminum in place of wood for climatic variations seems to be of practical use for those engaged in certain employments.

Finally, the ingenious combination Knife and Fork for the one-armed is highly commended. The medal of superiority was accordingly awarded.

1897. TENNESSEE CENTENNIAL AND INTERNATIONAL EXPOSITION, Nashville, Tenn.

The highest and only award for artificial limbs was given to A. A. Marks of New York.

The merits that received especial recognition were: Artificial Legs with Rubber Feet, Adjustable Knee Joints, Artificial Arms with Rubber Hands, and a Combination Knife and Fork for one-armed persons.

1898. TRANS-MISSISSIPPI AND INTERNATIONAL EXPOSITION, Omaha, Neb. Diploma and Gold Medal awarded to A. A. Marks, New York.

Marks' Artificial Legs with Rubber Feet and Artificial Arms with Rubber Hands are superior to all others in the following points:

Excellence of mechanical construction.

Minimum weight, maximum durability.

Noiselessness.

Motions that simulate nature.

Knee joints, adjustable and noiseless.

Suspenders, of variety adaptable to every condition.

Knee lock for short and enervated stumps.

Fittings that permit pressure at points of toleration, avoiding impact on the vascular parts, thereby preventing choking of blood vessels.

Rubber hands with ductile fingers, most accommodating and possessing the greatest range of utility.

1900. EXPOSITION UNIVERSELLE DE PARIS, FRANCE.

A. A. MARKS, New York.

DEAR SIR:—I am instructed by Commissioner General Peck to inform you that you have been awarded the

(GRAND PRIX) Grand Prize

for your exhibit in Class 16 at the International Exposition, Paris, 1900.

Respectfully yours,

J. H. GORE, Juror-in-Chief.

In competition with nearly fifty manufacturers from all parts of the world, A. A. Marks won over 20 POINTS OF MERIT, thereby earning the ONLY GRAND PRIZE FOR ARTIFICIAL LIMBS.

1901. PAN-AMERICAN EXPOSITION, Buffalo, N. Y. The points of merit and claims for superiority presented to the Board of Jurors, as follows:

First. The rubber foot with spring mattress.

Second. Knee joint with adjustable bearings and removable bushings.

Third. Hip joint for hip-joint amputations.

Fourth. Knee lock for short and enervated stumps.

Fifth. Suspenders arranged to minimize the burden and tax on the shoulders.

Sixth. Aluminum sockets for ankle-joint and partial foot amputations.

Seventh. Rubber hand with ductile fingers and palm attachment for holding implements.

Eighth. Wrist joint admitting of rotation, displacement of the hand and substitution of laboring implements.

Ninth. Elbow lock, holding arm in flexed and other positions.

Tenth. Humeral rotation, admitting the arm to rotate above the elbow joint, so that when flexed it can be brought closer to the person.

Eleventh. Artificial hand for partial hand amputation.

Twelfth. Artificial legs for bathing purposes that are absolutely waterproof.

Thirteenth. Artificial arms that are absolutely waterproof.

Fourteenth. Combination knife and fork designed for persons who are temporarily or permanently disabled in one hand.

Upon these points of merit the Gold Medal and Diploma were awarded to A. A. Marks.

1902. SOUTH CAROLINA INTER-STATE AND WEST INDIAN EXPOSITION, Charleston, S. C. Gold Medal awarded to A. A. Marks, of New York, for artificial legs and arms of superior construction.

1904. THE LOUISIANA PURCHASE EXPOSITION (WORLD'S FAIR), St. Louis, awarded to A. A. Marks, of New York, the only GRAND PRIZE for ARTIFICIAL LIMBS, the highest award given to any exhibit in any department.

The Grand Prize at St. Louis following the Grand Prix at Paris. 1900, prove beyond controversy the superiority of Marks' artificial legs, feet, arms, and hands, and the maintenance of their excellence not only in America, but throughout the entire world.

1905. THE LEWIS AND CLARK CENTENNIAL EXPOSITION, Portland, Oregon, awarded two Gold Medals (highest awards) to A. A. Marks, New York, manufacturers of the celebrated artificial limbs with rubber feet and hands.

1907. NEW ZEALAND INTERNATIONAL EXHIBITION, Christchurch, New Zealand, November, 1906, to April, 1907. The highest award of merit, Gold Medal, to A. A. Marks, New York, U. S. A., Artificial Limbs.

1907. JAMESTOWN EXPOSITION, Norfolk, Va., April 26th to November 30th. The highest award Gold Medal to A. A. Marks, Artificial Limbs, New York.

FOREIGN MONEY EQUIVALENTS.

The prices given in this book are in United States money. Parties ordering artificial limbs or supplies can make remittances in their own national money or any money that may be most available. The following table has been computed according to the rates of exchange August 2, 1910.

UNITED STATES.		BRITISH.			FRENCH.		GERMAN.		ITALIAN.	
Dollars.	*Cents.*	*Pounds.*	*Shillings.*	*Pence.*	*Francs.*	*Centimes.*	*Marks.*	*Pfennigs.*	*Lire.*	*Centesima.*
100	00	20	11	6	512	80	416	00	512	80
75	00	15	8	7½	384	60	312	00	384	60
65	00	13	7	6	833	30	270	80	330	30
60	00	12	6	11	307	60	250	00	307	60
50	00	10	5	9	256	40	208	30	256	40
40	00	8	4	7½	205	20	166	65	205	20
35	00	7	4	0½	179	50	145	80	179	50
30	00	6	3	5½	153	90	125	00	153	90
25	00	5	2	10½	128	20	104	15	128	20
20	00	4	2	4	102	60	83	35	102	60
15	00	3	1	9	77	00	62	50	77	00
10	00	2	1	2	51	30	41	65	51	30
5	00	1	0	7	25	65	20	85	25	65
2	00		8	4	10	25	8	35	10	25
1	00		4	2	5	15	4	17	5	15
	50		2	1	2	60	2	9	2	60
	25		1	0½	1	30	1	5	1	30
	10			5		52		42		52
	5			2½		26		21		26

CHAPTER XXXVII

TESTIMONIALS

Letters commendatory of the work we have done for the comfort of those with amputated or injured limbs can be numbered by the thousands. To print them in full would be impracticable. One hundred and forty pages are all that can be given to this subject and in order to make it interesting and far reaching we can take but a few lines from those letters only that cover the field, not only in the scope of industry, age of wearers, experience with limbs of other manufacture, but remoteness of residence, thus proving that our work is capable of every conceivable use not only in efficiency but strength of construction and endurance under every climatic condition.

Nearly every kind of amputation, as well as deformity, is shown; nearly every industry, and practically every part of the world, represented.

It will be noticed that most of the writers were supplied without leaving their homes. They had their measurements taken, and sent to us, and had artificial limbs constructed by them. Chapters XV and XXX enlarge on this feature.

*ALL TESTIMONIALS MARKED WITH AN ASTERISK (*) ARE FROM PERSONS WHO WERE FITTED FROM MEASUREMENTS.

It was customary in former times to give with each testimonial the full post-office address of the writer; but the frequency of complaints by the writers as well as the readers, has induced us to locate by counties and states only and furnish complete addresses when asked for. Artificial limb wearers move about the same as other persons. Among eight hundred, a large proportion change their locations every year and cannot be reached by the old addresses. For this reason it is better to give up-to-date addresses as they are needed and called for. Any person desirous of communicating or conferring with testimonial writers can make a list from this chapter and send it to us. Immediately upon its receipt we will send addresses that have been corrected to date.

* GEORGE ABBOTT—Railway Agent, Harbor Grace, Newfoundland. Below knee.

The leg you made for me is now ten years old and has given perfect satisfaction. June 10, 1909.

* JAMES A. ADAMS—Laborer, Northumberland Co., N. B. Partial hand amputation.

The artificial hand you made for me ten years ago is still in good order, and it is one of the best hands that is made. I would not be without it, I can do most any kind of work with it. March 23, 1910.

* MRS. E. E. ABEL—Housewife, Ontario. Knee amputation.
I am very thankful for the leg made me from measurements.
I do all my housework and a lot of walking and I have never

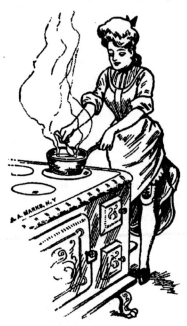

used a cane or anything, and I can walk without any trouble.
TOWNSEND ACKERMAN—Hotel keeper, Ulster Co., New York.
    Above knee.
The leg you sent me is O.K. I get along nicely with it. I keep
it on all day long and it does not trouble me at all. March 16, 1909.
* ANTONIO ALARCON—Merchant, Mexico. Below knee.
When I gave my order in 1887 I never imagined that an artificial
leg could form so perfect a substitute for the natural one in walking, riding on horseback, and even dancing; I supposed it would
merely serve to hide the defect. Experience has demonstrated to
me the superiority of artificial legs with the rubber feet. They
combine simplicity of construction with stability and ease in
walking.—Translated from Spanish.   April 24, 1910.
* WM. E. ALBEE—Stoker, Franklin Co., Mass. Below knee.
I have used the leg you made for me for six years. My work
is firing stationary boilers; it is hot and heavy. I believe that I
could not have done the work that I had to do with any other
artificial leg.   Oct. 10, 1909.
* D. A. ALLEN—Station Agent, Pike Co., Ark. Knee amputat'n.
The artificial legs furnished by you at different times have
given entire satisfaction in every respect and have all been perfect,
although made from measurements taken by myself. I am employed as R. R. agent and operator and attend to all the various
duties connected with the position.   May 30, 1908.
LEONARD D. ALPAUGH—Brakeman, Morris Co., N. J. Below knee.
On July 29th, 1903, I lost my left leg three inches below the
knee, and soon after purchased an artificial one from you, which

has given me entire satisfaction. The leg is a good strong one, and can be depended upon in performing all the work I have occasion to put upon it.   Oct. 5, 1909.

* ROBERT F. ALLEN—Carriage Painter, Livingston Co., Ill. Above knee.

I am still satisfied to wear the artificial leg you made for me in 1895. It is very comfortable.   Nov. 23, 1908.

* J. HENRY ALSTON M.D.—Dorchester Co., S. C.

The artificial arm I recently ordered for my patient was received and found to fit perfectly, and the patient is very much pleased with it. The mechanism and material are superb.   July 29, 1907.

ALICE ANDERSON—New Zealand. Above knee.

My friends say I have improved wonderfully in walking since I obtained your new style of artificial leg for thigh amputation. I am nearly as well as if I had never lost a leg.   Dec. 27, 1908.

RICHARD ANDERSON—Farm Superintendent, Somerset Co., N. J., Ankle amputation.

I have worn many makes of artificial feet, but there are none so satisfactory as yours. Work every day from 12 to 18 hours and frequently walk twenty miles. Cannot say too much in praise of your limbs.   July 17, 1909.

* VICTOR A. ANDERSON—Penobscot Co., Me. Above knee.

I am wearing one of your legs now that I bought fifteen years ago.   March 24, 1909.

* WM. ROBERT ANDREWS—Storeman, Auckland, New Zealand. Above knee.

The artificial leg I received from you eighteen months ago pleases me very much. It is a great blessing to me.   May 8, 1909.

* JOHN WESLEY ANDREWS—Clerk, Argentine Rep., S. A. Below knee.

I am acquainted with a Spaniard in need of an artificial leg. I have told him repeatedly that your make is the best in the world. The one you made for me in 1888 lasted for 18 years and the one you made in 1906 is still as good as new. You and I are old acquaintances and I think a good deal of you, although we have never met. You people are the only ones who know what artificial limbs really ought to be.   Oct. 10, 1909.

* MRS. JOS. ANTHONY—Conception Bay, Newfoundland. Above knee.

I have worn the artificial leg you made for me and am highly satisfied. I can walk to the Salvation Army Barracks without the aid of a stick. I am a member of that noble body of people.
                                                    April 8, 1908.

THOMAS APPLEBY—Farmer, Ontario. Below knee.

It is with pleasure I inform you that the artificial leg you made for me, nearly seven years ago, is being used satisfactorily and advantageously. I cannot give too much praise for your work, and doubt very much that the limb can be improved upon. I wear it constantly without the least discomfort.   Oct. 6, 1909.

MISS JOSEPHINE AREY—Penobscot Co., Me. Shortened leg.

I wish to express my continued gratitude for the apparatus made by you six years ago. At that time I could not get about the house without the assistance of a crutch. I walk now without the assistance of a cane. It seems as though I were living in a new world. It has done more for me than I ever dared hope for. I only wish all who are thus afflicted might be able to call on A. A. Marks, who will add much happiness to their lives and benefit them as much as he has me.   Oct. 13, 1909.

* F. S. ARMANTROUT—Clerk, Adams Co., Ind. Above knee.

I have worn artificial legs of your make for many years; the last one I have had a little over two years. It is giving the best of satisfaction.   Aug. 21, 1909.

A. J. ARMSTRONG—Train Dispatcher, Erie Co., N. Y. Below knee.

In 1891 I suffered the amputation of my right leg. After trying two different makes—one with cords and ankle joint and the other with hard rubber—I purchased one of your legs with sponge rubber foot in 1895. I wore it until November, 1903, with perfect satisfaction, and without one cent cost for repairs. In my occupation as train dispatcher for the New York Central R. R., I do not have to be on my feet as much as others, but my home is two miles from the office, and I walk both ways in winter and ride my wheel in summer. In fact I do the same as I would if both feet were natural. The one I purchased from you last gives the same perfect satisfaction. I think thirteen years of constant wear without a cent for repairs, must appeal with force to wearers of artificial feet with cords and ankle joints.   Oct. 8, 1909.

* WILLIAM J. ANGIER—Engineer, Richmond Co., Ga. Below knee.

I have no trouble with my artificial limb. It is the third of your legs that I have worn, and I am proud to say that I would

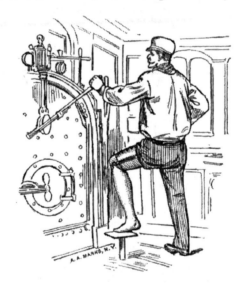

not have any other. My amputation is six inches above the ankle, left foot. I am running a locomotive every day, hauling passenger trains, and I am never inconvenienced in any way.   Oct. 9, 1909.

* MRS. J. W. ARMSTRONG—Bexar Co., Tex., son Freddie, aged 9.

I cannot estimate the comfort my little son has in the limb you made for him twelve years ago, when he was only two years old. It has enabled him to take part in all boyish pastimes and he goes from morning until night, running, walking, and playing the same as other boys, and without fatigue.   Oct. 13, 1909.

* JOSE A. ARRIGHI—Arg. Rep. Above knee.

I have the pleasure to inform you that the leg procured for me by Mr. Jose Anto. Orfila, over two years ago, has proved excellent, and the fit is perfect, even in the heat of this season of the year, and when the weather is temperate, I cannot tell that I am wearing it. I walk three miles a day, sometimes much more, with the greatest ease and comfort.—Translated from Spanish.

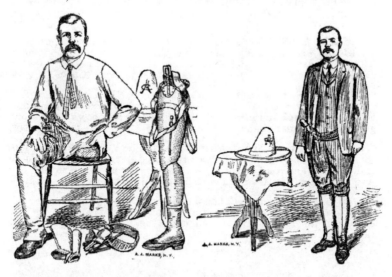

* ALFREDO J. J. AUSTIN, M.D.—Mier, Mexico.

In January, 1900, I ordered an artificial leg from you for Andres Cantu, Custom House Guard at this place. Mr. Cantu has a stump with only 1½ inches of the thigh bone. He duly received the leg and has used it ever since exposed it to all climatic variations,

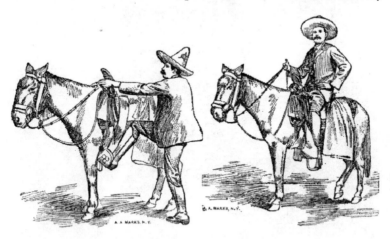

mounted and afoot day and night, ever on the lookout for smugglers on the Rio Grande River. He is considered one of the best officers in the service. He claims that his artificial leg fulfills all the requirements of the natural. I send you four photographs as follows:—1st, showing bare stump; 2nd, standing; 3rd, in the act of mounting, and 4th, mounted. They were taken Jan. 1, 1908,

* EMIL ASHE—Saw mill, Mora Co., N. M. Wrist amputation.
You made an artificial hand for me, right side, in 1892, fifteen years ago and I am still using that arm. Your artificial arms are without question the best in this and European countries. I have traveled abroad and there is nothing as good as yours there.
Dec. 22, 1907.

* AIME N. ASSELIN—Androscoggin Co., Me. Elbow amputation.
I had an arm made by you a few years ago and I am satisfied with it. I am now advising a friend of mine to get an arm of you.
March 2, 1910.

* DR. JURJUS AUN—Syria, Turkey. Below elbow.
I have received the artificial arm for Abraham Fadel; it fits and he is very much pleased with it. I congratulate you for your great help to mankind.
Jan. 28, 1908.

* MARTIN BAAL—Gardener, Dubuque Co., Ia. Ankle amputation.
I am so well pleased with the artificial leg you made for me so many years ago that I shall give you my order for another one just as soon as the Government will give it to me.   July 18, 1909.

* A. J. BABIN—Quebec, Canada. Below elbow.
I am wearing an artificial arm and hand you made for me. It has given me entire satisfaction and I do my work twice better than before.
Nov. 18, 1908.

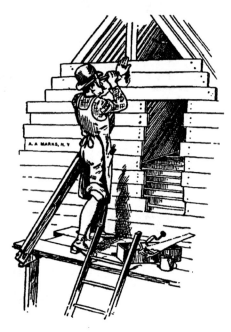

J. F. BALDRIDGE—Carpenter, Wyandotte Co., Kan. Above knee.
I still wear the leg you made me years ago. I am able to walk much better than before amputation, having been a cripple since the Civil War. I have built a house each year, four of which were two stories high, doing most of the work myself on every part of the building.
Oct. 9, 1909.

* FRANK E. BAIR—Laborer, Pettis Co., Mo. Above knee.
I received an artificial leg from you in 1906. After three or four
days practice, I got so that I could walk around without the aid
of even a cane. Walked down town at least a mile. A. A. Marks
artificial limbs are first-class and ahead of any I have ever seen.
Have compared notes with many others. Feb. 10 1909.

COL. JONATHAN BAKER—Elizabeth Co., Va. Below knee.
I am living at the National Soldiers' Home in Virginia. My leg
was amputated below the knee twenty years ago. Since that time
my experience with the Marks manufactured legs is most satisfactory. I can walk eight miles a day with ease and do laboring
work. Dec. 18, 1907.

* NORMAN COLE-BAKER—New Zealand. Above knee.
I have worn one of your legs since 1889, and have hardly had it
off in all that time for a single day, and the last four years I have
been living back in a new settlement where everything is very
rough. I have often been fourteen hours on horseback at a time
either stock riding or packing, and during the winter do my
share of bush felling. The rubber foot acts splendidly. Jan. 12, 1907.

* WM. H. BALL—Teamster, Osceola Co., Mich. Below knee.
I am well pleased with the artificial leg you made for me. I
have worn it every day since I got it. May 16, 1909.

* WM. L. BARNDEN—Laborer, Westmoreland Co., N. B. Below knee.
I received my artificial leg in good condition. It fits me in
every respect and I am very much pleased with it. A week after
I got it I was able to walk as good as any man I have ever seen
with an artificial leg. There are a number of men in this vicinity
with other makes but they all admire mine. You are at liberty
to use this testimonial if you desire. Feb. 19, 1910.

* PETER BARNES—Mill hand, Newcastle Co., Del. Wrist amput'n.
It affords me great pleasure to speak in the highest terms of your
artificial hand, which answers every purpose. I am proud to say
that I can do almost anything with it. March, 22, 1907.

* MISS C. G. BARR—Otago, New Zealand. Knee bearing.
I am very thankful to you for the leg you made me. It con-
tinues to be in perfect order and has been in use for nine years
and have never once had to have anything done to it. It is marvelous what you can do for creatures that have been maimed.
July 4, 1909.

* MISS EDIE BARRATT—Ravensthorpe, England. Below knee.
When Dr. Teale, of Leeds, advised me to apply to Mr. Barstow
for a Marks (American) Artificial Leg, I was very much worried
because it was so far away, but I am thankful I took his advice.
The artificial leg far surpassed anything I ever dreamt of. I
walk so naturally that nobody notices that I have an artificial
leg. I am a member of a tennis club and play nearly every evening
during the season, and I play as well as most people. Often I
walk six miles without a rest, and can do anything in house work
like other women. I like the stability of the rigid ankle, as the
steel mattress and rubber foot give all the spring required.
April 27, 1908.

* MISS ELFREDA BARRETT—Seamstress, Newfoundland. Above
knee.
I cannot praise your artificial legs too highly. I can do everything in the line of housework. I move about very quickly and
take long walks. I have surprised people with what I do since I
have been wearing your artificial leg with spring mattress rubber
foot. Oct. 12, 1909.

*JOSEPH H. BATY—Ship Caulker, Westchester Co., N. Y.

In 1865 I had the misfortune to lose my right foot and part of the left on the Harlem Railroad, and when it was healed I called on you to furnish me with a substitute for the lost member. I have been wearing one constantly for the last forty-four years,

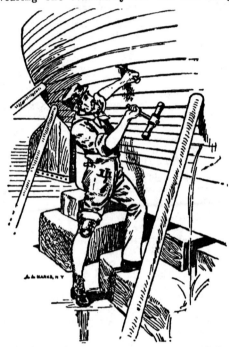

and can truthfully say that I am more than satisfied with it, not knowing what I could do without it, as my work is very heavy at times and keeps me either on my feet or moving about. My trade, as you know, is ship caulker.

* FLORIPE BARRIL—Chile, South America. Above elbow.

The artificial arm you made for me in 1897 is as good to-day as if I had only used it a year instead of ten years since I met with my misfortune, and no one can detect that it is an artificial arm.   Nov. 21, 1907.

* MANUEL BARRO—Weaver, Bristol Co., Mass. Below knee.

I take pleasure in telling you that the leg is a great success. I am highly satisfied. I walk naturally. I shall encourage everybody in need to get in touch with you.   Nov. 15, 1908.

*G. H. BARSTOW—Representative for A. A. Marks in Great Britain, Mexborough House, Ferrybridge, Yorkshire, Eng. Below knee.

I have worn artificial legs for the past 25 years, and have made a careful study of the subject. In my opinion there is no artificial leg made that approaches a Marks for durability, comfort, and natural appearance. I get about with comfort and ease, have visited all the principal towns and cities in Great Britain and Ireland, with frequent trips on the Continent. I have worn various types of artificial legs previous to the Marks, but none of them were made so that I could leave home for any length of time, on account of their liability to break down. My present leg has not cost me one pound for repairs during the years I have worn it. Am pleased at any time to give advice to anyone unfortunate enough to have lost a limb. I wore your leg for many years before I became your British representative.   April 6, 1909.

Persons in Great Britain in need of artificial legs or arms, feet or hands, are referred to Mr. Barstow, who will take measurements, attend to all details of ordering and apply them and give advice on all points.   A. A. MARKS.

* L. A. BASTIDAS—Colombia, S. A. Below knee.

My right leg was amputated a little below the knee in 1887. As soon as the stump was healed I was advised to order an artificial leg from you. I received one in 1889. The leg fitted correctly, and I handled it with extreme facility. Although it was only guaranteed for five years, it lasted me until the end of 1902, and was then in good condition. I, however, replaced it with another from your establishment, and in it I noted important improvements. My occupation is that of a merchant and farmer. I take trips on horseback over very rough roads of 36 to 60 leagues. I walk with ease and comfort.—Translated from Spanish.   Nov. 16, 1909.

* JUAN BECKER—Uruguay, S. A. Below knee.

I received the artificial leg with rubber foot which you made for me and I have been wearing it constantly ever since and can walk perfectly and do all kinds of work. I am compelled to be on foot, walking about from morning till night, and my stump never feels fatigued. I therefore tender you my most sincere thanks for sending me such a perfect apparatus.

DANIEL G. BECKWITH—Farmer, Chemung Co., N. Y. Above knee.

There is but one leg made that I would wear and that is the MARKS. I lost my leg in the Civil War and have worn artificial legs of your construction since 1876. The leg I am now wearing has been in use for fourteen years and has not cost me one cent for repair.   July 1, 1909.

* GILSON BELL—Reporter, Hawaii. Below knee.

The limb forwarded to me by express on the 22nd of August, 1907, has given me satisfaction. I must say I am exceedingly well pleased with it. The leg I got of you previously was put to active service for ten years.   Jan. 10, 1908.

* FRANK A. BENNER, M.D.—Montreal, Canada. Partial foot.

The artificial leg I purchased of you for a Chopart amputation has been put to the severest test. It has given me all the satisfaction possible.   Sept. 18, 1907.

* S. A. BENTON—Anson Co., N. C. Below knee.

The leg I got of you in 1896 is still in use and is in remarkable good condition.   May 25, 1908.

* V. BERNIER—Laborer, Quebec. Shoulder amputation.

I feel satisfied with my arm; everything goes all right. Have used it six years.   Oct. 20, 1909.

MONS. F. J. BERNIER—Montreal.—Below knee.

It affords me great pleasure to add my testimonial to the long list you already have. I am a professional prestidigitateur. When I lost my leg, I realized the importance of getting an artificial one that would imitate nature in shape and action as well as possible. I traveled a great deal and examined the works of most of the manufacturers, and finally concluded that I could get the best results by wearing one of your legs with rubber foot. I have worn the leg over five years. When I appear on the stage my steps

are elastic and never betray the fact that I wear an artificial leg.
After having worn your leg about six weeks, I invited the surgeon
who amputated my limb to witness my performance; he invited
in turn his medical class. When I was called upon to show my

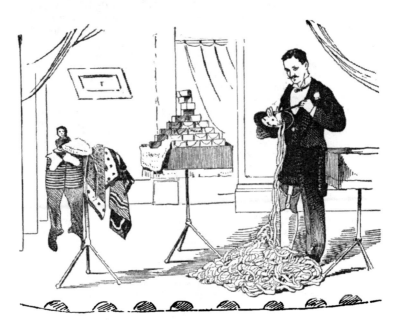

artificial limb, you should have seen the expression on those
students' faces—they could hardly believe it.

* MRS. JANE BIRD—Worcester Co., Mass. Below knee.

I take pleasure in recommending your artificial limbs. I had
the misfortune to have mine amputated half way between the knee
and ankle, the future looked dark until you furnished me with a
limb nineteen years ago. I wore it continually until you made
a new one five years ago. I have a large family and do all my
housework with ease.   Oct. 11, 1909.

* EDWARD T. BIRTLES—Saddler, New Zealand. Below knee.

I have had the artificial leg I received from you in use about
a year. I am well satisfied with it and find it far more satisfactory
than any I have previously used. It is very light and comfortable
to wear and so far is wearing well. The foot retains its shape
perfectly.

* HENRY J. BISHOP—Teacher, Newfoundland. Above knee.

My leg was amputated two inches above the knee in June,
1897. I obtained a substitute from you in July, 1898. I stand and
walk about for hours at a time without feeling the least fatigue.
I have on several occasions walked eight or ten miles in a day with
it. It scarcely ever occurs to strangers that I am wearing an
artificial limb. Hardly any expense for repairs of any kind have
been needed during the ten years I used it. Its successor made
by you a few years ago is at present in harness and giving the same
satisfaction as my old friend No. 1.   Oct. 30, 1909.

* DAVIS H. BISHOP—Miner, Indiana Co., Pa. Below knee.

I have used one of your limbs one year to-day. The rubber foot I am well pleased with, and I am satisfied with the fitting. My leg is off three inches below the knee. I am a coal-digger, and am working every day. I can walk one mile in twenty minutes. Your spring mattress rubber foot is the best out.

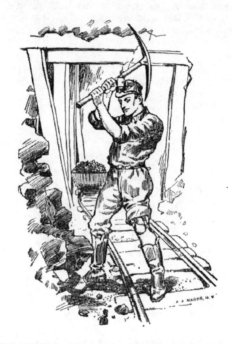

* ALBERT BLAKELY—Ravensthorpe, England. Below elbow.

Just a line to let you know that I am getting on splendidly with the Marks Arm. I am writing this letter with the rubber hand.
       July 8, 1908.

J. ANDREW BLAKER—Teacher, Monroe Co., W. Va. Shortened leg.

I have been wearing an appliance of your make for about seven years. My leg is six inches short and the ankle is very weak, but with the extension I can walk with ease. My occupation is that of a teacher, and as such, I must stand and walk a good deal. I can ride a wheel, skate, and in fact do anything that I could do with two natural limbs.   Oct. 13, 1909.

* O. F. BLEVINS—Registrar, Wilkes Co., N. C. Below knee.

I have been wearing one of your artificial legs for about six years and can say that it has given entire satisfaction. I live two miles from our court house and I walk to and from the court house every day. My occupation is registrar of deeds for Wilkes County, N. C. My leg is amputated just below the knee. I take great pleasure in recommending your make of limbs. Sept. 17 1908.

* H. L. BOLDRICK—Winnipeg, Manitoba, Canada.

I lost my right arm fifteen years ago and know the value of your artificial arms.   Aug. 24, 1907.

CLEOPHAS BOLDUC—Baggageman, Quebec. Below knee.

My occupation is train baggageman on the Canadian Pacific Ry. About fifteen years ago in an accident on the road my left leg was amputated. Shortly afterwards I purchased an artificial one from your firm and it was in constant use for ten years. My run on the road is 172 miles which occupies seven hours daily, and I have no difficulty in doing my work and have never lost any time and have had no soreness in my stump. The artificial leg recently purchased has the appearance of giving the same good service as the old one.

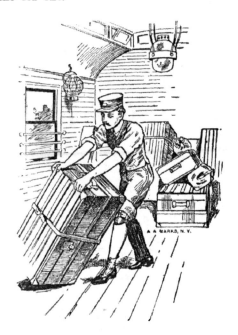

* H. E. BOLICH—Farmer, Medina Co., Ohio. Ankle amputation.

Your artificial legs are the best in the market. The one you made for me fits perfect.   Nov. 30, 1908.

* J. LALUNG BONNAIRE—Martinique, West Indies. Below knee.

My son thanks you very much for the artificial leg which he is now wearing for over a year. It enables him to go about and do things as other children of his age—he goes to school, runs, romps and plays. I extend to you my warmest thanks for the excellent artificial leg you sent me for my crippled boy.   Nov. 18, 1908.

* J. J. BOOTH—Miner, San Bernardino Co., Cal. Below knee.

The artificial leg recently made for me has been received, and I am wearing it with comfort. I have subjected it to the severest kinds of tests for over one month and it stands them all. In my work as miner I have to climb a 60 degree shaft, 110 feet deep, twice every day and have no difficulty in doing so. I have already made one walk of eight miles in an afternoon. You will remember that you made an artificial leg for me in 1883, when I was only eight years of age, and since then you have made two or three legs. All of these have given me the best of satisfaction.

Jan. 17, 1910.

JAMES G. BRADY—Lackawanna Co., Pa. Both arms amputated
below the elbows.

I am writing you a few lines to let you know how nicely I am
doing with the artificial arms you made for me. This letter is
written with the pen held in the right rubber hand. I have
worked for the Lackawanna Iron & Steel Co., I have been Alderman
of my own Ward, I have been registrar of voters, and in fact have
engaged in many occupations that have required a great deal of
writing, and I do it all with the artificial hands. Thanks to you.
The people in our Ward say your artificial hands are wonderful
when they see me writing.

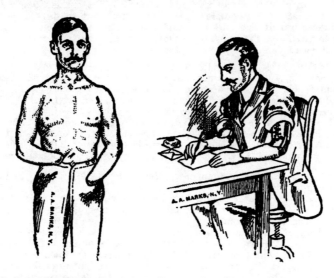

* C. C. BOSE M.D.—Bengal, India. Ankle amputation.
I am glad to inform you that I have great satisfaction in the
use of the foot you made. I agree with you that it is better not
to have a joint at the ankle.   May 19, 1908.

* GEO. B. BOWDEN—Merchant, Transvaal, Africa. Below knee.
I am feeling confident with your artificial leg. I wear it constantly at business. I like your limbs so well I shall send on
some of the old ones to be reconstructed.   April 5, 1909.

* L. BOUTINON—France. Below knee.
I have been wearing the artificial leg you made for me constantly, and it is with the greatest pleasure I can certify that I
never felt as comfortable before while I wore other patents. The
main objection I made against your system was the absence of
the ankle joint, but now I can say, this is the chief merit of your
limbs. I am now able to walk much longer distances than ever
before.

* FRED BRADLEY— So. Wales, England. Instep amputation.
A year ago you made an artificial foot for my instep amputation.
I have worn the leg in a most satisfactory way.   Jan. 10, 1908.

* ALLEN T. BOWIE—Court Clerk, Adams Co., Miss. Knee bearing.
In 1883 my leg was amputated below the knee. Have used several
makes of artificial limbs and now wear A. A. Marks knee-bearing
one with the most satisfaction.   Oct. 8, 1909.

* DR. CARL B. BOYD—Gila Co., Ariz.
The Indian, Andrew Pat, for whom you constructed an artificial leg from measurements which I took, is able to get around nicely.
March 17, 1909.

* DAVID BOYTER—Shoemaker, Algoma Co., Ont. Both below knee.
I am satisfied with the comfort I am getting from the artificial legs you made for me over a year ago. There is no trouble for me to get about and I have been told by persons that I can walk as well as anyone with their natural legs.   Nov. 9, 1908.

* HAROLD BRADY—Farmer, Cass Co., Mich. Above knee.
In January, 1903, I had the misfortune to lose my left leg, as I was troubled with necrosis of the bone and had to have my leg amputated about six and one-half inches from my body. I got your leg in July, 1903, and have worn it with great satisfaction. I can ride a bicycle and get around with ease.   Oct. 11, 1909.

* LUIS BRAVO—Lawyer, Portugal. Below knee.
The artificial leg I obtained from you two years ago, made from measurements which I sent you is of admirable construction. It is light and easy to walk with and I am satisfied with it. I take pleasure in recommending your work to others.
For eighteen years I was tied to an artificial leg made in Lisbon after some French system. It never was really useful. I feel that the artificial leg you made for me is very much better, lighter and more efficient.   Oct. 20, 1909.

A. BRIDGEMAN—Mill Inspector, New Haven Co., Conn. Below knee.
My leg is amputated below the knee, leaving a stump of about six inches. I have worn artificial legs for over thirty-five years. I have worn two different legs with ankle and toe movements, also three legs of your manufacture, and it gives me great pleasure to state that I have always found your style of leg capable and able to do all that I require of it. My vocation compels me to do considerable walking and am on my feet almost continuously twelve out of twenty-four hours. The last leg you furnished me is giving as good satisfaction as those of the past, and I can express myself no better than by saying that I know your make of leg to be the best substitute for nature in the world.   Oct. 8, 1909.

* BASIL S. BRIGGS—Solicitor, Wakefield, England. Above knee.
I found it awkward to walk on the limb Mr. Barstow ordered for me at the start, as I had fallen into peculiar habits acquired during my three years' experience with London legs. I had one day to hurry to catch a train. I did catch it, somewhat to my surprise and did not feel exhausted at all.
Walking is wonderfully easy with the Marks Rubber Foot Leg. I have no longer the severe headache which used invariably to follow any considerable amount of walking with the London hardwood foot leg, and I am looking forward to greatly improved health as a result of the change.
I do not think it too much to say that the new leg has given me a new lease of life, and it has certainly made the future much brighter.   June 10, 1909.

* C. ELLWOOD BRIGHT—Farmer, Caroline Co., Md. Above knee.
I have a leg of your make and I like it very much; have been using it ten years. I have a six-inch stump from the hip joint. The leg works all O.K. I am farming and trucking, and I do my own work. I have plowed new ground. I believe the Marks rubber foot cannot be beat.   Oct. 20, 1909.

* J. W. BROCK—Traveling Salesman, Boone Co., Ind. Below elbow.

The arm I bought of you about six months ago is a perfect fit in every way. It gives me a great amount of service, such as using a knife or fork or brush, holding my paper when writing, driving a horse, holding my newspaper while reading. When traveling I carry two valises, and the heaviest one in the

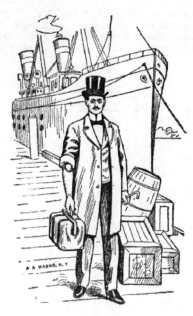

artificial hand. It is a great help to me in walking; it balances my whole body and helps my looks, and by its use my stump has become stronger.

WALTER C. BROOKS—Boston, Mass. Below knee.

The artificial leg you made for me is better than any other I have ever worn. I walk naturally and am highly pleased.

A. J. BROWN—Station Agent, Franklin Co., Vt. Both below knees.

There are quite a number of different makes of legs in and around this place, but none that have stood the wear and usage that yours has. I have worn a pair of your legs for twelve years constantly. Anyone knowing what a station agent's duties are will know to what work my artificial legs have been subjected. There are none like the Marks for me.   Oct. 11, 1909.

* GEO. BROWN—Painter, Nelson, New Zealand. Below knee.

The artificial leg I received from A. A. Marks is working all right. I never use any assistance in walking, as I walk just as well as I ever did. I am very well satisfied.   March 13, 1909.

* THOMAS P. BROWN—Farmer, Saskachewan, Canada. Below knee.

I am indeed well pleased with the artificial leg I bought of you in 1907. I have not lost an hour's work since I got used to it.

Before I received the leg my stump was in very bad shape. My physician told me that I would have to undergo another amputation. This I would not submit to, but got your artificial leg and commenced to wear it. Gradually my stump started to improve and in comparatively a short time it was entirely healed. No treatment or medication did as much good as the wearing of the leg. Your manner of fitting so as to avoid pressure on blood vessels caused an early healing.

If this recommendation is of any use to you, you may put it in your circulars and I will gladly answer any correspondence.
                                                                    March 1, 1910.

* J. H. BROWN—Steamboat Pilot, Ohio Co., Ky. Below knee.

I am pleased to say that I find great satisfaction in wearing your leg. I am a steamboat pilot, and sometimes stand on my feet for eighteen hours, walking a bridge or climbing a ladder just

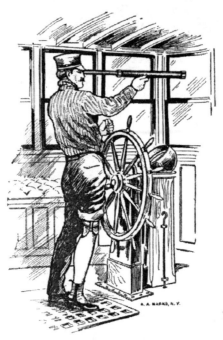

the same as I ever did. I would not be without one for ten times the cost of a leg, and I am ready and willing to give any information I can to anyone in need.

* W. R. BROWN—Farmer, Lawrence Co., Ark. Above knee.

I wish to thank you for the leg you made for me. I am so proud of it I cannot express my gratitude. I can go anywhere I want to with it.   Oct. 9, 1907.

* JEAN BAPTISTE BRUN—Merchant, France. Above knee.

It is with pleasure I acknowledge that your artificial leg is excellent. I am no longer a young man, am seventy years of age, and quite heavy. I am well pleased with the leg, and get around satisfactorily.—Translated from French.

SYLVESTER H. BUBB—Lycoming Co., Pa. Both below knees.

The artificial legs you made for me in 1893 (sixteen and one-half years ago) were of unquestionable material and durability. I have had a great amount of satisfaction in using them. The qualities of your leg are very important to anyone of limited means who wear artificial limbs.   Nov. 15, 1909.

* EDWIN BULPIN—Telegrapher, Ventura Co., Cal. Below knee.

I have worn your make of artificial limbs since 1880. The experience I had previously with limbs of other construction than yours makes me a fast advocate of your methods of constructing limbs.   May 28, 1908.

* MRS. CHAS. A. BURK, York Co., Pa. Below knee.

I cannot help but speak highly of your work as I am wearing an artificial limb made by you sixteen years. Other makes of limbs, a number of which I wore before I got yours, lasted on an average of less than five years.   Oct. 25, 1909.

* JOHN BURKLEY—Dancing Teacher, Hamilton Co., O. Below elbow.

I have worn your artificial arm now for five years, using it at the factory for three years. I worked around the factory like

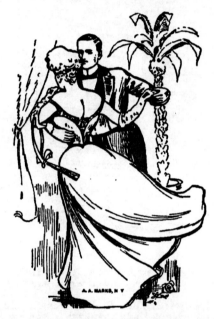

any ordinary man. Since I left the factory I have given my attention to teaching dancing. My artificial arm is so natural that the dancing people do not know which is the artificial one until I tell them—which I don't do very often.

DAVID BURROWS—Dutchess Co., N. Y. Above knee.

Nine years ago I had the misfortune to have my right leg cut off above the knee. Seven months after I got one of your artificial legs and from that time to this I have never had any trouble with it. It operates so well and fits me so perfectly that I almost forget that I am wearing an artificial leg.   March 5, 1910.

JAMES BURTON—Weaver, Oneida Co., N. Y. Below knee.

I think more of the Marks Leg than I did five years ago and then I thought it was the best in the world.

For the last two years I have been in Virginia, roughing it on the Blue Ridge Mountains. I was with a party and went with them every place they went. I have looked over many other makes of limbs, but the "Marks" for me every time. Oct. 9, 1909.

* JOHN BYRNE—New London Co., Conn. Below elbow.

We all know an artificial arm can't be expected to do the same amount of work as the natural one. When I first put your arm on it felt heavy, but now it feels fine, it balances my shoulders so that lots of people whom I have spoken to since I got your arm hardly know me, they say it looks so real, my friends many times ask me which is the real one. I am in the grocery business for myself. I can do up bundles with the aid of the rubber hand.

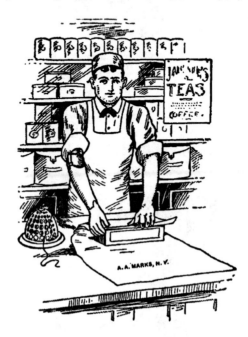

My arm has been amputated since July 7th, 1897, my stump healed in good shape, it feels much better when wearing the arm.

* EPIFANIO BUSTAMANTE—Barber, Mexico. Below knee.

I am very much pleased and thankful to you for the last leg you sent me. I always recommend you, stating that your make is the best in the world, and whenever I see persons in need of limbs I always advise them to apply to you. Words fail to state my thanks for the construction of this last leg. I was always suited with the first one, but I am very much better pleased with this. The reputation of your manufactory is known all over the world. If I were in good circumstances I would not hesitate to take the journey solely for the pleasure of knowing my benefactors, and to give them an embrace as a proof of my gratitude.—Translated from Spanish.   Oct. 8, 1909.

* JAMES BUTLER—Fisherman, Newfoundland. Elbow amputat'n.

With much pleasure I send these few lines to you to tell you that I am greatly pleased with the artificial arm you sent me. I am deriving good satisfaction from it. It is a great help in my daily labor, it has been very serviceable and I hope and believe it will be so as long as I live.   Oct. 16, 1909.

* JOHN BUTSON—Farmer, New Zealand. Above knee.

In September, 1899, I was so unfortunate as to lose my right leg above the knee, leaving about six inches of a stump. I was advised to get one of your patent artificial limbs with rubber foot. I have now used it for eighteen months. My occupation is a farmer. I can use it much better than I expected. I think anyone in need of a limb could not do better than use one of your make.

* A. H. CAMERON—Teacher, Alberta, Canada. Above elbow.

I am grateful to you for manufacturing and supplying me with an arm which I wear with comfort, pleasure, and satisfaction. The amputation is above the elbow. I would not be without it, it establishes an equilibrium of the body, it has developed my shoulder, by giving it exercise. For these reasons, coupled with the excellence of workmanship, naturalness of form, and superior quality of material in your limbs, I recommend them to all who may need such.

* D. CAMPBELL—Horse-dealer, Ransom Co., N. D. Above knee.

In regard to your leg, must say it has given me good satisfaction. I have only about an eight-inch stump. I am a farmer and horse-dealer, and find it necessary to be on my legs from twelve to sixteen hours a day. Have not run across anyone wearing an artificial limb that could be on it more hours a day than I. Oct. 15, 1909.

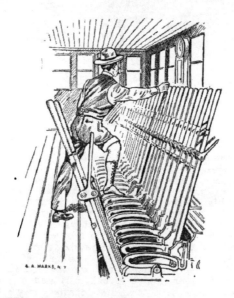

W. L. CANFIELD—Towerman, Orange Co., N. Y. Instep amputat'n.

The artificial foot you made for me February 1st, 1903, is giving good satisfaction, and I would wear no other make. Have been wearing artificial limbs for over fifteen years, and find your patent to be far the best for ease and comfort, and to work on. I can do my work as well as though I had my own foot. I work in a tower throwing twenty levers for twelve hours a day, and am on my feet all the time. My foot is amputated in the instep. Cannot recommend your patent too highly. I have worn other makes, but could get no comfort out of them, and one caused another amputation.   Oct. 27, 1909,

* CHAS. J. CAMPBELL—Farmer, Worcester Co., Mass. Below elbow.

I received my arm. It fits perfectly—just as well as the old one which you made for me over twelve years ago. I go in the woods and chop two cords of wood a day. Would like to have anybody that is in want of an arm call and see me and I will show him that I can do just what I say.   Oct. 28, 1907.

JOHNNY CAREY

On the evening of June 7, 1888, stole into the yards of the railroad depot at Utica, N. Y., with an armful of papers. It was his intention to board an express train which was about due. The train

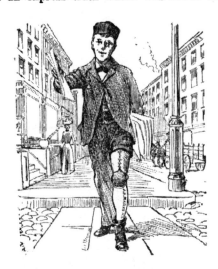

was late. Johnny sat upon the platform step and fell asleep. When the express came it ran over his leg and mangled it in a frightful manner. Johnny's first thought was that the yardmaster had got hold of him and that he had better get out of the way. In his efforts to get up he was brought to realize the fact that he had been run over. The depot men picked him up and took him to a neighboring hospital where the surgeons amputated the mangled leg. Johnny made a quick recovery, and soon got about on crutches. A few sympathizing friends contributed enough money to buy one of Marks' artificial legs. Johnny soon learned to walk, and resumed his newspaper traffic. Ever since then he has been going about so naturally and comfortably that nobody suspects that he is the same Johnny Carey who met with the frightful accident in 1888; he is able to run, walk, jump on and off cars just as well as other boys, and he manages to sell as many papers as any of his fellow-newsboys.

* C. G. CARD—Carpenter, Essex Co., Mass. Below knee.

My artificial leg is perfect. I am much pleased with it. I put the limb on two months after amputation, and have worn it ever since for six years. I am a carpenter by trade, and do the work of carpentry in all its branches. I would advise anyone in need of an artificial limb to select yours in preference to all other kinds. They are light, strong, and reliable.   Oct. 19, 1909.

* MRS. FRED. CARDINAL—St. Lawrence Co., N. Y. Below knees.

I have worn a pair of artificial legs since December 5, 1903. I have never used a cane or crutch since I got them. My husband runs a big farm. I milk eight cows nights and mornings. I am on my feet from six o'clock in the morning until eight and nine at night, and am not any more tired than I would be if I had natural legs. I do all my housework, have three children, a hired man and my husband, that makes six in the family. I do my own sewing on a sewing machine and can run the machine as well as any woman with her own feet. I do a good deal of work in the garden. I had my limbs taken off about fifteen years ago by the cars, one is seven and a half inches below the knee, and the other four and a half inches below the knee.

* A. A. CARNEAL—Baltimore, Md. Above knee.

I purchased an artificial leg from you eighteen months ago for my little daughter, aged five years. Dr. Rumsey conducted the transaction for me. I am glad to say the leg has given perfect satisfaction. She walks surprisingly well, never using a crutch or cane.   May 13, 1909.

* CELANIRA CARRASPO—Chile, South America. Below knee.

To-day I give you my most profound thanks for the artificial leg which you made. Can walk well with it.   Nov. 21, 1907.

* LAWRENCE CARRINGTON—Drug Clerk, Shelby Co., Tenn. Above knee.

The artificial leg Dr. Hayes ordered for me for which he took measurements and sent them to you has been in use for five years. I put it on the same day I received it, and have been wearing it continuously since and have had no trouble whatever. My stump is only eight inches long from the body.   Oct. 16, 1909.

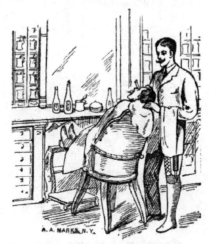

* L. A. CARROLL—Barber, Monroe Co., Miss.

I suppose you are aware of the fact that I have been wearing one of your artificial legs for over four years. I think myself the best one-legged man in Mississippi, from the simple fact that I am wearing one of your artificial limbs. I am a barber by trade; I stand at my chair fourteen to sixteen hours each day, and work hard. I have won two races on my bicycle; I can ride as fast as any man in town, and just a little faster. This is my first opportunity to tell you what I think of your limb.

* THOMAS CARROLL—Cook Co., Ill. Ankle amputation.

In regard to the artificial limb which I purchased of you, I wish to say that I cannot praise it too highly. As my work requires me to be on my feet all day, the leg gives me no trouble, but is easy and comfortable.

* JOHN E. CASE—Farmer, Mason Co., Ky. Below knee.

As the artificial leg I bought from you so many years ago has given me such good service, I would rather have your make than any other I know of. Your leg has never given me any trouble notwithstanding the hard work I have done on it.   Nov. 6, 1907.

* JACOB CASE—Mason Co., Ky. Below knee.

I bought an artificial leg from you for my boy in the year 1902. I sent you measurements and had it constructed by them, as soon as the leg was received I had it applied, and the young man walked on it, and has never been without it one day since. He went to work the Monday after he received it. Those that saw him before the leg was applied did not know him when he walked around on two legs. He can run, skate, and walk as well as any boy.
Dec. 6, 1907.

* GEORGE CASTLETON—New Zealand. Above knee.

I am now working for the same firm I worked for when I met with the accident, engineering and engine driving. I walk very well, indeed. I think the rubber foot is a great thing, as it does not jar, and the leg is so strong that it is not easily broken. I give it severe tests at my work.

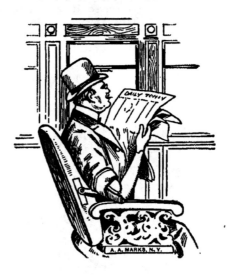

* DOLPH CHEEK—Salesman, Alamance Co., N. C. Below elbow.

It gives me great pleasure to say that the artificial hand made and fitted from measurements is perfect in every respect. People do not suspect me to be a one-armed man, as the "artificial hand" looks so natural. I can hold a book or paper in my rubber hand. With the hook and ring attachments I can do most any kind of work. People are surprised to see how well I get along. I can write with my hand, hold a knife to trim the finger nails on my left hand. I have now worn the arm for ten years. Oct. 12, 1909.

SERAFIN CAULA—Clerk, Cuba. Above knee.

It will soon be five years since I was at your establishment in search of relief. My deplorable condition was caused by an amputation in the upper part of the right thigh, leaving a stump only four inches in length. I had a leg made by another manufacturer, but was unable to walk on it, in spite of having practiced assiduously for more than six months. Completely disheartened I believed that I should never walk. I resolved, however, to go to your manufactory as a last resort. In ten days you furnished me with a limb so perfectly adjusted that I have used it constantly with ease and comfort. Although my occupation as a Government employee obliges me to sit most of the time, I take plenty of exercise and walk perfectly.—Translated from Spanish.　　　　April 30, 1909.

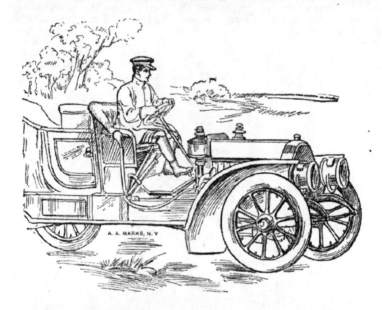

GEORGE L. CHILDS—Chauffeur, Essex Co., N. J.

I have been wearing one of your legs for years and have found it the best in the world. I have been chauffeur for nearly two years, and have been driving a large motor car with good results. I can recommend your limb to anyone in the world, and I will be glad to do so.

* F. A. CHEESBROUGH—Saginaw Co., Mich. Above knee.

I received my limb alright and am well pleased with it. It fits well. I am able to walk and go up and downstairs and can sit down nicely. I am greatly encouraged and will certainly speak well of the Marks limb. My stump is very short, only three inches from the body.　　　　March 11, 1910.

* A. C. CHENOWETH—Photographer, Lane Co., Ore. Above knee.

I have worn the artificial leg you made for me six years ago. I have done everything with it I would require of the natural leg and am perfectly satisfied.　　　　Aug. 15, 1909.

* W. R. CHEVES—Supt. Sawmill, Berrien Co., Ga. Partial hand.

I lost four fingers and the palm of my right hand in 1896, about a year afterwards I bought from you an artificial hand. This hand

has never given me any pain by reason of contact with the stump,
Besides being of considerable service, it hides the evidence of
maimedness. I would advise anyone in need of an artificial limb
to go to you.   Oct. 7, 1909.

* JOSE TEMISTOCLES CHIRINO—Soldier, Venezuela. Above knee.

The duty which my gratitude imposes upon me compels me to
make the following statement.

I was wounded in the leg in one of the battles of the last war
by a Mauser bullet. The projectile smashed the bone in such a
manner that my leg was hopelessly injured. Lack of means and
medical attention occasioned many complications, and after six
months of great suffering, I came to this city where they performed the operation, as the only means of quieting the pain.
Shortly afterwards my physician, Dr. Pedro Leon, A., advised me
to write to you for the purpose of procuring an artificial limb which
would .replace the one I lost. In truth you sent it, and it has
greatly exceeded my expectations. I have only used it a very
short time, and I walk without any trouble and am again engaged
in my usual occupation. It is not heavy, neither does it tire me,
nor pain my stump and does not inconvenience me in any way.—
Translated from Spanish.

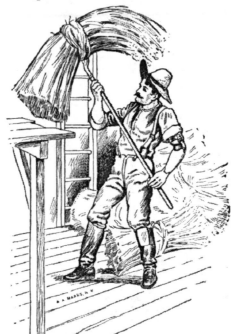

* HARRY T. CLARK—Farmer, Belmont Co. O. Below elbow.

In regard to the artificial hand I got of you, I received it the
first of April, 1902, and have worn it constantly, and find it of
great use in the different works that I have to do. I work on the
farm until the fall of the year, then I have a steam hay press
with which I travel around the country baling hay for the farmers.
The first year I received the hand I pitched wheat for three wagons.
To make a long story short, I get along with the hand nearly
as well as I did when I had both of my own hands.

* ED. CHIPMAN—Newfoundland. Above knee.

My leg was amputated in November, 1908 and I obtained an artificial one from you in the spring of 1909. I have been wearing it ever since and I am happy to say I have every satisfaction with it. I can walk around anywhere. Would not be without it for any money. You will please add my name to your long list of testimonial writers and I trust you will live long and continue your good work. March 18, 1910.

* ED. H. CLAIR—Millhand, Penobscot Co., Me. Below elbow.

I have one of your artificial hands and I assure you that I cannot get along without it. I am training for a musician and play the slide trombone. Nov. 7, 1908.

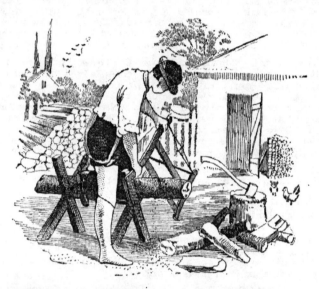

* J. D. CLUCK—Farmer, Muskogee Co., Okla. Above knee.

In July, 1884, I accidentally split my right knee-joint with an ax, which limb, three days later, was amputated four inches above knee-joint, leaving an eight-inch stump. In January, 1886, I purchased my artificial leg of you by sending measurements taken by one of my neighbors and myself. I am now compelled to say that, after about ten years of constant use, I feel confident I made no mistake in taking your patent. I often walk to church, over a mile, in company with others. My chief occupation is farming. I often saw wood all day, or I can pick a hundred pounds of cotton in a day, and that is about the amount I picked before my leg was amputated. Oct. 4, 1909.

* W. A. CLARK, M.D.—Bryan Co., Okla. Above knee.

The leg I bought of you for myself sixteen years ago was worn continually for twelve years. I then bought another of you which I am now wearing and have worn for five years and it is still good. I was formerly in the lumber business, had to handle lumber and ride horseback. A great many people making my acquaintance did not know that I used an artificial leg. I am now a practicing physician. Oct. 10, 1909.

J. HENRY CLARK, M.D.—Essex Co., N. J.

I cheerfully and fully indorse the Marks rubber hands and feet. I have several patients using them, and with perfect satisfaction.

REV. I. N. CLEMENTS—Madison Co., N. Y. Knee-bearing.

I have worn an artificial limb of your make for about twenty-three years. Previously I had worn one of a different manufacture, but I did not like it. Since wearing your make I have walked more easily, and with no noise.

* FRED CLOWES—School Teacher, Australia. Both below knees.

I have much pleasure in recommending your artificial limbs to all who are afflicted as I am. Your legs have made such an improvement in my appearance that strangers cannot tell that I have lost both of my natural ones until some person tells them. The legs felt a little awkward the first fortnight, during which time I was forced to use two sticks, but before long I could walk without the aid of them. This may be considered very good progress seeing that I never used my knee joints until I got your artificial legs.

FRANK COLE—Railroader, Ulster Co., New York. Below knee.

It is with pleasure I write this letter to you in regard to the artificial leg you furnished me. It is certainly a wonder how you people can make such an artificial limb and have it fit so perfectly and enable one to walk so well. It does not seem possible that an accident ever occurred to me. You can refer anybody who wishes to know something about artificial limbs to me. I never have a sore stump, the leg fits so perfectly. You deserve every medal you ever received from the Expositions. Sept. 27, 1909.

JAMES COLE—Farmer, Crawford Co., Pa. Below knee.

The leg you made for me is the best artificial leg that I ever wore, and I can't speak too much in praise of it. The rubber foot is a great improvement over any other make. I shall get your make of limbs hereafter. I lost my leg in the Civil War.
Oct. 14, 1909.

* CHAS. S. COLLINS—Telegraph Operator, St. Lawrence Co., N. Y. Above elbow.

Have worn one of your arms above elbow amputation for twenty-three years; am well pleased with it.   Feb. 14, 1908.

* ISAAC COLLINS—Fisherman, Newfoundland. Below knee.

I am thankful for my artificial leg. I am able to walk three miles over ice, and do my work the same as when I had both natural legs. I am able to take my gun as usual and go shooting. I am able to go in my boat as I did before. This artificial leg with rubber foot can't be excelled unless you get the blood circulating in it.

J. D. CONGER, M.D.—Wood Co., Tex.

You can refer anybody to me. The leg I got from you for Mr. Smith, after he had tried two other kinds, fitted him perfectly. He can dance in a quadrille and no one ever can detect that he wears an artificial leg.   March 3, 1908.

FRED W. COLSON—Elk Co., Pa. Knee joint amputation.

I am still wearing the leg you made for me in 1901, it has proved satisfactory, I do not wear any suspenders to keep it on, I have been firing and working on railroads and boilers since I got it. Aug. 2, 1912.

CHAS. COLBATH—Luzerne Co., Pa. Arm amputated below elbow.

The arm I obtained from you in 1895 is all that I could expect. It is a great help to me, although the arm was made sixteen years ago, it is still in good condition.   Aug. 30, 1911.

* JAMES W. COPELAND—Musician, New Brunswick. Below knee.
Your artificial limb has given the very best of satisfaction, and
it is impossible to tell that I wear one at all. I am a musician,
and leader of a band, and sometimes have to walk long distances,
as at parades, a person has to be pretty well supplied with limbs to
stand that, the routes of parades being about five or six miles, and

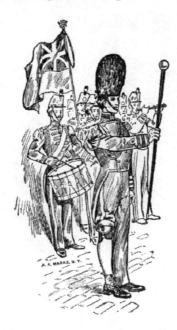

sometimes more. Well, the Marks leg just suits me, and my
artificial limb is just as good as the natural for that purpose.

* HAROLD CORNES—Salesman, Auckland, New Zealand. Above
knee.
It is now three years since I received the artificial leg which
you made for me from measurements and I have worn the same
every day since. There is not the slightest doubt as to the merits
of your work. Your make is undoubtedly the best in the world and
a great deal of it rests in the spring mattress rubber foot.
June 30, 1909.

JAMES A. CRANDALL—Clerk, Philadelphia Co., Pa. Below knee.
I have been wearing your patent artificial leg for some years
and in my opinion your leg is far superior to any other made,
because of its ease, elasticity, and stillness. These are obtained by
the use of the rubber foot. Also because of the durability. I have
no trouble in the least to get around. I can ride a bike, play ball,
in fact I go in for all out-of-door sports. I cheerfully recommend
your legs to all needing them. Oct. 8, 1909.

* MRS. LUCY CROMARTIE—Columbia Co., N. C. Below knee amputation.
I write you a few lines to let you know that the artificial leg that
I got from you in 1907 has given me much pleasure and comfort,
and I don't see how I could do without it. May 15, 1911.

W. T. COREY—Rutland Co., Vt. Above knee.

For about two years I suffered from diseased bone in my knee-joint. On the 13th of May, 1903, my surgeon found it necessary to amputate above the knee, leaving an eight-inch stump, and on the 15th of July following I came to your factory and purchased

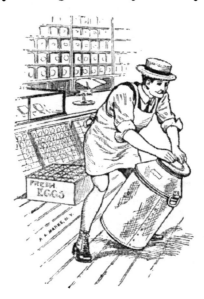

an artificial limb with rubber foot, which I am wearing now. I began work on the 27th of August, 1903, and since then have not missed wearing the leg a single day. I have heavy barrels, boxes, and milk cans to handle daily.

* J. COSTELLO—Tel. Operator West Australia. Ankle amputation.

I am very much satisfied with the artificial leg for ankle joint amputation you made for me a year ago.   Sept. 4, 1908.

* ESTEVAO COTTA—Miner, Brazil. Below knee.

It is a satisfaction for me to be able to state that I am wearing an artificial leg made in your accredited house. The leg is well constructed. I got used to it in a few days and am now able to walk naturally, and as the result of your success I have interested two other parties of this locality to order from you.   June 29, 1909.

* DANIEL COYLE—Welland Co., Ont. Below knee.

I have received the leg and I am greatly pleased with it. I like it better than the first you made for me, although that was satisfactory. I walk very naturally and in fact as well as a man does in possession of his natural legs. I wish you every success in your business.   Jan. 2, 1909.

* JOHN CRAWFORD—Miner, Athens Co., Ohio. Below knee.

This is the second artificial leg I have bought of you and can say that both have given the best of satisfaction. I have worn four artificial limbs. The first I got was worth about ten cents. The next was nearly as good. The third one was from you and it gave such good satisfaction that had it not been for a fire in which my leg and nearly myself were burned up, I dare say I should have been using it yet. My occupation, that of a miner, requires an artificial limb that is nearly indestructible.   March 22, 1909.

* W. L. CORGAN—General Store, Jackson Co., Mo. Both legs.

I have worn a pair of Marks legs for about eleven years. My left leg is off about five inches above the knee, and the right is off five and one-half inches below the knee. My legs were made from measurements taken one thousand miles from New York by myself, assisted by a friend. I have never seen New York or Marks' factory, and they have never seen me. In ten years I don't think I have spent ten dollars for repairs. I have seen lots

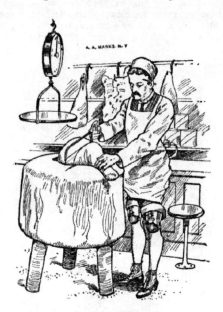

of wearers of other legs, and have yet to see any in my condition that could walk with me. I am in the general store business, and work in all the departments, not now and then, but every day in the year from early until late. My first pair of legs lasted a little over nine years. Am now wearing my second pair. Therefore, brothers, don't be discouraged if you get a leg or two cut off, for if you are the right kind of stuff, there is lots of fun here for you yet. I belong to the Improved Order of Red Men, am on the degree team and help do the work, and also an Odd Fellow.

* JAMES P. CROSBY—Worcester Co., Mass. Below knee.

Having worn an artificial leg procured from you I can say that after an experience of over thirty years with different makes, yours with the rubber foot is the most comfortable I have ever worn, and as it was fitted from measures, and without any alterations whatever, I thought it phenomenal. I have not expended a cent for repairs, and it is as good as the first day I put it on eleven years ago. I am on my feet most of the time.   Aug. 19, 1909.

* CHAS. R. CROW, M.D.—Stewart Co., Tenn.

The leg for Miss Lulu Vick came in good shape, fits well and is giving entire satisfaction. Has been without her limb about seven years, been on crutches all that time. On third day after receiving leg she walked to school. You cannot imagine how proud she is.   Nov. 12, 1907.

* ENRIQUE P. CORTEZ—Sonora, Mexico.   Right foot at ankle and
    left foot in instep.

I am pleased to inform you that I have used the artificial leg and
part of foot you made for me.   They enable me to mentally lay
aside the sad fact that I am a cripple.   I am a captain in the
Federal Army of the Mexican Republic.   My right foot and toes of
the left were frozen and became gangrened in 1893, when I was
caught in a severe snow storm in an expedition to the Sierra Madre.
You made a right leg for me in 1893 and with slight repairs in
1903 made the leg as good as new, promising at least to last ten
years longer.   For this I am very grateful to you.   My right leg was
amputated at the ankle joint.   The end sloughed and I have no flap

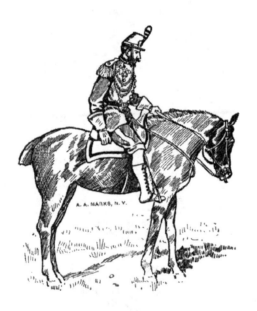

A. A. MARKS, N. Y.

or cushion on the end of the bone.   Therefore, I do not or cannot
bear any weight or pressure on the end, but the leg which you constructed applied weight and pressure some distance above the
end, and inconvenience is not felt in the least.   I walk perfectly
over rough ground, ride well on horseback, and in short, although
I have lost one foot and part of the other, I am enable to continue
in the service of my country.   I certainly feel very grateful to
you for the good work you have done in the way of repairing
me.—Translated from Spanish.

* JUAN COVARRUBIAS—Bank Clerk, Chile, So. Am.   Above knee.
    You have already made three artificial limbs for me and I am
about to order the fourth and await your reply before I order it.
The limbs you have made for me have lasted on an average of
ten years which I think is a great satisfaction and I take great
pleasure in remarking that to everybody I meet in Chili.   We
have French, German and Belgian manufacturers here but their
products are so inferior to yours that there can be no comparison.

JOHN CROWE—Truck Driver, Washington, D. C. Below knee.

Permit me to extend to you my congratulations on attaining such a high state of perfection in artificial limb making. I lost my left leg about three inches below the knee by reason of a gunshot wound in the Civil War. I resorted to the use of an artificial leg and though I wore several other makes, none pleased me till I had a trial of yours which far surpasses all others, and the rubber foot improvement I consider ideal, not only on account of its noiselessness but also for its elasticity and safety. I have worn several of your make all to my entire satisfaction and though I do some heavy work, in all cases they sustain the strain which many times is very severe. Weigh over 180 pounds, get about quite actively and attend to my daily duties with ease and comfort.

* REV. H. L. CRUMLEY—Fulton Co., Ga. In charge of an orphan asylum, in behalf of an inmate he wrote:

We have found the artificial limb you made for "Leona Miller," a small girl in our Orphans' Home, durable, serviceable, and with the occasional lengthening very satisfactory. She is now nearly grown and finds the leg indispensable.

* HENRY CURTAIN—Canvasser, New Zealand. Below knee.

Twelve years ago while loading wheat on my cart at Auckland wharf a full sack fell on my leg. After suffering some time it was discovered that gangrene had set in, and as a result my leg had to be amputated just below the knee. I obtained an artificial leg with patent rubber foot from you and after giving this four years' hard and satisfactory wear I decided to obtain another. My object in so doing was to make sure that I should not be left without, were your firm to retire from business. I have been wearing both legs alternately for the past twelve months without discomfort. My present occupation, which I have followed since my recovery, is that of a tea canvasser. This vocation necessitates a well fitting leg and one that can be relied on. I have already recommended your firm to unfortunate fellow sufferers, and will continue to do so in future.

* MRS. LUCY M. CUNDALL—England. Below knee.

I am pleased to say that the Marks Artificial Leg I got last year through Mr. Barstow is a splendid fit, and I am able to walk comfortably and like other people with it. Since I got it I have quite lost some very nasty stump corns, which gave me a lot of trouble before. I have almost given up taking a stick with me even when I go for a long walk, and I can really do just as well without one, only I got so used to one with my other leg that I sometimes feel I want something to carry.

Please use this letter, if you think it will be the means of making anybody else as happy and comfortable as I am.

March 5, 1909.

B. CYR—Tailor, New Brunswick. Hip joint amputation.

I must say that I am perfectly satisfied with my artificial leg. As you know, it is a hip joint amputation. I can walk in the house without a cane. Of course on the street I use one.

* HARMON DAILY—Farmer, Essex Co., N. Y. Both below knees.

In the fall of 1891 I lost both of my feet by slipping between two coal cars on the D. & H. R. R., my right leg was cut off one and a half inches below the knee and my left about four inches below the knee. After the stumps got healed, my doctor recommended to me A. A. Marks as the best limb manufacturer in the country. I purchased a pair of legs from him and put them on the same day. My occupation is that of clerk and farmer. I have to be on my feet sixteen hours out of every twenty-four. I can follow a plow or hoe and can do almost anything that I did before I lost my legs. I can climb a ladder no matter how tall and when I get to the top I feel as safe as I would be on the ground, for there is no ankle joint in the Marks leg to get out of order. The limbs I am now wearing I got over thirteen years ago and they will last me sometime yet. A year ago I purchased another pair of the Marks legs with some improvement over the old ones, made from my own measurements and are very satisfactory.

WM. T. DALBY, M.D.—Apache Co., Ariz.

I have had various opportunities of testing the merits of the Marks artificial limbs with rubber feet and hands and can cheerfully recommend them to be superior in every respect to any which have come under my observation.

REV. C. H. DALRYMPLE—Butler Co., Neb. Above knee.

After wearing a limb for eighteen years I know how to appreciate one. Your foot movement is so noiseless and easy that I'd not think of going back to my old style. At first thought I never could use it, but in a very little while I found I could. It has grown better and better right along and is now comfortable and works naturally.

* PAULINA DANERT—Nurse, Germany. Partial foot.

I always take pleasure when opportunity presents itself to recommend your firm, and have been the means of inducing quite a number of persons in Germany to patronize you, as I have had so much comfort and satisfaction in wearing the artificial leg you made for me in 1897.   Feb. 26, 1908.

* JACOB P. DARIO—Station Master, Mexico. Above knee.

I am very much pleased with the leg which you made for me four years ago.   Dec. 9, 1907.

* WM. R. A. DAVIDSON—Engineer, B. C., Canada. Above elbow.

The artificial arm you made for me fits fine. I am greatly pleased with it. I wear it constantly and have no trouble with it whatever. It helps me very much.   Aug. 6, 1909.

* MISS ALPHA A. DAVIS—Bergen Co., N. J. Below elbow.

The arm I purchased from you last May gives me such comfort and satisfaction that words are not capable of expressing my pleasure. The hand is natural in appearance, so much so that I am constantly deceiving people. If I ever have the opportunity to direct anyone, I will surely send them to you.   Oct. 25, 1909.

WILLIAM B. DAVIS, M.D.—Westchester Co., N. Y. Above knee.

I had the misfortune to lose my right leg when I was six years old. At the age of eight I tried my first artificial limb. My profession compels me to be on my feet the greater part of the time. I feel no fatigue whatever. I can say this, that having used one of Marks artificial limbs I feel I can never get along without one.

* HARRY S. DAY—New Zealand. Below knee.

I have used one of your artificial legs for the last nine years and a half and I have found it most satisfactory. I consider that the state of perfection that you have reached with artificial limbs is wonderful. I can work and do almost all the things I could do before my accident. I work principally in my butter factory, but also ride a great deal and use many farm implements. I have much pleasure in recommending your artificial limbs to anyone.

* PETER M. DEANS—Signalman, Ontario. Below elbow.

I am pleased to state that the artificial arm you sold me about fifteen months ago, which was fitted from measurements, I have worn it day and night without pain, ache or mark on the stump.

I have seen a number of other patents but I do not think they can be compared with your rubber hand in any respect. I am employed as signalman and can attend to my duties without the least trouble.

* Z. T. DANIEL, M.D.—Physician, Sheldon Co., Neb.

In September, 1899, I performed the operation of amputation of the left leg on Ceca Yammi (Peter Three Thighs), a Sioux Indian. He was suffering from necrosis of the tarsus, and a complete invalid, absolutely unable to stand. I did not succeed in getting his consent to operate until I told him about your excellent limbs, how he would be enabled to walk, run, ride, work, etc. In due

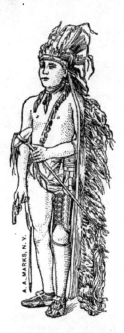

time the stump healed, and I sent you measurements for his leg. It came by express, and I immediately adjusted it. To my surprise it fitted him perfectly, and at this writing he is going about among the Indians with as much ease and comfort as could be desired. Inclosed is a photograph in war costume which he sends you with his compliments, with a hope that it will be interesting to his race, and an example of what the "White Medicine Man" can do for his people. Oct. 10, 1909.

A. C. DEDRICK, M.D.—Bristol Co., Mass.

I certainly advise the application of artificial legs to growing children as soon as their stumps are properly healed. John Kershaw, a young growing lad, has worn one of your legs for some time. He plays football, baseball, and indulges in all other sports.

* IGNACIO C. DE ALMEIDA—Sac Paulo, Brazil.

With pleasure I inform you that the artificial leg which I got from you over thirty years ago has given me the best possible results. It substitutes the leg which I lost in every respect. Your limbs are in comfort as well as strength, lightness and durability, simply perfect. June 27, 1909.

* DAVID DAY—Millard Co., Utah. Above knee.

Six years ago I put on one of your artificial limbs. I can truthfully say it has been a great help to me, and I am confident that
there are none better. I get along without any other assistance,
and am able to attend to an acre and one-half of garden. In fact,

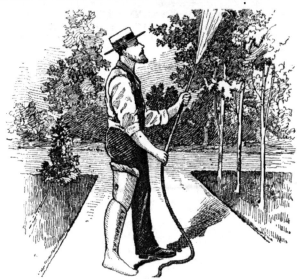

to make a long story short, everything is as you said it would be,
and I am satisfied.

MRS. J. W. DeREVERE—Wyoming Co., N. Y. Above knee.

I have worn your make of artificial leg for a little more than
nine years, and I cannot speak too highly of the rubber foot. Although my work is not laborious I walk a great deal. I would
recommend your make in preference to any other.

* BERNARD DETERS—Farmer, Clinton Co., Ill. Above knee.

I am wearing one of your artificial legs, and am getting along
fine. I wear it every day and do almost any kind of work on the
farm. Last winter I went to school and one morning was obliged
to walk through fourteen inches of snow.

PACIFICO DIAZ, M.D.—Argentine, S. A. Both above knees.

I am extremely pleased to salute you, and to enclose with these
lines the order made by my friend, Mr. Raul Cordeiro, for an artificial leg to replace the one he has lost. I have taken the measurements for him, and hope that your firm will make a leg for him as
perfect and as useful as those made for others whom I have sent
your firm in the same manner. Those I am wearing myself continue to give excellent service.

* JOHN A. DICKSON—Telegrapher, Assiniboia. Above elbow.

It is seven years since I lost my arm. I was railroading at
that time and got caught in a coupling, causing amputation above
the elbow, leaving a stump six inches long. I decided to get one
of your arms, and had my measurements taken. When I received
it I put it on. It proved to be a splendid fit. I advise anyone
who has lost an arm to purchase one of yours, and am sure that
he will never regret it. I am now working for the railway company as agent in one of their offices, and have not the least
trouble to do my work.

* C. C. DIDIER—Grocer, Cook Co., Ill. Below knee.

Fifteen years ago I lost my foot in an accident with a mower. I then purchased a limb, thinking that it was the best in the market, but it did not give satisfaction. I then heard of A. A. Marks limbs with rubber feet. I purchased one and in all the years that I have worn it, I must say that it is the best on earth. I have a grocery store, and do as much work in walking and lifting as anyone. I am on my feet all day, and I could not do it with any other limb than yours with rubber foot.

F. C. DIEFENDORF—Brakeman, Jefferson Co., N. Y. Below knee.

I have been going to write to you for some time to let you know that I am highly pleased with the artificial leg I got of you. I walk without a crutch or cane, wear the limb all day without the least bit of suffering or inconvenience and travel over all kinds of rough grounds. Oct. 8, 1907.

WILLIAM DIETZE—Machinist, New York City. Below knee.

I lost my leg below the knee from gunshot wound received in the late war. As soon as my stump healed the United States Govern-

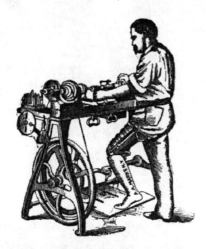

ment presented me with one of ———'s legs with an ankle joint. I wore it for a short time, and thought I liked it, but when I had one of your rubber feet applied to it I at once discovered that I had bettered my condition. I have worn your rubber foot now about twenty-eight years, am a machinist, and work at the lathe and forge. For ten years I worked on a foot lathe, doing the treading with my rubber foot.

* MRS. AGNES A. DILLON—St. Johns, N. B. Below knee.

My leg was amputated below the knee in 1882 and three years later I got one of your artificial legs. I do all my own housework, I run a sewing machine and do considerable walking with ease and comfort. Jan. 11, 1908.

C. J. DINEEN—Glass Cutter, Steuben Co., N. Y.—Below knee.

In July, 1902, you constructed an artificial leg for me, my leg having been amputated above the ankle joint in 1883 on account of railroad accident. I am pleased to state that your leg has proved serviceable and satisfactory. I use it constantly and do anything that I want to. I cannot help but speak well of your work as the leg has always given me good satisfaction.

* JAMES D———— Plasterer, Woodward Co., Okla. Below knee.

I have used artificial legs for over twenty-nine years, and I think I ought to be a good judge. I can walk easier with your leg and rubber foot attachment than with any other leg I have ever tried,

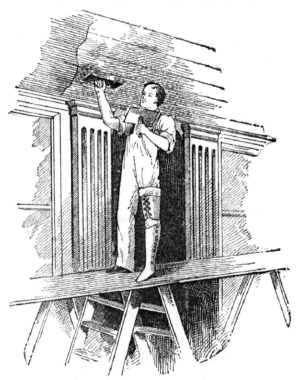

and I have tried four different kinds. I am a plasterer by trade, and work on the scaffold every day now. It fits me better than any leg I have ever tried, and it was made from measurements.

* J. H. DINGMAN—Oil Producer, Crawford Co., Pa. Below elbow.

For the past ten years I have worn two of A. A. Marks artificial hands, one for dress, the other for working. They both have given me the best of satisfaction. I am an oil producer, and do a great deal of work about my wells. Can do nearly as much as any of my men. My left hand was amputated about three inches below the elbow.   Oct. 10, 1909.

* W. A. DIXON—Tailor, New Zealand. Above knee.

In 1903 I received an artificial leg from you to replace the left one, which I lost by being caught in machinery in Victoria. I had previously used a Colonial made leg, which gave me much pain, and chafed the stump if I walked any distance, but since I have used your manufacture I have had ease and comfort, and I can walk long distances without any inconvenience. It has far surpassed my expectations. The leg was made by you from measurement, and could not be more perfect in any way. In my travels I have met many other makes, but have always heard yours spoken of as the best, and I only regret that I had not got you to make me one years previously.

* BETTY DOUGHTY—Vocalist, England. Below knee.

I have much pleasure in stating that I consider the artificial limbs with rubber feet, made by you, to be second to no other make on either side of the world. My left leg was amputated when I was four years old, from which time till about four years ago I had various limbs fitted as I grew. Since wearing your limb I am able to not only go about easily and naturally, but also to appear on the stage in opera, playing Erminie, the Countess in Olivette,

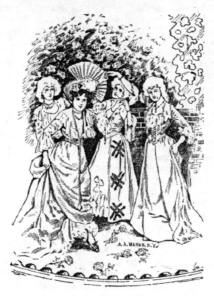

Dolores in Florodora, and other parts necessitating quick movement and short dress, which I wear without anyone being able to detect that I am at all lame. I shall be pleased to communicate with anyone who would like further information.

* E. C. DOULL—Clerk, Alameda Co., Cal. Instep amputation.

The artificial foot for instep amputation you made for me is more than satisfactory. I have worn it for seven years. I walk perfectly with it and a person could not tell that I had an artificial foot. I can skate on roller skates and dance as well as any of them with good feet.   Oct. 18, 1908.

* JOHN DOWNEY—Engineer, Gogebic Co., Mich. Ankle amputat'n.

I am using the third artificial foot received from you. It is perfectly satisfactory in every respect.   Oct. 15, 1909.

* GEORGE DOYLE—Barber, Lewis & Clark Co., Mont. Above knee.

I wish to state the limb I received of your firm is satisfactory in all respects. As you know I have but a ten-inch stump, but there are very few people who know I have a limb off. I have seen several people here wearing limbs, but I can walk better than any. I have recommended your limb to many.

JOHN F. DOZIER—Farmer, Norfolk Co., Va. Above knee.

I have just received the third artificial leg you have made for me and it is a perfect fit and is just right in every respect. Hope you success. The two previous legs you made for me lasted over twenty-eight years. I spend most of my time in fishing and hunting.   Nov. 25, 1909.

A. S. DRAPER—Commissioner Dep't of Education, Albany, N. Y.

Seven years ago I was so unfortunate as to lose my right leg at the knee, and since then you have made two artificial legs for me (the second is reserved in case of emergency that I might not be without a limb) which are giving very good satisfaction. The mechanism is ingenious,. and I am able to get about with considerable facility and very comfortably.

* D. DRUMMOND—Farmer, Ontario. Ankle joint amputation.

Artificial limb received and fitting satisfactory, although the measurements were taken ten years ago, this one fits as well as the old one. My leg was amputated at the ankle joint in 1879, used three wooden artificial limbs with ankle-joints, but when visiting Columbian Exposition, in 1893, was measured and procured one of yours, and have no hesitation in saying that it has lasted nearly as long as the other three and given better satisfaction. I am a farmer by occupation, and can perform all the work of a farm.

A. DUDDENHAUSEN—Real Estate, Jefferson Co., Wash. Below knee.

After wearing your artificial leg for six years I have pleasure to state that the expense incurred in maintaining it has been but a few cents and that for oil. The leg has given me good service every day all these years, without the least bit of trouble.

If you can do business making legs that last forever or as near so as you do your customers cannot complain.   Oct. 14, 1909.

M. A. DUMOND, M.D.—Tompkins Co., N. Y.

You can rest assured that I shall do all I can for your artificial limbs, as I consider them the best in the market.

W. DUNCAN, M.D.—Chatham Co., Ga.

I endorse Marks artificial limbs with pleasure. My associate, Dr. T. I. Charlton, who rendered me very valuable assistance in taking the measurements for the last two legs ordered from A. A. Marks, also endorses them. No complaint has been made to me by any person for whom I have procured the Marks artificial limbs, and they seem fully adapted for all that is required of them.

* H. A. DUNLAP—Carleton Co., Ont. Both partial feet amputat'ns.

I have received the two artificial feet you made for me and find them in good condition. They fit perfectly and I am well satisfied with them.   March 15, 1910.

* WM. H. DURHAM—Bookkeeper, Windsor Co., Vt. Below knee.

Somewhere about nine years ago I got, through Dr. Woodward, one of your artificial legs, and have been wearing it constantly ever since, and without one cent spent for repairs or alterations.
          Oct. 9, 1909.

* MISS C. DYSON—England. Above knee.

The Marks leg, obtained through Mr. Barstow, is admirable. I walk comfortably and follow my usual employment. This is wonderful, as it is only eight months since the amputation. My doctor considers the leg perfection. I will always recommend anyone in need of an artificial limb to you.   Jan. 29, 1909.

* WM. EAGLESON—Providence Co., R. I. Below knee.

I purchased an artificial leg of you eight years ago. It has given me perfect satisfaction. I honestly would not exchange this leg for any other.   June 11, 1908.

* JAMES EARL—Laborer, New Zealand. Above knee.

To say that the artificial leg you made for me pleases me would but inadequately express my gratitude. When your readers understand that my leg was amputated close to the hip, they must acknowledge the perfection of the artificial limb, which enables me to get about naturally.

W. E. EDGERLY—Brooklyn, N. Y. Both legs amputated.

In October, 1897, I met with a railroad accident that deprived me of both my limbs. My right leg was amputated a few inches below the knee and my left in the knee joint. In two months after the amputation I ordered of you a pair of artificial legs.

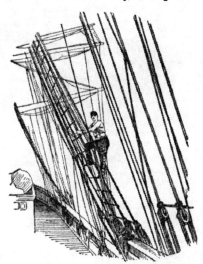

You fitted me neatly, and in a short time I was able to get about and mingle among my friends, go to my club, and engage in business. I am part owner of the bark "Obed Baxter," and as I am very fond of the sea, I occasionally take long cruises, and have but recently returned from a cruise covering two years, which carried me around the world. I am sending you a picture of myself at the wheel, a position I frequently occupy. I also send you

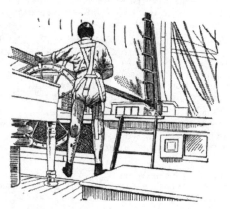

a picture of myself in the shrouds, taken off the coast of Japan, Although I do not make a practice of going aloft, I have done so on a number of occasions, and have found very little difficulty on account of my artificial legs. I also send you a photograph of myself on horseback while in the Hawaiian Islands, near the city of Honolulu,

The artificial limbs of your manufacture are marvels. They are light, simple in construction, and thoroughly efficient. I have not had occasion to send my limbs for repairs since they were

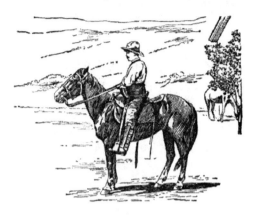

made, and from all appearances it will be a long time before any repairs will be required.

If this letter pleases you, you can publish it among your testimonials when occasion arises.

* AARON ECKER—Farmer, Frederick Co., Md.   Below elbow.

I would not take double the cost for the arm you made for me. I have loaded farm wagons, plowed and laid off corn ground. I even tie my shoes with the hook and my other hand. Nov. 1, 1909.

* ALLEN J. ECKLES—Grocer, Genesee Co., Mich.   Ankle amputat'n.

For years I had a diseased foot. It was finally amputated in 1907. In three months after I sent you my measurements and cast and had an artificial limb made. I received it and have worn it since with the best of results. I ride a bicycle and get about as I had hardly ever hoped to. I have never enjoyed such good health as I have since my foot was amputated.   Jan. 10, 1910.

WM. P. EDDY—Manufacturer, Brooklyn, N. Y.   Partial foot.

I have used your artificial foot for thirty-five years and ought to know something about it. I have worn many different kinds. There is no one who has solved the problem of applying an artificial leg to Chopart's amputation except yourself. I feel exceedingly grateful for the good work you have done for me for so many years.   Feb. 16, 1909.

* ADOLPH EDQUIST—Laborer, Sweden.   Ankle amputation.

I wish to express my entire satisfaction with the artificial leg for ankle amputation you made for me two and one-half years ago.
Nov. 16, 1909.

* LEE EDWARDS—Brass Worker, Vernon Co., Ill.   Above knee.

I thought I would write a few lines and let you know how I am getting along with my leg. It works fine, cannot find any fault with the fitting.   March 3, 1903.

* R. E. EDWARDS—Coal Miner, Campbell Co., Tenn.   Below elbow.

I received the artificial arm ordered for me by Dr. Beasley and I am pleased to state that it fits perfectly and I am delighted with it. I regret now that I did not get one earlier and I shall take great pleasure in speaking good words for you. Dec. 2, 1908.

* T. S. EDWARDS—Ireland. Above knee.

The leg you made from the measurements I sent you fits admirably, and leaves nothing to be desired. I feel myself a new man, and the limb has turned out to my expectations, nay, far beyond. The rubber foot is a great improvement over the old articulating ankle joint.

ADAM E. EHRLIN—Car Repairer, Erie Co., O. Below knee.

I wish to inform you that the artificial limb you made for me in 1903 has proved to be a fine piece of workmanship. I am well pleased with it. It exceeds my expectation. I can walk better, straighter, and have gotten rid of that squeak at last. After wearing an ordinary ankle joint limb for eighteen years, I can truthfully say yours is the best, and the fit is perfect. Oct. 29, 1907.

* REV. S. H. EISENBERG—Centre Co., Pa. Above elbow.

I have used an artificial arm made by you for twenty years. There was no difficulty in obtaining correct size from your system of measurements. My arm is off above elbow.   Oct. 23, 1909.

* EDWIN ELDRIDGE—Clerk, New Zealand. Below knee.

It is now four years since I received my artificial leg from you which has given every satisfaction and as regards wear, it is first-class.   Sept. 30, 1908.

* JAMES W. ELDRIDGE—Farmer, Hamilton Co., Tenn. Above knee.

I am always ready to speak a good word for your make of artificial leg. I am now wearing the second leg you made for me, and this has been in use for six years.

I lost my leg when I was a mere lad, but with the aid of the Marks leg I have been able to earn my living. I have done everything from punching cattle to keeping a set of books. Oct. 14, 1909.

* J. H. EMORY—Mill Operator, Spartanburg Co., S. C. Below knee.

There are two hundred hands working in the same room with me, all able-bodied men and I am the only one maimed, and I have won the prize this month for quantity and excellency of work. This makes me think that the Marks leg is really better in one sense than the natural one as I led the way in my room.

I would not exchange this leg for any that I have ever seen. I have been wearing it for nine years.   Jan. 29, 1908.

* MISS LIZZIE ENDERSBY—Yorkshire, England. Below knee.

Nothing would give me greater pleasure than to tell everyone who needs an artificial leg of Mr. Barstow, of Ferrybridge, who ordered the leg for me. My heart is full of gratitude and I cannot speak too highly of his ability and the care and interest he takes in his patients after the fitting of the artificial leg, so as to secure perfect ease and comfort. I have so much confidence in his ability that I would tell my friends. If I were 1,000 miles away and needed another leg, I would wish him to supply it. You see I have had the discomfort of an ill-fitting artificial leg and know the difference, and how to appreciate a good fitting leg in full.
April 20, 1908.

* ISAAC ESCALANTE—Mexico. Below knee.

I take pleasure in informing you that I am getting on very well with the artificial leg you made for me in 1909, so well do I walk that nobody knows that I wear an artificial leg except those who are intimately acquainted with me. I seldom use a cane, although I carry one with me. I am greatly admired on account of my dancing. I can go up and downstairs without help. I ride horseback as well as anyone.   March 2, 1910.

* ANTON H. EXNER—Farmer, Saskatchewan, Can. Above knee.

I am very much pleased and satisfied with the artificial leg you made for me four years ago. I am a farmer and do almost all my own work. During the last summer I worked for eight weeks on a thrashing machine without getting tired. I could not do without the leg. My stump is only five inches long from my body. I wish you all the success possible.   Nov. 20, 1909.

* THOS. EZELL—Salesman, Jasper Co., Ga. Below knee.

I have used your artificial foot and leg continuously for eleven years, and it gives perfect satisfaction. The fit by measurements was perfect. I had no repairs done, although I was in active

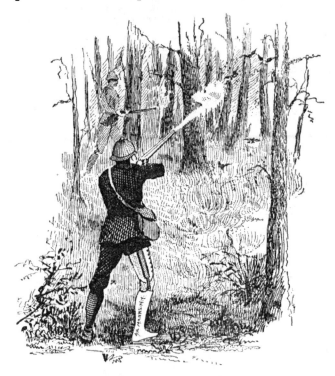

business, such as a salesman in retail dry goods and grocery store, and have walked the old field, bird-hunting, for one-half day at a time. The rubber foot seems as good to-day as when first bought.

* MRS. ELIZA A. FAIRFIELD—Missisquoi Co., Que. Below elbow.

I received an artificial hand from you about six years ago. My hand was taken off two and one-half inches above the wrist; unfortunately it was my right hand that I lost. Your hand was fitted from measurements at home. I am satisfied with it. I would not like to be without it.   Dec. 30, 1908.

* MRS. W. A. FAIRWEATHER—New Brunswick, Canada.

My son, Asa, had his leg amputated on account of typhoid fever. The amputation took place when the lad was five years old. He walked on a crutch for about one year, at the end of which time we procured from you an artificial leg. We put the leg on immediately, and a few weeks after he walked about without the aid of a cane or crutch. In September, 1902, he began his schooling, and has continued it to the present time. He walks, runs, swings, jumps, plays ball, and enjoys himself as well as other boys. We

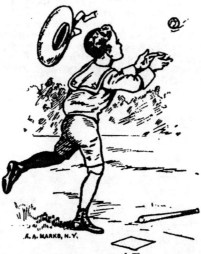

were advised by many not to procure an artificial leg, as it was not supposed that he could use one, but we were afraid that the child might receive some injury from using crutches, and therefore determined to get the leg. We do not regret having done so. The results attending the case make me feel it a duty to recommend every person who has a child, no matter how young he may be, who has lost a limb, to provide the child with an artificial one of your make as soon as possible.   **Oct. 21, 1909.**

J. W. FARILL, M.D.—Cherokee Co., Ala.

I have experienced the worth of the A. A. Marks artificial arm, and would say it is a perfect Godsend, and worth its weight in gold.

* J. C. FARLOW—Prison Guard, Randolph Co., N. C. Partial foot.

I have worn one of your limbs with aluminum socket for the past twelve years. Think they are the best for partial foot amputations. I can get around so well that many of my acquaintances do not know that I wear an artificial limb. Although my heel was allowed to drop backwards while healing, the aluminum socket holds it in place. I rode a bicycle seventy-five miles over rough country roads in one day. My occupation at present is prison guard on the public roads, which compels me to stand on my feet nearly all day. I have worked at house painting since I have been crippled, and I have no trouble in climbing ladders.   **Oct. 15, 1909.**

* JOSE M. FIDANQUE—Jamaica, B. W. I. Below knee.

I am delighted with the new system of limb and I feel certain that all those who have worn it must report similarly to you. It is a wonderful improvement on the other models and I have to thank you for the great comfort it has brought to me as I have never felt so at home in any other leg since my amputation five years ago. I have the highest admiration for your ingenuity in this your latest invention and I take pleasure in expressing my gratitude to your firm for the ease, comfort and relief of the new pattern.

                              June 2, 1910.

FRANK FAUST—Fireman, Schuylkill Co., Pa. Below knee.

I wish you to know how many days the leg you made for me worked in one year. You see that it exceeds more working days of ten hours each than there are working days in the year. If you know of anybody, with an artificial leg, who has turned out more days' work than I have firing a big coal engine, remembering that I have to walk two miles to work and two miles from work, making four miles every day in addition to my work, let me know who he is, that I may compare time with him. During the month of January I worked 407 hours; February, 292; March, 358; April, 325; May, 280; June, 316; July, 337; August, 376; September, 337; October, 391; November, 375; December, 337. . . . If you will add up

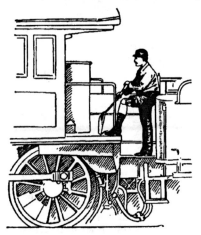

the number of hours, you will find that it amounts to 4,131, or more than 413 days for the year, and you know there are 313 working days in the year, so I have worked a year and one hundred days in the year 1899, wearing your artificial leg every hour of that time, and it has not cost me one cent for repairs. It is as good now as

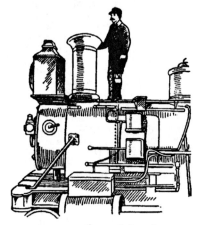

it ever was. The engine that I am firing is one of those big ones that haul coal from the mines to Pottsville, No. 148. I inclose a photograph of my engine, where you will see me at my post of duty. I get all over her with the same ease that I ever did. Sometimes I climb on top of the boiler while in motion. I can tell you more about what I am doing with my leg if you want it. The hard use I am giving your leg and the excellent wear it is giving prove it to be the best in the world. Jan. 10, 1909.

THOS. FERNEY—Signalman, Quebec. Below knee.

I take great pleasure in recommending your artificial limbs, especially for their durability. My leg is amputated six inches below the knee joint. I have worn one of your limbs since 1888.

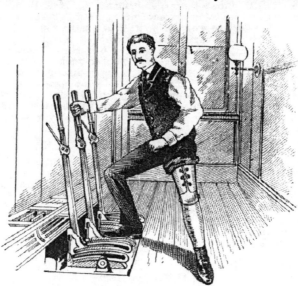

I am employed as signalman, and attend to my duties without the least trouble.

* R. S. FETTERS—R. R. Agent, Chicago, Ill. Below knee.

I purchased an artificial arm from you in 1894. It has given perfect satisfaction. Fourteen years of hard service is a good test. Feb. 8, 1908.

* EDWARD FLEMING—Torbay, Newfoundland, Fisherman. Both below the knees.

In 1888 you constructed a pair of artificial legs for my brother Peter, also a pair for myself. We both lost our legs from exposure and frost-bite, having been driven by wind off the banks of Newfoundland. It might surprise you to know that I am still wearing those legs, only think of it, twenty-one years. I do a great deal of work on them. I never thought that artificial legs could stand the test as these have. Oct. 24, 1909.

J. D. FLEMING, M.D.—Muskingum Co., Ohio.

Edward Buchanan has used an artificial hand made by you with entire satisfaction. He has nothing but praise for your mechanical aid. March 20, 1908.

* ANTONE FLINT—Railroad, Waco Co., Ore. Partial foot.

I received my leg which Dr. Dumble ordered for me and I must say it fits perfect. I can walk miles, in fact four days ago I walked four miles over a rough road. I expect to go back to train service in a short time. June 12, 1909.

H. J. FOLLWEILER—Bookkeeper, Lehigh Co., Pa. Below knee.

I purchased my artificial leg from you December, 1903, for an amputation below the knee. It is giving perfect satisfaction, in fact I could not do without it. It is light, strong, and well made.

I am a bookkeeper by profession, but spend much of my time on the farm, where I have to walk much.

There is very little wear and tear of your legs, and I heartily recommend them to all who are contemplating purchasing. The rubber foot and non-articulating joint give me a firm, natural, and graceful walk.   Oct. 15, 1909.

* JOS. M. FORD—Stone Cutter, Baltimore Co., Md. Below knee.

I take great pleasure in recommending your leg as the best I ever wore. Previous to wearing yours I had worn four ankle-joint legs made in different parts of the country. But I never had the comfort and feeling of security I have had since wearing your right ankle, spring mattress, sponge rubber foot. I am a stone cutter, and my business requires me to stand among broken stone much of the time; while wearing ankle-joint legs either ankle joints or toe joints were always getting out of order. All this has been done away with since wearing the rubber foot and stiff ankle. The leg I am now wearing is the second you have made me, and neither one has been any expense to me. Aside from comfort, I walk better, travel farther, and am in every way better satisfied than I ever was with any other make.

There are many that are now wearing ankle-joint legs, if they only knew the comfort of the stiff ankle and rubber foot, would discard their old legs and try the rubber foot. It took me a long time to make up my mind to try it, but I never regret that I did, and never expect to wear any other kind.   April 28, 1907.

* T. F. FORSTER—Blacksmith, Lake Co., Colo. Above knee.

I am one of those who have to resort to artificial legs. I am thankful to say that I am well pleased with your make. My

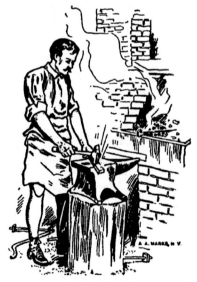

amputation is seven and a half inches from my body; applied leg March 28, 1903, and have worn it every day since. I do blacksmith work.

* W. H. FORREST—Builder, South Africa. Below knee.

I am much pleased with your artificial leg. It is a perfect fit. I have made up my mind never to wear an ankle joint foot again. I was eighteen months a member of the Town Guard, during the Boer War, and was never off duty, when the Guard was in active service, and to this day the commanding officer is not aware that I walk on an artificial leg. The doctor who has assisted me in measuring, is so pleased with your work that he is turning all his work your way.

THERON C. FOWLER—Farmer, New Haven Co., Conn. Wrist amp.

I have worn one of your artificial arms for the past seventeen years and could not do without it. I find it of great help in riding

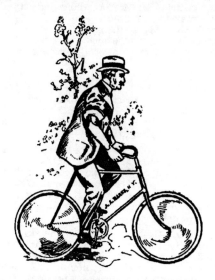

a bicycle, which I use in my business. I have ridden on an average over 3,000 miles per year for five years. I simply place the hand on the handle-bar the same as the natural one.   Oct. 13, 1909.

* FRED FOX—Farmer, Crawford Co., Ill. Below elbow.

I am a farmer and have worn one of Marks artificial arms for six years. It is a great help to me. I do most all kinds of work on the farm. I lost my hand in a corn shredder and the amputation was three inches above the wrist.   Oct. 16, 1909.

* JOHN FREY—Laborer, Brevard Co., Fla. Below knee.

Mr. Joseph Reddick, in our employ, is using one of your artificial legs and has been since last December. It is surprising to see how well he is getting along. We believe he is just as good in his work as before he lost his leg.   Oct. 4, 1907.

ROBT. L. FRYER—R. R. Engineer, Middlesex Co., Conn. Below knee.

Taking the limb in general which you made for me in April, 1905, I must admit it has been a success. Within a month of its receipt I was working at my trade as a machinist and handling some heavy machinery. I have only been required to leave the leg off one day and that from no cause of the leg. No one knows of my crippled condition except those that are intimately acquainted with me.   March 14 1910.

CHARLES A. FULLER—Lawyer, Chenango Co., N. Y. Above knee.

My leg was amputated within eight inches of the body at Gettysburg. For many years I wore a leg with an ankle joint which gave me no little vexation. Whenever the spring that kept it in place weakened, the foot would drop and the leg trip, and I would lose my natural sweetness of temper. I have worn the Marks leg for the past nineten years and have had no such trouble with the rubber foot. I am now wearing my second leg, and it looks as if it might do good work for the next dozen years.   Oct. 12, 1909.

* CHAS. A. FUREY—Essex Co., Mass. Below knee.

The artificial leg you made for me suits me in every respect. Your work is the best and I cheerfully recommend everyone to you. You made an artificial leg for a young lady in this place some time ago. She married and now resides in Newfoundland. She is getting along fine, has no trouble and praises your work ·very highly to everybody. In fact everybody I have met wearing your artificial legs has the same story of contentment to repeat.
                                                      Sept. 8, 1907.

I. C. GABLE, M.D.—York Co., Pa.

I have recommended the A. A. Marks very valuable patent artificial limbs to a number of my patients, who are wearing them with perfect satisfaction, and I have no hesitancy in saying in my judgment they fulfill their purpose better than any others that have come under my observation.   Oct. 13, 1909.

* MISS MARY A. GALLAGHER—Tuscaloosa Co., Ala. Below knee.

I am wearing the second artificial supplied by you. I get along without any assistance; lost limb six or seven inches below the knee in 1886, bought one of your manufacture in 1887, used constantly for six years, and at the present I am wearing the second, bought in 1903. I would never be without one. It is the talk of all my friends how active I am with it.   Oct. 16, 1909.

* HECTOR GARCIA—Cashier, Peru. Below knee.

I take pleasure in informing you that the leg constructed by you has turned out very well, in fact so well it can hardly be distinguished from the natural member. I take all kinds of exercise, dance with great perfection and can hardly be beat in a running match.   May 17, 1909.

REV. RUFUS P. GARDNER—Merrimack Co., N. H.

It gives great pleasure to assure you that the apparatus made by you in 1876 has answered my expectations, enabling me to walk in a natural manner and leave the crutch.

My parish work calls for a great deal of walking, which I can do with great ease. Hoping many others may find, as I have, the value of your great work.   Oct. 15, 1909.

* FREDERICK GARLAND—Trinity Bay, Newfoundland. Below knee amputation.

I have been wearing one of your artificial legs for the last three years. I am convinced that there is no better leg made. I have been in company of people who never suspected that I was wearing an artificial leg. I attend to my work every day which is fishing in the summer and working in the lumber woods in winter.   March 10, 1910.

* C. H. GASQUE—Telegraph Operator, Hampton Co., S. C. Above knee.

In 1891 I bought a leg from you and wore it every day for ten years. Then I purchased another and liked it even better than the first. The last one I got has been in daily use for more than seven years. I am greatly pleased with your make of limb. Oct. 19, 1909.

R. A. GAULT—Locomotive Engineer, Otsego Co., N. Y. Below knee.

September 28, 1897, my right leg was amputated at the middle third, below the knee. I am a locomotive engineer, and in just six months from that day I was back on the road at work. I have worn your artificial limb for over ten years, and have never had a spot as large as the head of a pin on my limb caused by chafing. I have stood on the engine beside the boiler with the heat at one hundred and ten degrees, and it did not affect the leg at all. I have tested it in every way. I can climb around the engine as well as I could with my own limb, can run and jump, and my weight is two hundred and twenty-five pounds.   Oct. 16, 1909.

HENRY P. GEIB, M.D.—Fairfield Co., Conn.

The persons to whom Marks has furnished artificial appliances for amputations of the feet (one Smyes' and other Pirogoff's operations) express themselves as being perfectly satisfied.

The appliances are light, easily applied, and do not produce excoriation or tenderness at the end of the stump.

I consider that Marks' appliances fulfill all the indications called for in providing artificial support after amputations.

* JAMES T. GIBSON, M.D.—Highland Co., Ohio. Below elbow.

On the fifteenth day of October I took the measurements for B. F. Puckett, Jr., for an artificial hand and part forearm. He has submitted it to-day for my inspection. The fit is perfect. Could not have been better had you had him at your place of business to fit personally.

G. H. GLIDDEN, M.D.—Herkimer Co., N. Y.

For many years I have considered Marks artificial limbs the very best in the world. I cannot recommend them too highly. In every case they have proven better than expected. Oct. 15, 1909.

THEODORE GOBLE—Signalman, Suffolk Co., Mass. Below knee.

I have worn one of your artificial legs with rubber foot for over eight years, and it has given complete satisfaction. I would not exchange it for any other make. I have worn it constantly since I got it. My work is in a railroad signal tower throwing levers. I work twelve hours a day.   Oct. 18, 1909.

* GARLAND GOHAGAN—Jefferson Co., Ky. Below elbow.

I am very much pleased with my artificial arm. I am doing considerable work with it, in fact could not get along without it.
     April 29, 1908.

IRVING GOLDFARB—Stenographer, New York City. Below knee.

The artificial leg you made for me in 1898 is still in good service. It has proved to be a remarkably strong leg. In July 1905, while boating on the Long Island Sound, one of my party fell overboard; I jumped in after him; he was rescued by another person. I became exhausted and it was necessary to drag me out also. Some time later while camping on the Palisades, I fell off a cliff, the leg striking against a rock. A few months after that, I was run over by a delivery wagon, the wheel passing over the artificial leg. It is now two years since these accidents occurred and I am still wearing the leg. I am a young man, love to engage in athletic sports and find the leg ready for anything.   Nov. 8, 1907.

* CARLOS GOMEZ—Havana, Cuba. Knee bearing.

I received a package containing the artificial leg I ordered from you, for which I sent measurements taken at my home. I was agreeably surprised to find that the leg fitted perfectly, and can suggest no alterations that could possibly improve it. The rubber foot is perfection, I doubt very much that there can be anything better.—Translated from Spanish.   June 6, 1908.

* RAFAEL GONZALEZ—Manufacturer, Silas, Mexico. Below knee.
I thank you for the artificial leg. It fits perfectly. I extend to you my gratitude.   Jan. 22, 1909.

* R. S. GONZALEZ—Army Officer, Lara, Venezuela. Below knee.
I am still using the artificial leg you made for me ten years ago. It fits perfectly and I have met with no inconvenience whatever. I have used artificial legs nine years constructed by many different manufacturers, and I can assure you that your make is the best of all.   May 25, 1909.

* JAMES W. GOOCH—Shelby Co., Tenn. Instep amputation.
In my opinion there is but one artificial leg in the market and that is Marks'. I have been wearing one for Chopart's amputation for over five years. I cannot see why I should not wear it for the next ten. So far as walking and getting about is concerned, I can see no diffrence between my artificial foot and my natural one. I have seen a great many makes of artificial limbs, but they do not attract me. I clearly understand the requirements of a limb and I know that Marks is the only person who has anything that will meet that requirement.   March 22, 1909.

DR. JOEL M. GOOCH—Bell Co., Texas.
In every case in which you have furnished artificial limbs under my orders, the results have been perfectly satisfactory. Oct. 18, 1909.

* JOHN GORDINE—Laborer, New Zealand. Above elbow.
I have been wearing your artificial arm now close on eight years and it has given me much satisfaction in every way. I always recommend anyone who has had the misfortune to lose a limb to you.   Dec. 5, 1909.

THOMAS GORMAN—Clerk, Westchester Co., N. Y. Both legs.
I am pleased to tell you that my artificial legs are perfect in every respect, and a great success. I walk about, go on cars, work in the store all day, wait on customers, tie up packages, and all the work required of an able-bodied man. I cheerfully recommend your rubber foot. I do not in any way consider myself incapacitated on account of the loss of my legs.   Oct. 16, 1909.

CHARLES W. GOULD—Lock Tender, Albany Co., N. Y. Below knee.
I write you these few lines to let you know that I am very much pleased with the leg. My occupation is lock-tending on the Erie Canal, and I get around just as good as anyone that has two good legs. I have been wearing your leg about twelve years.
                                                    Oct. 14, 1909.

MRS. JOHN F. GRAHAM—Worcester Co., Mass. Below knee.
I find pleasure in sending you this testimonial. My foot is amputated four inches above the ankle. I went on crutches for two years, then I purchased one of your artificial limbs. I do my own housework, and walk from five to six miles every Sunday through the country. I danced at a lawn party given by my friends six months after receiving your limb seven years ago. Oct. 19, 1909.

* JOHN N. GRAHAM—Mechanic, Grand Traverse Co., Mich. Above
    knee.
The artificial leg I got of you in 1903 has given satisfaction. I have never gone a day without the leg since I got it, and am doing work around a sawmill all the time.   Oct. 16, 1909.

* THOMAS GRANT—Telephone Operator, New Zealand. Wrist.
I can manage all the work in the post and telephone office. I manage very well in tying up the mail bags, I hold the receiver of the telephone in the rubber hand and take off messages with the other.   Jan. 19, 1910.

* PRIS. A. GRANT—Wauganui, New Zealand. Above knee.

The artificial leg for Miss Janie Scott came to hand some time ago. Miss Scott is managing with the limb very nicely. She uses a treadle sewing machine, walks to church, and in fact does every-

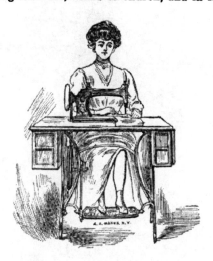

thing and goes everywhere the same as persons with natural legs. April 12, 1909.

* MISS EMMA C. GRAY—Student, Richmond Co., Ga: Above knee.

It is with pleasure that I testify to the good that the artificial leg has done me. It has been a Godsend. I have been wearing it since 1904, at which time I was only thirteen years old. I advise all who have had the misfortune of losing a leg to purchase one from you without delay. I am sure they will say the same as I do, that the Marks' artificial limbs are Godsends. Nov. 25, 1909.

PATRICK GREGORY—Priest, Montreal, Can. Above elbow.

The artificial arm I purchased from you five years ago has proven satisfactory. Sept. 13, 1907.

* C. E. GRAVES—Clinton Co., Ind. Partial hand.

I am employed as a life insurance solicitor and collector. The four fingers of my right hand were amputated, leaving the thumb with very little support. However, I find that I am able to handle books and papers to a much greater extent by the aid of the artificial hand than I could without it. It restores the hand to almost its natural appearance, which is a great advantage in dealing with the public.

DAVID GREEN—Driver, Suffolk Co., N. Y. Knee bearing.

My left leg was amputated just below the knee on September 14, 1903, and on March 25, 1904, I was fitted by you personally with an artificial leg which has given me splendid satisfaction. Oct. 23, 1909.

D. M. GREEN—Mechanic, Oneida Co., N. Y. Knee bearing.

I lost my leg in the Civil War and have worn artificial limbs since then. In 1871 the Government furnished me with a leg made by you. Since that time I have had renewals on the Goverment allowance four times. I have the highest praise for your work. Have always had ease and comfort, but I am now getting along in life, having reached my seventy-first birthday. Oct. 4, 1909.

* WM. W. GRANT—Engineer, Latimer Co., Okla. Above knee.

I'm still wearing your make of legs and won't wear anybody's else till you or I die. I have tried a cheap leg, I got it from Fort Smith; there wasn't a wagon in this town that could carry it.

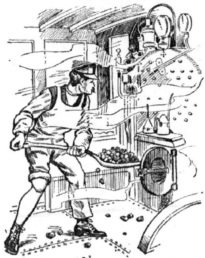

I have for years tended to the fire-pot of a boiler. I run a hoisting engine in a coal mine and do all kinds of hard work.   Oct. 18, 1909.

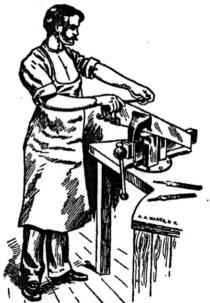

* J. D. GRAY—Saw Filer, Hillsboro Co., N. H.   Below elbow.

I have worn a hand of your make for more than ten years, and could not get along without it. I am a saw filer, and work every day. My hand is amputated about half way between the elbow and wrist.

* FRANK O. GREEN—Antrim Co., Mich. Instep amputation.
I have received your aluminum socket rubber-foot leg for partial foot amputation. I am pleased to say that the change from the old one is greatly to my advantage. The socket of the leg holds my foot in the right position at all times.   Aug. 27, 1908.

* MISS E. M. GREGORY—Wellington, New Zealand. Below knee.
I have worn an artificial leg supplied by you for the last five years, and found it a great comfort. I can do ordinary housework, walk distances and do not know what I should do without it. I recommend your limbs.   Nov. 10, 1908.

* CAPT. T. M. GRIFFIN—Farmer, Hinds Co., Miss. Below knee.
About five years ago I had my left leg amputated four inches above the ankle. Four months after I applied for an artificial leg with rubber foot of your construction. I have been wearing the leg ever since. I would not be without it for any consideration. I am a farmer, and can do nearly everything a man of my age (84) ought to be expected to do.   Oct. 16, 1909.

WILLIAM GRIFFIN—Washington, D. C. Above knee.
With reference to the artificial leg you furnished me seven years ago, I take great pleasure in saying that of all the limbs that I have worn during the last forty-five years, it is the best and most satisfactory in every way. Every limb I have gotten from you is better than the previous one. This shows that you are progressing. The former leg made by you was worn uninterruptedly for twenty-two years. As you know I am employed by the Government and my home is about a half mile from my place of occupation. But I walk to and from the latter all the year round with entire ease and comfort. I have repeatedly walked out in the suburbs of the city for miles, sometimes up and down hills, without any difficulty.   Oct. 14, 1909.

* J. C. GRIMIT—Farmer, Cullman Co., Ala. Knee bearing.
I have had no occasion to complain about your leg. It is now eight years since it was made. I would not give my artificial leg for a cart load of crutches or peg legs either. There is nothing on the face of the earth more valuble than A. A. Marks' artificial legs. My life was a misery before I got one.   Oct. 19, 1909.

MISS DESSIE GROSS—Blackford Co., Ind. Elbow amputation.
I am well pleased with my arm which you made for me three years ago, and the service it has given me has been very great.
               Aug. 24, 1908.

* J. L. GUTHRIDGE—Storekeeper, Franklin Co., Ohio. Below knee.
I have worn the artificial leg you made for me every day since I got it. While it is of entirely different construction from that which I have been wearing I am well pleased with it and am satisfied and enjoying the best of success.   Dec. 6, 1908.

JAMES E. HADLEY—Carpenter, Norfolk Co., Mass. Below knee.
My leg was amputated April 16, 1902. I returned to my work just eleven weeks after the amputation. I walk without a crutch or cane. I am employed by the N. Y., N. H., H. R. R., as a wood machinist. I can get about as well as any man in the shop, and do as much work as ever I could. I would recommend your leg to anyone needing the same.   Oct. 13, 1909.

* ALEX. HAGAMAN—Blacksmith, Watauga Co., N. C. Below knee.
On the 11th day of August, 1879, I had the misfortune to lose my left leg below the knee. I went on crutches eighteen months, then I made, with my own hands, a wooden leg, and wore it about

twenty-two years with much pain and difficulty. In 1890 I procured one of Marks' manufacture, on which I have been walking with comfort. I would not do without it for twice what it cost. My occupation is blacksmithing. I also do some farm labor and get about with ease.   Oct. 30, 1909.

JOSHUA HALL—Laborer, Monmouth Co., N. J. Railroad. Below knee.

I have never been able to find any fault with the artificial leg with rubber foot you made for me six years ago. Through the influence of some agent who happened to be around in our vicinity, I placed an order with a Western concern who made a speciality of the slip socket. It is to my regret that I did this, as I have not had a day's comfort with it. As soon as I can afford I will get another one from you and throw away this miserable imposition.   Oct. 13, 1909.

* W. E. HALL—Grocery, Shelby Co., Tenn. Below knee.

I am well pleased with my new leg, it fits all O. K. I have worn your make of artificial limbs since 1892, and in all my rounds have never seen anybody get along as well as I do. I can do anything, go as far as anybody. Am in the retail grocery business. I stand and walk all day.   July 26, 1906.

* A. A. HAMLING—Fireman, Calcasieu Co., La. Below elbow.

I am more than satisfied with the artificial arm you recently made for me. It is much better than the one that I bought from another firm which cost me more.   March 7, 1908.

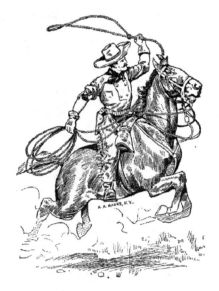

* L. H. HARKEY—Stock Farmer, Atoka Co., Okla. Wrist amput'n.

About four years ago I lost my right hand at the wrist joint. In about three months I ordered an artificial hand from you, which I have been wearing ever since. It has given me the best of satisfaction. Has never hurt me. I could not get along without it. I do most of my writing with it. I am a stock farmer. I hold my coil in my artificial hand and throw the loop of my rope with my natural one. Could not praise my artificial hand too highly. This letter was written with it.

JOHN HARMON—Coremaker, Cayuga Co., N. Y. Above knee.

I got my second Marks leg April, 1903. I had been wearing one for seven years. Never had any trouble with it. My limb is off above the knee. When I received my second leg, I laid the old one aside, put on the new one, and have never taken it off except at night. I have looked up all other manufacturers of artificial limbs, and I can safely say that the Marks leg is the only one that can be worn with solid comfort. It is hard to tell a Marks leg, going along the street, from the natural.   Oct. 13, 1909.

* L. V. HARMON—Farmer, Greene Co., Tenn. Below knee.

I have been using one of your make of artificial legs since August, 1904. I am a farmer and am now pulling corn and can pull as fast as any man on two good legs.   Nov. 20, 1907.

* JOHN HARRIS—Messenger, Augusta Co., Va. Below knee.

It affords me much pleasure to let you know that the leg I bought from you I am getting along very well with. I have worn it every day for six years.   Oct. 19, 1909.

* IRA F. HARROLD—Whitley Co., Ind. ·Below knee.

I have not heard from you in a long time. Will write, however, and let you know that I am still wearing the Marks leg which you made for me over six years ago. I am well plased with it and do not use a cane and do all kinds of work on a farm. Dec. 22, 1907.

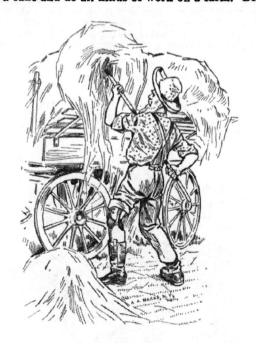

* GEO. W. HART—Farmer, La Grange Co., Ind.   Below knee.

I can recommend your artificial leg as the easiest of any that are made. I lost my leg in the Civil War, in 1863, and have worn a great many different kinds since then, but yours, with rubber foot, gives me the greatest comfort and best results. I am a farmer, and have a great deal of walking, heavy work, lifting to do, and I do it all without any difficulty.   Oct. 23, 1909,

WM. HART—Engineer, Clinton Co., N. Y. Above knee.

I have worn one of your artificial legs for the last five years and find it satisfactory in every respect. Have to walk one-half mile to work every day and back again, and stand on the leg all day. I am running a hoisting engine. I do not use a cane or crutch and have but three and one-half inches of stump from the body.
                                                              Dec. 8, 1908.

* O. GEO. HARVEY—Bookkeeper, South Africa. Ankle joint.

During the latter months of 1898 I ordered of you an artificial foot to fit a Symes' operation. The limb has given me the greatest satisfaction, so much so that I have determined to have another in case of accident to the first. The artificial leg was perfect, and in my case has done away with the pain caused by a misfitting, cumbersome one of the other make.   July 30, 1907.

* HERMAN S. HASTINGS—Clerk, Kings Co., Wash. Above knee.

When a boy of sixteen years I measured myself at home and bought one of Marks' artificial legs with rubber foot, amputation four and one-half inches from the hip. I wore that leg for fifteen years continuously. The repairs, including the expense of lengthening, was a matter of only a few dollars. The leg, in my younger days, was given very hard usage in teaming, lugging, lifting, etc. Still having confidence in Marks limbs, I bought another, with improvements, in 1903. My position now being a clerical one I am not so hard on my limb, and expect it to last as long as the former one. I desire to say further, that from the fact of having the artificial limb I obtained several prominent positions, which otherwise would have never been opened to me.
                                                             Oct. 20, 1909.

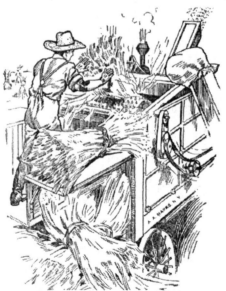

* G. L. H——Engineer, Juniata Co., Pa. Below elbow.

I have worn one of your artificial arms for over two years, and I have never had any trouble whatever with it. I run a steam thresher, and can get along almost as well as before. I can say to anyone in need of an artificial limb, that he will find A. A. Marks a comfort giver.   Aug. 1, 1909.

W. C. B. HASBROUCK—Watchman, Ulster Co., N. Y. Above knee.

I am wearing one of your artificial legs for above knee amputation and have been since 1903. I find it all, one in my condition should wish, and any time I can speak for your work I will cheerfully do so. Jan. 25, 1908.

* THOS. LAFAYETTE HATCH—Farmer, Alberta. Above knee.

The artificial leg purchased for Sylvester Hatch a year ago is giving entire satisfaction. Dec. 7, 1907.

* MRS. STANLEY HEATH—Housework, Aroostook Co., Me. Below knee.

I am a farmer's wife. I do all my own work, take care of three children. I can stand on my feet all day quite easily. I think your artificial limbs a blessing to anyone deprived of their natural ones. Oct. 20, 1909.

* F. HEITZ—Germany. Above knee.

Your leg satisfies me as well as an artificial limb can possibly do. It is very much lighter than the legs which I used formerly, and surpasses them also in carefulness and simplicity of construction. I thank you for the comfort which your ingenuity has procured for me. Oct. 27, 1909.

Speaker's Room,
House of Representatives,
Washington, D. C.

To H. M., Esq., Nov. 10, 1900.

My dear Sir:—The leg I wear was made by A. A. Marks. Amputations at or above the knee need better care in the matter of legs than those amputated below the knee. It takes more wisdom and experience to make legs for the former than the latter. For years I had a stump running down to within eight inches of ankle, but about three years ago I had to have it amputated at the knee. I tried many leg-makers and found none who could make a leg for me without taking a part of the weight on the end of the stump. Chicago utterly failed me in that direction. The moment I exhibited my stump to Mr. Marks, he told me that weight could not be taken on the end of the stump, and this before I told him of my experience in Chicago. I gave him an order at once, and his work has given me splendid satisfaction. I think they have better facilities for treating all kinds of amputations than any other leg-maker in the country.

Very respectfully,

I. L. HELM, M.D.—Fayette Co., Ky..
I have ordered several of your artificial legs. They have all given satisfaction.

N. M. HEMENWAY—Farmer, Kennebec Co., Me. Below knee.
It would be selfish of me if I did not say a word of the experience I have had with Marks leg and the treatment I have always received from that establishment. After having worn one of Marks legs for six years I went in 1908 and had another one made and fitted. Mr. Marks voluntarily kept the old leg, fixed it up and sent it to me without charge. I wear the old leg and the new one alternately and believe I will not have occasion to buy another as long as I live. The Marks limbs have never developed a fault. I know I am no exception as I am acquainted with others who have been treated by Mr. Marks and report the same. Oct. 25, 1909.

* JOHN HENDERSON—Laborer, Davidson Co., Tenn. Below knee.
I am pleased with the leg you made for me six years ago. I have done hard labor on it. I am on my feet ten hours every day. Jan. 20, 1908.

* PAUL A. HENSEL—Sawmill, Prince Edward Co., Va. Above knee.
A little over eighteen years ago I was run over by a horse car, and lost my right leg above the knee, which left me a stump of about six inches. At the time of the accident I was a boy six years old. Soon after I got a leg from you. I have been working

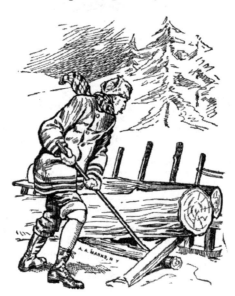

at a sawmill, and can do most anything in that line, I can haul logs from the woods, load and unload them, I can ride horseback as good as anyone, and when hunting season commences, I go and walk around through the woods and over fields. The new leg I got from you a few months ago is all O. K., and does not give me any trouble at all. I can go anywhere I want to with it, and wear it from early in the morning till late at night.

* FRANCIS HERCKENRATH—Holland. Above knee.

I take much pleasure in certifying that the two legs you furnished me from measurements, give me great satisfaction in every respect. I have never seen legs of better construction, and I do not believe that any other kind would need less repair. The rubber foot, and the knee-joint are far superior to all others I ever saw; hence, I can strongly recommend your highly respectable firm to all others. I lost my left leg in the year 1872.

* WILH. HERLTH—Manufacturer, Germany. Above knee.

I wish to inform you that the artificial limb furnished by you twelve years ago has turned out to my greatest satisfaction. I have previously also ordered limbs from several European firms, the execution of which, however, left something to be desired. I can therefore recommend your manufactory very highly. Translated from German.   Oct. 28, 1909.

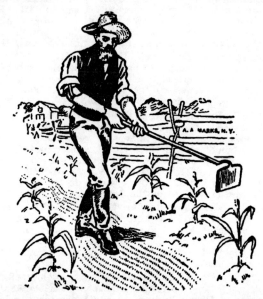

* WILLIAM HERMANN—Farmer, Bates Co., Mo. Below elbow.

I will try to write you a few lines to let you know that I am well pleased with the hand and tools. I am a farmer, and can do most any work with my artificial hand. I could not do without the artificial arm at all. I have worn it two years. I am writing this letter with the rubber hand.

* DOLORES HERNANDEZ de LAUREIRO—Cuba. Knee joint.

I thought after my amputation that I should not be able to walk except with the aid of crutches, which would make it impossible to attend to my household work. Thanks to your invention it has not been so, as to-day I can do all my work and attend to my children. I walk well with the artificial leg. Persons who do not know anything about my misfortune are astonished when told that my right leg is artificial.—Translated from Spanish.

JACOB F. HERTZOG—Farmer, Berks Co., Pa.

I have a resection of the right arm caused by a wound. I have thus far used five of your apparatus for the same, and each one gave ease and comfort, and entire satisfaction. I had two apparatus from different parties before I used yours, but they were not as easy nor as comfortable. I am a farmer by occupation, and with the use of your apparatus I am able to do all kinds of ordinary farm work.   Oct. 20, 1909.

* PATRICK HICKEY—Student, Harbor Grace, Newfoundland. Above knee.

I am wearing one of your artificial legs and am doing remarkably well with it, and shall recommend your work to anyone in need.
                                                              Jan. 19, 1909.

* OTIS L. HIGBY—Machinist, Whitman Co., Wash. Below elbow.

I have been wearing one of your artificial arms for three years and indeed it is very satisfactory.   Jan. 16, 1909.

* REV. E. B. HIGGINBOTHAM—Clergyman, Elbert Co., Ga. Both below knees.

I heartily endorse the several testimonials I have heretofore sent to you. The first pair of legs you made for me in 1880. I wore them thirteen years, then I got a new pair which I am now wearing. I am seventy-one years of age and without your artificial limbs could not do the ministerial labor I have done.   Oct. 18, 1909.

THOS. HIGHAM—Lorain Co., Ohio. Below knee.

The foot I got of you five years ago is giving the best of satisfaction. I have worn it steady, and it don't make my leg the least sore. I surprise everybody the way I walk. I don't think I could have got as good a fit anywhere else.   Oct. 20, 1909.

* JOSEPH HINKS—Engineer, Schuylkill Co., Pa. Below knee.

The leg I purchased of you over twenty-one years ago contiues to give entire satisfaction. It is almost as good to-day as when I bought it. The change of the old style of rubber foot for a fiber spring mattress foot, is a decided improvement. I am wearing it now, and am delighted with it. It is very easy to walk on, and I believe my walking is better, as there seems to be more strength and support in the spring from the toes.   Oct. 18, 1909.

* GEO. C. HOBBS—Merchant, London England. Below knee.

I have worn one of Marks rubber foot legs for twenty years, before that I had seven years' experience with other makes.

I am convinced that Marks is the best and that there are none anywhere near his in the line of efficiency and durability. You can refer anyone to me at any time.   July 21, 1908.

* MOSES HODDINOTT—Sailor, Newfoundland. Below elbow.

My arm was amputated in 1905. I purchased a Marks arm in 1906 and have found it satisfactory. I could not manage without it at all. I am a sailor and the arm with hook helps me in many ways. I can chop wood and do any carpenter work on board the boat.   Dec. 13, 1908.

* GEORGE A. HOLLAND—Merchant, Hochelaga Co., Quebec. Above knee.

In September, 1897, I first tried one of your artificial limbs. I had previously used the articulating ankle and had often considered the advisability of making the ankle rigid. Naturally when I heard of your rubber foot I saw you had solved the problem.

I have now used your make of limbs for twelve years and am more thoroughly convinced than ever that the rigid ankle gives the nearest approach to the natural motion, besides a safer and surer footing.

In October, 1902, I got a second leg from you as a reserve one, thus expressing in a practical way my appreciation.

For sure footing, safety and comfort in walking, I recommend the rigid ankle and rubber foot first, last and all the time.
                                                              Oct. 27, 1909.

* ROY HOLT—Clerk, McIntosh Co., Okla. Ankle joint.

In regard to the leg I purchased from you in 1903, I must say that I am very well pleased with it. I put it on the day I received it, and have worn it constantly ever since. I cannot say

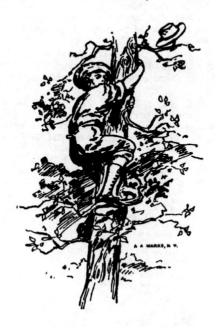

enough in praise of it. I run, jump, climb trees, and participate in all the sports of the season, and am at no inconvenience.
Oct. 17, 1909.

* T. E. HOLDEN—Farmer, Buffalo Co., Wis. Below knee.

I have worn artificial legs for twenty-one years. My limb is amputated six inches below the knee.

The first leg I got had an ankle joint. I will not have another of that kind unless I want an artificial leg and music box combined. The ankle joint breaks down so often that you have to watch every step you take.

The first leg I got of you was in 1893. It is still in good condition. I am hard on artificial legs, as I am a hard worker on the farm.

I ordered another leg of you in December, 1903. It is giving me great satisfaction in every respect. I believe your make of artificial legs is far superior to any other, because of the ease, elasticity, durability, and noiselessness. These are obtained by the use of the rubber foot. Oct. 20, 1909.

* NEWTON HOPTON—Sacramento Co., Calif. Below knee.

I take pleasure in writing to you pertaining to my new limb. I am very glad to say that it is an excellent fit in every respect.
Sept. 21, 1908.

H. R. HOSFORD—Farmer, Columbia Co., N. Y. Below knee.

I am a farmer, which has always been my principal business. For the past thirty-eight years or more I have worn the rubber foot constantly. The elasticity of the rubber foot no doubt added much to its durability, and at the same time gave a more natural movement in walking, obviating the disagreeable thumping that attended the other foot I had used, and at the same time the jar to the natural limb, making it more comfortable and easy.

Oct. 20, 1909.

* U. M. HOUSEL—Jeweler, Somerset Co., Pa.   Above knee.

I am getting along fine and recommend your work to all in need. My leg was amputated in 1875. I got your leg in 1898 and my second in 1908.

Feb. 3, 1909.

* JOAQUIN HOYOS—Lara, Venezuela, South America.   Above knee.

I am a great walker. My friends often ask me which is the artificial leg. I tell them to find out or ask Marks. Wore Marks leg since 1897.

Jan. 1, 1908.

* H. A. HOWARD—Farmer, Caswell Co., N. C.   Below elbow.

I have been intending to write to you for some time. I am pleased to report that the arm fits nicely and surpasses my expectations as to usefulness. I can plow and use a hoe far better than I had any idea that I would be able to. The ring and hook are very useful in loading and unloading wood, in carrying anything that cannot be carried with the hand. The fork and brush do their part with satisfaction.

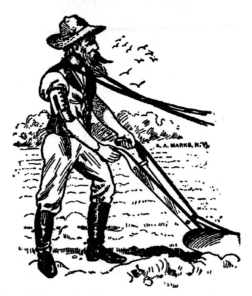

The rubber hand is very useful in nailing, as I can hold the nail between the finger and thumb; without the rubber hand I could not nail at all.

My stump is six inches long, and since using the arm it has improved very much, and does not pain as it did before.

* ED. HOWELL—Telegrapher, Williamson Co., Ill.   Below knee.

At the age of eleven I suffered the amputation of my left leg about one inch above ankle-joint. Two years later purchased an artificial leg from St. Louis. The limb was the ankle-joint style. After thirteen months' usage the joint became so worn that the foot was allowed to turn over, all attempts to repair substantially were useless. November 7, 1892, I purchased a limb from you, wearing it continually until September 21, 1903, when a double

barrel hammerless shotgun fell, discharging both barrels through my artificial leg and stump, four inches above the ankle-joint, necessitating re-amputation. I was so near the gun that both shot and wads passed through, making a clean opening one and one-half inches in diameter entirely through the leg. After recovering I again brought the old leg into use, with the expectation that it would be so weakened as to render it useless, but to my surprise it served me for another year. In 1906 I bought a second leg from you which further confirms me in my belief in your superiority.
Oct. 26, 1909.

L. P. HUBBARD—Brass Worker, New Haven Co., Conn. Both feet.
In 1896 I had a double amputation at the ankle joints. I procured a pair of artificial legs with ankle joints, which gave me a great deal of trouble. My stumps would get sore. In April, 1902, I received one of your artificial legs with a rubber foot, which has given entire satisfaction. In March, 1904, I received the mate to the one I got two years before. Both legs are giving entire satisfaction. My occupation is bench work in a brass manufactory, sitting or standing. I consider that I have as good a pair of artificial limbs as is made.
Oct. 18, 1909.

* G. H. HURST—Huddersfield, England. Below knee.
Dear Mr. Barstow:—I just sit down to remind you that it is just twelve months since I came to your house for my Marks Artificial Leg. And I am very pleased to say that I have never had cause to regret it. I have followed my usual employment, and I think I have done remarkably well, to say that it is only eighteen months since my accident happened. I watched you very minutely when you took my measurements, which I have found since that, they were taken with exactness.
The way which you receive people at your house and the hospitality you show them, is enough to show the sincerity you have in them. In my firm opinion, Mr. Barstow, there is only one kind of leg to beat the Marks and that is a good natural one.
Feb. 16, 1911.

* THOMAS HUNT—R. R. Porter, Hamilton Co., Tenn. Below knee.
I am wearing one of Marks' legs, and it has given me satisfaction in every respect.
Dec. 8, 1908.

* G. L. HUME, M.D.—Quebec. Below knee.
The artificial leg sent by you to Geo. Beausoleil eight years ago, made from measurements, I am pleased to state has given entire satisfaction. My patient can walk without aid of cane or crutch, and very few people are able to detect any difference. The arm you made for Fred Ball is equally as suitable. Oct. 20, 1909.

* JOHN H. HYNES—R. R. Man, Hartford Co., Conn. Below elbow.
I am wearing my arm constantly and it does not give me any trouble. My co-workers are very much surprised to see that I get along so well.
Sept. 22, 1907.

F. C. HUNTLEY—Builder, New York City, N. Y. Above knee.
In 1892 I had my left leg amputated a little above the knee on account of gangrene following an injury that I received in my knee. In the following July I applied to you for an artificial leg. I superintend the laying of artificial stone in new buildings. This compels me to go up and down half completed stairways without balustrades and very frequently up and down ladders. I never use a cane or crutch and walk so well that very few persons suspect that I have a wooden leg. I weigh 200 pounds and am enjoying the best of health and never miss a day from my work.
I consider your rubber foot the most valuable invention in artificial limb construction that has ever been made. Oct. 21, 1909.

CHARLES HUNT—Private Policeman, New York City, N. Y. Wrist.

Before I placed an order with you, I visited other firms and came to the conclusion that you made the best and most practical hand; the results have justified me in my decision. I am a policeman and

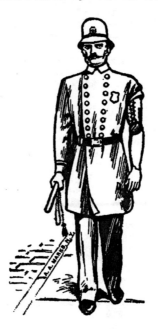

have been for the last eight years. I have on several occasions been obliged to use violence in order to hold my man.

C. P. HUTCHINSON—Dauphin Co., Pa. Instep amputation.

I am glad to testify that your appliance for my foot, a Chopart's amputation, is the finest article in the market. I am a fireman on the P. R. Road and do my work every day.

W. H. IRVINE, M.D.—New Brunswick, Canada.

Mr. McLeod got his leg two months ago, and it works satisfactorily.

G. L. ISBISTER—Farmer, Columbia Co., New York. Below knee.

My limb was amputated when I was a boy of eight years, leaving me a stump of five and one-half inches below the knee. For over twelve years I continually wore an artificial leg of your make which has given perfect satisfaction. My occupation is a farmer, requiring me to do all kinds of labor, plowing, hoeing, etc. I also ride a wheel.

D. E. ISHAM—Carpenter, Chautauqua Co., N. Y. Ankle amputation.

For fit, lightness and strength, your metal socket leg for ankle joint amputation is far ahead of any other leg I have worn. I know the requirements of an artificial leg, having worn one for forty years.

* G. LAVIN ISLA—Merchant, Mexico. Below knee.

Every day that passes makes me more and more content and satisfied with the artificial leg you made for me a year ago. I dance, ride horseback and do everything just as if the leg was natural.

Feb. 25, 1907.

* GEO. V. JACKSON—Hartford Co., Conn. Below elbow.

The artificial arm you recently made for me is satisfactory in every respect. I just advised a friend of mine who is in need of an arm to go to you.

* P. C. JACKSON—Engineer, Alaska. Partial hand amputation.

The artificial hand I received from you, constructed on the plan of P-38, fits perfectly and I am greatly pleased with it, much more so than I expected to be. It is of great use to me in engineering, as I can hold almost any instrument with the fingers. Feb. 28, 1909.

PROF. F. E. JACOBY—New Haven Co., Conn. Below knee.

When I met with the misfortune of losing my right leg, I felt that all the sunshine had passed from my life. Fortunately I came in possession of one of your books, and as I perused its pages, I received much encouragement. Some tried to dissuade me from obtaining an artificial leg inside of four or five months, but I was so determined to get about on two legs again, that I procured an artificial leg from you in exactly nine weeks after my natural leg was amputated. Five days after I received the leg my doctor saw me skating on the canal. He was amazed; he told me that I beat anything he had ever seen.

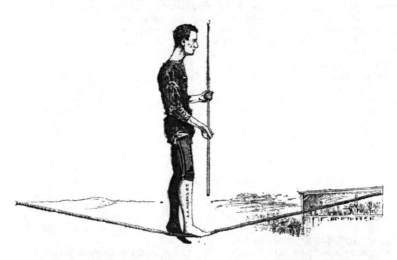

I was a professional tight rope walker and aeronaut before I lost my leg, and I did not propose to allow the loss of a leg to compel me to seek another occupation. I can walk a tight rope nearly as well as ever I could. The rubber foot enables me to balance with safety. When I am dressed, without exposing my limbs, no one would suspect that one of my legs is artificial.

While walking on the ground I never feel the necessity of looking out for uneven or bad places. I feel safe and sure on my rubber foot, no matter where I place it. I consider your invention of the rubber foot with spring mattress the most valuable and important.

Note.—The above illustration has been made from an instantaneous photograph taken of Professor Jacoby while performing on a tight rope. He is balancing entirely on his artificial leg; his natural foot is off the rope in the act of passing forward to take the next step.

* LUCY JAMES—Cook, Madison Co., Va. Below knee.

The leg you shipped to me in 1903 is still in good order. I began wearing it as soon as I received it. I attend to my household duties without the least inconvenience. I must say that it is a God-send, for I never expected to get around with as much ease and comfort as I do now.   Nov. 1, 1909.

* J. A. JARRATT—Blacksmith, De Soto Co., La. Below knee.

I had the misfortune to lose one of my legs in 1857, and have been wearing artificial limbs made by you since 1864. The last leg I got was made in 1892. It has given me such good service I do not wish to throw it aside for another one. However, if you will guarantee another one to last as long as this one has and then guarantee me to live until I wear it out, I have the money to pay for it. I have had several to try to sell me a limb of their make, but I always put up the above proposition to them and that ends the matter.

I do not believe that the artificial leg of your make, which I have worn for seventeen years, has been out of use more than two months in that time and that was not caused by any trouble with the leg, and all the repairs that I have been put to during that long period have not amounted to $10.00. I have shod horses, worked in a blacksmith shop, built wagons, built houses and painted one church all alone, with no help to raise my ladders, and made my scaffolding. I am now nearly seventy years old and if I live long enough to need another artificial limb you will make it for me.   Nov. 8, 1909.

MICHAEL J———Hungary. Above knee.

Nearly ten years ago I was furnished with an artificial leg by A. A. Marks of New York. I have had no trouble with it whatever and walk with it in the most natural way. It gives me pleasure to speak favorably of Marks artificial limbs. I have seen a number made in Europe and different parts of the world, but none of them have shown the worth and merits of those constructed by Marks. I am on my artificial leg all the time and it has to be a good one to hold me up and meet the demands I make upon it.
                          Oct. 29, 1909.

* ARTHUR JOHNSON—Farmer, Twigg Co., Ga. Below knee.

I received the artificial leg you made for me January 9th and found it to be all right. I can plow, cut wood, and do all my own work, such as shoeing horses, mules, and general repairing.
                          May 18, 1908.

* C. C. JOHNSON, M.D.—Aiken Co., S. C.

I have ordered several of your artificial limbs for different persons in this State. All of them are now being used with utmost satisfaction. The leg recently secured for a young patient of mine is so natural and useful that the acquaintances of the gentleman cannot realize that he has been maimed and is wearing an artificial leg. He and at least two others of the wearers of Marks legs in this section are expert bicycle riders, having learned to ride since procuring your legs.   Oct. 19, 1909.

ELI W. JONES—Farmer, Marion Co., Ill. Above knee.

I lost my leg March 16, 1865, in the Civil War, thigh amputation. Have been wearing artificial legs since with more or less trouble, until sixteen years ago when I got one of yours with the rubber foot. Wore it with great comfort for nine years. Seven years ago you made me a new one which is as near perfect as an artificial leg can be. I walk with perfect ease. The main objection I made against your system was the absence of the ankle joint. I now find that to be the chief merit of your limbs.   Oct. 27, 1909.

* O. W. JONES—Barber, Bertie Co., N. C. Below knee.

I take very great pleasure in recommending your house after you having given me perfect satisfaction. Jan. 22, 1909.

W. R. JONES—Clearfield Co., Pa. Above knee.

The rubber foot is a grand success. I am much swifter on this limb than the one I have been wearing from another firm. I heartily recommend your work. Oct. 17, 1909.

DR. G. H. JUILLY—San Francisco, Calif.

The leg you made for L. Roy has given excellent satisfaction.

* F. H. KAPPA—Machinist, Jefferson Co., Ky. Above knee.

The first artificial leg ordered from measurements at Pensacola, Fla., October, 1884, has given me great satisfaction and good service. May, 1902, I ordered the second, which is superior in construction, especially the spring mattress rubber foot is an improvement which I cannot praise enough.

I am a machinist by trade and experience no difficulty in following my occupation, and only experienced people can tell that I am wearing an artificial leg. Oct. 21, 1909.

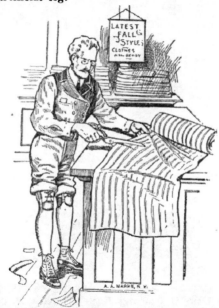

* SYLVANUS J. KEITH—Tailor, Nova Scotia. Both below knees.

Twenty-three years ago I had both of my legs amputated below knees and had been wearing artificial limbs with ankle joints for twenty years with much trouble and dissatisfaction. One year and a half ago I purchased a pair of your artificial limbs with rubber feet attached and since then the trouble so common to me for so long has disappeared. I am engaged in the tailoring business and do all the cutting, which means that I am on my feet most of the time. I go about the store up and downstairs and out for short walks without the use of a cane and without the unpleasant squeaking and rattling of joints which used to annoy me so much. The rubber foot does not produce that wooden leg sound so often noticed from less modern appliances and I have no hesitation in recommending your artificial legs with rubber feet as being the very best on the market.

SAMUEL M. KATZ—Machinist, Luzerne Co., Pa. Below knee.

The leg I bought from you three years ago has given me entire satisfaction. I have not lost one day from work since wearing it.
Dec. 11, 1907.

THADDEUS S. KAUTZ—Conductor, Dauphin Co., Pa. Partial foot.

Having made a study of three makes of artificial feet, I came to the conclusion that the Marks foot is the most practical of all. I have made a thorough test, using your foot in the capacity of a brakeman for eight years.   Oct. 9, 1909.

JOHN KELDER—Machinist, Queens Co., N. Y. Below elbow.

The artificial arm I received from you eight years ago has proved satisfactory. I am an engineer and have to run locomotives and do all kinds of engine work. I am able to do all this with the aid of your artificial arm. I would not part with your hand for $500.00.   Oct. 19, 1909.

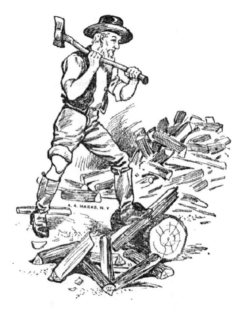

SAMUEL P. KEMP—Farmer, Lawrence Co., Pa. Above knee.

My artificial limb is working fine. I have had more comfort in the six years I have been wearing A. A. Marks leg, than I have had in all the time before, about thirty-three years.

My stump is just eight inches long and I can walk good without a cane and I can do almost any kind of work on a farm. I can plow, plant corn, dig and shovel clay or pitch hay and chop wood and other kinds of labor as well as any other man. Oct. 18, 1909.

STEPHEN KELSEY—Essex Co., N. J. Above knee.

It gives me great pleasure to be able to say that the legs you have made for me have been most satisfactory and comfortable. As you know I have worn them for fourteen years. I have gotten so now that it never occurs to me that I am lame. I have no difficulty in running automobiles or riding motorcycles.

I advise any young person with diseased or shortened limbs to have them amputated and get one of your artificial legs.
Nov. 15, 1909.

DR. E. J. KEMPF—Dubois Co., Ind.

The arm and hand of Joseph Goetz were received, and Goetz is well pleased, and even more than that, he is tickled. He can write his name and do any kind of light work.

* JOHN KEMPER—Grayson Co., Texas. Instep amputation.

I have been wearing your artificial foot for instep amputation for nearly fifteen years, and it has given me perfect satisfaction at all times. I can cheerfully recommend the same as the best made.
Oct. 24, 1909.

JAMES J. KENNELLY—Produce Clerk, Brooklyn. Below knee.

On the 15th of November, 1893, I began to wear one of your artificial feet. I continued my studies and graduated from the High School without any of my fellow students knowing that I wore an artificial foot. I am a member of the Royal Arcanum and there are not three members of my lodge know that I wear an artificial foot.

* REV. J. H. KENT—England. Above knee.

After nearly two years' use of the Marks artificial leg I can speak well of it. I cannot speak too highly of the careful way in which Mr. Barstow took my measurements, and which proved so satisfactory.
April 15, 1908.

* T. M. KEOGH—Musician, England. Below knee.

The new leg is a great success. I can walk fast with perfect ease and no friction, and it works well when cycling. I am a member of the Liverpool Masonic Motorcycling Club, and I have often ridden from eighty to one hundred miles a day. I can never understand any person requiring an artificial limb, and who has had " Marks " brought before their notice, going elsewhere for one, and at any time any of your prospective clients would like to see "Marks" leg in use I shall be pleased to show them how I ride a bicycle, run, and do things any ordinary person with both their natural limbs do.
May 9, 1909.

* THOMAS KILLGOUR—Auckland, New Zealand. Below knee.

The artificial leg which you made for me eleven years ago has proved of the greatest comfort and satisfaction, and although the usage I have given it has been rough, it will unquestionably last me several years longer.

In the course of my occupation as a bush contractor, I have to travel continually over many miles of heavily timbered mountainous country, both walking and riding, often covering forty miles a day. The timber for the most part grows on very rough and broken country and on the sides of precipitous gulleys, and I experience only a little difficulty in getting over such country.

The rubber foot enables me to walk much more easily and comfortably and the leg is considerably lighter than what I previously wore which had an ankle action.
Feb. 26, 1910.

* GEORGE OSCAR KINARD—Packer, Bibb Co., Ga. Below elbow.

The arm I got from you was the cause of my securing a better position than I have ever had. I have been in the company of strangers for several hours at a time and they did not discover that I had but one natural arm.
Oct. 21, 1909.

* W. F. KLECKNER—Car Checker, Schuylkill Co., Pa. Below knee.

The artificial leg you made for me has given so much satisfaction that I would not part with it for any consideration. I have been traveling with friends that did not know I had my leg off until they were told. This goes to show that I walk well. I shall recommend your make of legs at all times.

GEO. D. KERNS—Jefferson Co., Mont. Knee bearing.

In regard to my experience in using an artificial leg will say that I have worn one thirty-one years.

The first rubber foot I wore for twelve years, and the second I am still wearing. I am a stone mason and builder. My work is on rough ground, with spall, fragments, and rubbish as usually seen about stone buildings while under construction. This is the place to test an artificial leg. No other leg ever did so much good. It has a stiff ankle joint which is really its charm.

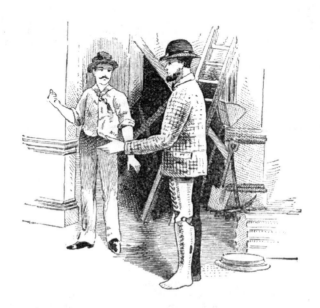

I can stand on the heel or toe at will; this gives me great advantage in turning about and getting around lively.

If on a sidehill, roof, or ladder the ankle-joint foot is not safe, but the rubber foot is always safe.

* LENA KLEIN—Jennings Co., Ind. Above knee.

The artificial leg you made for me in 1896 is still in good condition. I wear it continuously. It cannot be beat by any leg that is made.   Jan. 27, 1910.

REV. J. W. KNAPPENBERGER, A.M.—President, Allentown College for Women, Lehigh Co., Pa. Above knee.

I have been wearing A. A. Marks artificial limb since 1890. I have found it satisfactory in every particular and I consider it the best in the market. It is comfortable, easy to manage, wears well, and protects from injury.

* WILLIAM KNEIPP—Cattleman, Australia. Below elbow.

The hand I got from you gives every satisfaction. I can use the knife to cut my food quite well, and I hold the reins in the artificial hand when driving and riding. It is worth double the money for looks only.

* VERNON KNOWLES—Clerk, England. Below elbow.

I am writing again to show my appreciation for the artificial arm purchased of you. I have worn the same continuously ever since. I camped three weeks on Horse Shoe Island. I have used the hand for paddling a canoe, carrying minnow pails, holding fishing rod, digging bait, washing myself.

I have just completed a trip through England and the Continent, during which journey I used the hand constantly for carrying my suit case, cutting my food, etc.   Sept. 25, 1909.

G. FRED KOHLER, JR.—Bergen Co., N. J. Below knee.

I have been wearing one of your rubber feet now since March 9, 1904, and have not had any chafing of the stump or any other difficulty. I do not limp at all.

* CHAS. KORTE—Mora Co., New Mexico. Below knee.

In the twenty-one years that have passed since I bought an artificial leg of you, I have worn the leg continuously. I have been very much satisfied and thankful to you, for I have done my work same as though I had my natural leg.   Feb. 25, 1910.

* L. KRASKER—Pearl Worker, England. Below knee.

After wearing an artificial leg (made in France) I met a friend in Australia who wore a Marks leg, and he strongly recommended me to have one. I am thankful that I took his advice, for I never felt so comfortable before. My order was put through Mr. Barstow.   Jan. 25 1909.

* W. L. KUHN—Cigar Store, Frederick Co., Va. Above knee.

The new leg I got from you two years ago fits nicely and I expect it will last as long as the other one, which I had worn continuously for twenty-two years. The leg was constructed by you in 1886.   Feb. 2, 1910.

GEO. W. KUTCH—Boatman, Schuylkill Co., Pa. Below knee.

I am wearing your make of artificial limbs since 1886. I am what is commonly called a waterman, and work upon a barge. Your leg gives entire satisfaction. It gets damp, occasionally wet, but no ill effects result. I can perform my work as well as those who have their two natural legs. In winter time the barges are often covered with ice, which makes walking very uncertain, but I can get around as well as most who have their natural legs.   Oct. 16, 1909.

* PETER KUTCHERA—Marathon Co., Wis. Below elbow.

The artificial arm I got from you some time ago has far surpassed my expectations. The rubber hand is certainly a good invention. I can carry a grip or bundle with it, I can also close and open my latch door. My right arm being amputated two inches below the elbow. I had no idea that I would have any control of the artificial arm.   Oct. 19, 1909.

* FRANCISCO LABORDE—La Plata, Argentine Rep. Below knee.

I am entirely satisfied with the almost perfect construction of your leg. I walk almost naturally.   Aug. 8, 1908.

* E. L. LAIRD—Crawford Co., Kan. Above knee.

It is with pleasure I inform you that the limb purchased for my daughter when she was six years old is giving the best of satisfaction, far better than I supposed it were possible, considering the location of the amputation—her stump is a very short one above the knee. I heartily recommend your work.   Dec. 14, 1909.

* H. M. LAIRD—Drug Clerk, Monmouth Co., N. J. Below knee.

I have given the limb you sent me a thorough trial. I can say that I am well pleased with. It seems to be what I want. Last week I walked half a mile and was no worse for it. I want to thank you for the satisfaction you gave me. You may use my name as reference.   Nov. 1, 1909.

* RODOLPHO LAMBEA—Farmer, Cuba. Below knee.

I am well pleased with the artificial limb you sent me. I am working on a farm and use your artificial leg to great advantage. I thank you for what you have done for me.—Translated from Spanish.   Sept. 29, 1909.

* THOMAS LANGTON—Herbalist, England. Above knee.

I have received the leg you made for me and having now worn it for the last five years, I have much pleasure and satisfaction in testifying to its qualities, which are in every particular as good as one could wish. It is comfortable, light, strong and safe, the finish and mechanism are a great improvement on those I have previously worn. I desire also to express my gratitude to you for your patience, persistence and unfailing courtesy in bringing about this most gratifying result. Shall recommend your firm whenever possible.   Oct. 25, 1909.

NORMAN A. LAMPMAN—Laborer, Columbia Co., N. Y. Below knee.

I think you would like to hear from one of your artificial legs. I am wearing mine right along every day. The leg is alright. I have always been very thankful that I have a leg of your make and get along so well.   March 4, 1908.

* R. M. LANIER—Tax Collector, Ware Co., Ga. Below knee.

About twenty-five years ago I lost my right leg just below the knee, and since that time I have used three of your artificial limbs. In 1902 purchased the last one. I have always found them to be comfortable and durable in my work. I am tax collector of Ware County, Ga., which occupation carries with it considerable walking, and I get around with all ease and comfort. I don't think your class of work is surpassed by any.   Oct. 17, 1909.

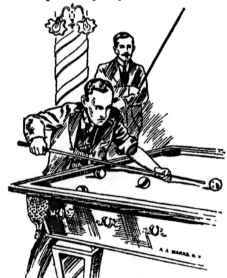

* EDWARD W. LASLEY—Laborer, Antrim Co., Mich. Below elbow.

I lost my arm below the elbow last October. I had one of your artificial hands made by measurements, and have worn it every day since. I am greatly pleased with it. It fits perfectly, and with the glove on one could not tell it from the natural hand. I do most anything with it. I can punch the bag, play pool, and box with it. I find it very useful, and I wouldn't be without the hand for anything.

* MRS. MARY LANO—Todd Co., Minn. Below knee.
I have worn one of your artificial limbs for the last fourteen years, the first one I wore seven years, the second I got eight years ago, both made from measurements. I am well pleased with them. I am sixty-six years old, and can do all my house-work.   Oct. 18, 1909.

* JOSEPH LAROCK—Sawmill, Carleton Co., Ontario. Above knee.
I guess I am the best walker in Canada. I have worn the leg you made for me now six years. The rubber foot is great to walk on.   April 27, 1908.

* J. B. LEBOIX—France. Above knee.
After wearing your artificial leg with rubber foot for seven years, I am pleased to recognize all the merits your make deserves. The leg is comfortable, and construction is simple. I have as yet had no need for repairs, and have subjected it to hard tests every day.— Translated from French.   Oct. 27, 1909.

* C. L. LEDLIE—Chatham Co., Ga. Ankle amputation.
I am still wearing the artificial leg you made for me in 1907, and am glad to state that I have been complimented by several good doctors who know of my case. I highly recommend your limb whenever I get a chance to do so. I am at present employed by the Southern Cotton Oil Company as operator. Am on my feet all day and I think that tests my stump and your foot pretty well.   Feb. 7, 1910.

* MISS FLORENCE M. LEE—Washington Co., R. I. Below knee.
It is seven years this month that you made for me the leg, and I am doing nicely with it; the former leg made by you was applied when I was four years old, and I wore it eight years. I work and walk every day. I have no trouble whatever with it, and have worn it all the time since you made it for me.   Oct. 20, 1909.

* PATRICK W. LEE—Trooper, New Zealand. Above knee.
I was a member of one of the New Zealand Contingents, in active service during the Boer War, and lost my right leg as a result of injuries received in the Western Transvaal. The amputation is about five inches above the knee. Acting on the advice of a clergy-man, who is himself wearing one of your limbs, I obtained one, and have worn it every day since.
It is a wonderfully good substitute, and to a great extent removes the disability imposed by the loss of the natural limb. I am not engaged in any particular vocation at present, but do a lot of walking, and can get about with but little inconvenience

* WILLIAM LEES, M.D., C.S., L.S.A.—Chester, England.
The arm for Williamson has arrived safely and fits him perfectly. I am highly pleased with it, and intend to show this patient and his arm, and also Mr. Howson and his leg, at our Chester Medical Society. I consider them triumphs of mechanical art.

* ANTONIO LEONARDO—Fruiter, Oriente, Cuba. Below knee.
I am enjoying the artificial leg you made for me a year and a half ago. It makes a young man of me. Everybody admires your work. I am engaged in the fruit business. I am never tired of praising your skill.   April 25, 1909.

* H. E. LEWIS—Grocer, Washington Co., R. I.—Below knee.
I have been using the artificial leg you made me twelve years ago continuously, and am up and down a step-ladder a great deal, and feel perfectly safe. My weight, at the present time, is 214 pounds. I never use a cane, as I can walk better without it.
                                        Oct. 18, 1909.

PETER L. LEE—Watchman, Worcester Co., Mass. Below knee.

Your leg is all that you claim for it in fact it is much more. I am night watchman in a large worsted and carpet mill, which requires my walking up several flight of stairs every night. I am twenty-five minutes on the go winding clocks. I also have two large boilers to take care of, and have to wheel fourteen to sixteen

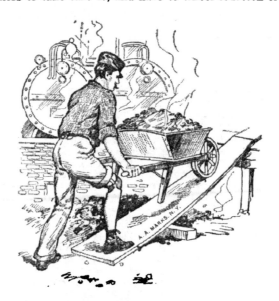

large wheelbarrows of clinkers and ashes every night up an incline two and a half feet in ten, which I do without trouble.

The artificial leg that I wore before I got yours gave me much trouble, and kept my stump sore and irritated nearly all the time. It compelled me to undergo a second amputation.

* C. G. LINDAHL—Snohomish Co., Wash. Below elbow.

I have now used the artificial arm which you manufactured for me for eight months, and I am glad to say that it is a perfect fit and that I am very satisfied with the outfit.   March 28, 1910.

J. S. LINDLEY, M.D.—Indian Agency, Okla.

I deem it due to you to say that the artificial leg you furnished the Indian Department for Joe Chilchuana, the Apache Indian, gives the utmost satisfaction in every respect. The young man wears it with the greatest ease, satisfaction, and comfort, and is delighted with it. One who does not know that he is wearing an artificial limb would not detect it in his walk. You are to be congratulated upon the satisfaction your work gives.

* ARCHIE LIVINGSTONE—Laborer, Cassia Co., Idaho. Both below
    knees.

I got my legs amputated in December, 1901, and received artificial ones from A. A. Marks, June, 1902. I have been wearing them ever since; they were made from measurements, and fit right. They have not bothered me at all. I am a rider, and can get on a horse quicker than many that have not lost their limbs.   Nov. 15, 1909.

JAMES LIVINGSTON—Railroad, Perry Co., Ill. Below knee.

I have worn one of your artificial legs since 1891 (seventeen years) and it has given entire satisfaction.   Nov. 27, 1907.

ENOS LINCOLN—Saline Co., Kansas. Above knee.

After having worn your artificial leg with rubber foot for more than thirty years, I have no hesitation in saying it is the best leg in use; it is simply the most durable of any of the many I have seen. The rubber foot with stiff ankle is unquestionably the best and softest leg made; it never drags at the toe from weight of

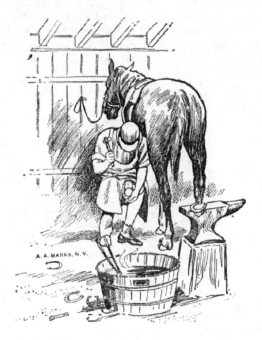

mud. It is so simple a child can adjust it. I have worn artificial legs since 1862, and do all kinds of work. I am a blacksmith, and shoe horses. I have dug wells, and quarried stone and other heavy work. I can walk farther in a given time than any man on any other kind of a leg, with the same length of stump as mine; it is only three inches from center of hip joint.

JULIO LLUBERES—Conductor, Santo Domingo. Above knee.

A month after amputation I had an artificial leg applied at your establishment, and upon my arrival here I filled the position of conductor of a passenger and freight train for three months, and for the past five years I have discharged the duties of station agent at Bajabonico, both of which I have performed satisfactorily. I can put the leg on in two minutes. I walk a great deal, both for work and pleasure. I have got on the train when the locomotive was under very rapid headway. I can assure you that I am well satisfied with the leg, and believe it the best in the world—Translated from Spanish.   Nov. 10, 1909.

* FRED LORD—Paper Hanger, York Co., Me. Wrist amputation.

The artificial hand you made for me some time ago is doing good service; it has stood up under very severe work. It has proved a great deal better than I expected an artificial arm would. I have had it five years and it looks as though it would be good for five years more.   Sept. 18, 1908.

* GIROLAMO LORENZONI—Lawyer, Italy. Above knee.

In September, 1895, after thirty years of suffering, I had my right leg amputated, above the knee, leaving a very short stump. I obtained an artificial leg made in Padua. I walked very badly with it, and was in despair, when fortunately one of my friends made me acquainted with your firm. In 1897 you furnished me with a magnificent artificial limb, which I have worn ever since. I am most contented with your system, especially the construction of the foot, which is unimprovable in every respect.   March 17, 1910.

* MRS. S. F. LOVELACE—Pittsylvania Co., Va. Below knee.

I have worn one of your artificial legs nearly ten years. It was made from measurements. I do all kinds of housework, walk to church and a mile or so to see my friends None but those that are afflicted know what a blessing an artificial leg is. I would not be without it for double what it cost.   Oct. 1, 1907.

GEO. J. LOWERY—Printer, Boston, Mass. Both below knees.

I bought a pair of artificial legs from you in 1899. They have given me perfect satisfaction. I have worn them continually since.
    Jan. 31, 1908.

* EBEN P. LOW—Rancher, Honolulu, Hawaii. Below elbow.

It is seventeen years since I got an artificial arm from you and ten years since I got a duplicate. Both have served me with wonderful help, considering the class of work I am engaged in. I have had several falls from my horse landing on my artificial arm which has suffered no injury. I have made a record that stands to be equaled or beaten, that is a record of one minute and twelve seconds for roping and tying a wild steer after the steer has been given sixty-five feet start. I know that I stand before the world as " The champion one arm roper." I enclose a photo of myself in my cowboy outfit in preparation for the catch of the steer in the contest before the public, where fourteen of the most expert cowboys of the kingdom participated, so much for the help of your artificial arm.   Jan. 15, 1910.

* M. F. LUCAS, M.D.—Lincoln Co., Ont.

A few years ago I fitted a young man with one of your arms and legs in the city of Victoria, B. C. You will no doubt be glad to learn that his limbs have given the greatest satisfaction.
    Oct. 20, 1908.

* THOMAS F. LUSH—Teacher, Lycoming Co., Pa. Knee bearing.

I am now wearing my second artificial leg, both made by you, and I can truly say that they have both been satisfactory in every respect. Your artificial limbs are a combination of lightness, durability, and strength, which makes them superior to any other artificial limb that I have ever seen. I wear a knee-bearing leg. The last one that I purchased from you I took my own measurements, which almost anyone can do by your system. Oct. 22, 1909.

* J. N. McCUTCHEON—Clerk, Hamilton Co., Tenn. Above knee.

I consider your limbs the most simple, durable and comfortable I have ever seen or worn. I have worn one for twenty-four years with not more than $1.50 expense. The rubber foot is the next thing to nature, it protects my stump from sudden jars.
    Oct. 19, 1909.

* MATTHEW B. McGOVERN—Railroad, Levis Co., Quebec. Below knee.

The artificial leg you made for me in 1901 has recently had some repairs. It is now in the pink of condition and giving all round satisfaction. Expect it to last another nine years.
    Feb. 2, 1910.

* ALEX McDONALD—Engineer, Nova Scotia. Below knee.

I am happy to say that I have worn one of your legs for the last ten years. I feel convinced that no better can be made. I have frequently been in the company of people who never sus-

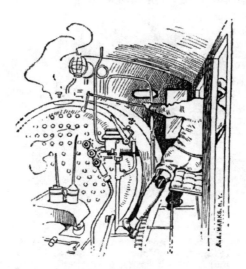

pected that I was wearing an artificial leg. I attend my work every day, which is engine driving. I had my leg taken off five inches above the ankle joint. Oct. 22, 1909.

* A. W. McEWAN—Secretary, South Africa. Above knee.

The artificial limb you so skillfully made for me, to accommodate an amputated thigh two and one-eighth inches from the crotch, has arrived here in good order, and after a fortnight's wear, I am enabled to use the limb with the greatest of ease and comfort. I consider it a wonderful arrangement in every particular, especially noting the easy, noiseless, and reliable knee mechanism, and the delightful natural suppleness of the rubber foot, which gives one a great amount of impetus in walking.

Previous to getting your limb, I had been wearing one with articulating joint at the ankle. I was forced to use two canes to assist me in walking; now I am able to walk with the greatest ease and comfort without canes.

J. H. McFADZEN—Lawyer, New Brunswick, Canada. Above elbow.

The artificial arm I purchased from you while in New York, in 1903, has proved satisfactory. I find it of great assistance, very comfortable, and it has developed the muscles of my arm and side, got them back into their normal and healthy condition, and besides it is of great benefit to my appearance. I have very much pleasure indeed in recommending same, my only regret now is, that I had not purchased it sooner.

My amputation took place twenty years ago, above the elbow. My profession is that of a barrister. On account of the mechanism of the rubber hand, I find no difficulty in holding papers, books, etc. I also find it very useful in driving a horse, carrying a valise, and in fact were it not for the wearing of a glove, it would often be hard to detect the artificial from the real. As I am a bit of a sport, I often engage in lawn tennis, billiards, etc. Oct. 18, 1909.

JAMES A. McDONALD—Westchester Co., N. Y. Both below knee.

Over twenty years ago I met with the misfortune of having both my legs crushed by the railroad cars, which necessitated amputation below the knees. I was then a mere lad, and did not fully realize the gravity of my misfortune.

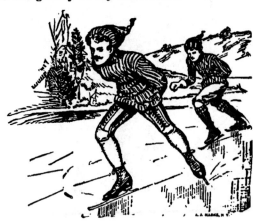

By the advice of my surgeons and others, I placed myself under your care for restoration. Your reputation as the one most competent in the land had so impressed me that, from the first, I felt that I was soon to realize the most that skill and ingenuity could possibly do for me. In this I have not been disappointed, for your labors have restored me to my feet, and I am for all practical purposes, myself again. I well remember how proud I was when your genius placed me in a position in which I could indulge in

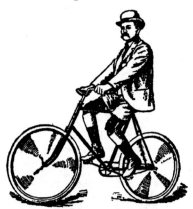

youthful sports, how I availed myself of every advantage, playing ball, boating, fishing and hunting in summer, and skating in winter. I even went so far as to swing my partner, on several occasions, at rural dances. I have always felt that your artificial legs were wonders and ought to be known throughout the land.

My latest fad is that of riding a bicycle. I found the task difficult at first, but I succeeded after repeated attempts, to ride well and to enjoy it.

* CHAS. McDOWELL—Farmer, Oneida Co., N. Y. Above knee.
The several artificial legs I have obtained from you have all
proved satisfactory, they all have lasted an unusual length of time.
I would not have an ankle joint no matter who I had to make my
leg. I can rely on the stiff ankle. The rubber in the foot is of
course necessary and your way of combining it with the mattress
is the thing. I work hard and never think of anything happening
to the leg.   Feb. 10, 1910.

C. D. McGEHEE—Railroad, Henrico Co., Va. Ankle amputation.
In 1890 I was in New York and had you make an artificial leg
for my ankle-joint amputation. I wore it six years with entire
satisfaction, then got another which I am now wearing. I consider the make of your limbs the best in the country. Dec. 21, 1907.

* WM. D. McINTYRE—Painter, Mercer Co., Pa. Below knee.
I purchased an artificial leg of you in August, 1903. I have
done many kinds of hard work since, from cow punching to coal
teaming, have put the artificial limb through what I am positive
no other kind of leg would have stood. I worked for a while as a
pile driver on the coast of Michigan. I was in water waist-deep
many days. The leg seemed to suffer no bad effects from the
soaking. I do not consider that I am handicapped in the least on
account of having lost my natural limb.   Oct. 8, 1909.

* SAMUEL McKEE—Belfast, Ireland. Below knee.
I got an artificial leg from you some time about the end
of June, 1875, and I have been wearing it ever since. I would
like to get another just like it. The limb I have has a rubber
foot for amputation below the knee. It is a pity you have not an
agent here, for there is only one party in this city who makes
artificial legs, and they are not to be compared with yours for
durability, neatness and comfort.

* S. B. McKEE—Lawyer, Alameda Co., Cal. Both below knees.
I take great pleasure in testifying to the merits of your artificial
limbs. I have used them since 1875.
They were fitted from measurements. I have worn them con-
stantly without any trouble. I am by profession a lawyer.
Your legs are the best made.

* VERNE McLAUGHLIN—Telegrapher, Saline Co., Ark. Wrist
   amputation.
I have worn one of your artificial arms since February, 1900, and
during all these eight years I have been a telegraph operator
and station agent. The hand has been tested to its utmost and has
proved itself valuable, useful and satisfactory.   Sept. 9, 1908.

ELLENA R. McLEAN—Teacher, Tolland Co., Conn. Above knee.
I am delighted with my success with the artificial leg you made
for me. Am teaching school every day.   Oct. 15, 1907.

* MRS. JANIE McLEAN—Robeson Co., N. C. Below knee.
I guess you will be somewhat surprised to hear from me. I
have been married two years and I have gotten along fine with
the artificial leg you made for me in 1903. The leg is still in
good condition and I do all my housework, washing, ironing and
sewing. Everyone says that they do not see how I get along so
well.   Dec. 3, 1909.

MIGUEL R. MACARIO—Railroad, Chihuahua, Mexico. Below elbow.

I will soon purchase another arm from you. The one I have been wearing for five years has given me the best of service. I can do most anything with it.   Aug. 25, 1909.

* HECTOR MACFADYEN—Scotland. Above knee.

I had my leg amputated above knee over twenty years ago.

I tried two artificial limbs by other makers for a time, but had to discard them both as unsatisfactory.

I am twelve and one-half stones in weight, and I can walk with ease and comfort with the Marks leg, which I have worn constantly for the last nine months.

It is a perfect fit, and I have every reason to thank Mr. Barstow personally for care and attention.   Feb. 5, 1910.

* JOSE DOMINGUEZ MACHADO—Engineer, E de Minas Gerals,
    Brazil. Below elbow.

The artificial arm I ordered of you gives me the greatest comfort. I want to do all I can to encourage your good work.— Translated from Spanish.   July 9, 1909.

* J. MADDEN—Watchman, New Zealand. Below knee.

My leg was amputated below the knee on August 2, 1887. In the following March I got my first artificial leg with ankle joint, which I wore until April, 1891, when I got one of your celebrated artificial legs with rubber foot, which I am still wearing, now over nineteen years, on an average of sixteen hours a day. During that time its expenses were nil except a little for bushing the knee-bolts, whereas with the ankle-joint leg I was continually putting my hand in my pocket.   Feb. 8, 1910.

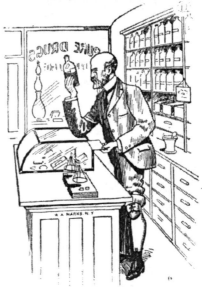

* A. E. MAGOFFIN—Druggist, Shawnee Co., Kas. Below knee.

I was a soldier of the Civil War when I was crippled in 1863, resulting in amputation of left leg below the knee. I immediately ordered a Marks leg, and have worn no other since. I get around very well, and have attended to my drug business for fifty-three years. The legs have given full satisfaction, and I have no desire to change for any other make.   Oct. 19, 1909.

* B. W. MAKKINK—Holland. Above knee amputation.

I received, in best condition, the artificial leg you sent me. It is a great pleasure to write to you of my perfect contentment. Up till this time the three legs I have worn were all of leather and steel, and so I could never make a correction at the spots that hurt my stump or abraded my skin. Now while the socket is of wood, I am able to form the borders just as I find from time to time necessary to prevent pressure. Marching and cycling is much easier than before and I am sure your rubber foot is a great improvement. It is a fact that walking with the rubber foot without ankle articulation is much easier and quicker than when there is an articulation. I am thankful you have helped me so very well, and I shall recommend your work everywhere I can.   June 6, 1912.

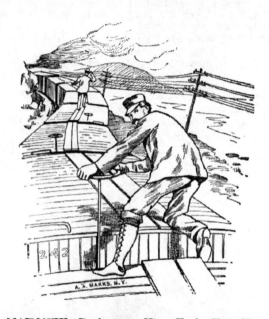

DANIEL MAHONEY—Brakeman, New York City, N. Y. Instep.

I have used one of your artificial legs for the last fifteen years, and found it all right. My foot was taken off at the instep. In my position as a brakeman I can do my work without any trouble whatever.

From my experience in using your leg, I verify all you claim for it.   May 7, 1909.

* WM. O. MAIN—Laborer, Washington Co., R. I. Above knee.

I have worn artificial legs of your make for sixteen years with greatest success.   March 10, 1908.

REV. E. L. MAINES—Clergyman, Wayne Co., N. Y. Below elbow.

A little more than a year ago I had my left arm amputated about five inches below the elbow. Two months and a half later I went to the Marks establishment, in New York, to investigate their artificial limbs. I had been advised to get an all-willow hand, but thinking of the advantages of rubber over willow, I decided to personally investigate the matter, so made a special trip to the city. I am glad to say that so far I have found much comfort in wearing the Marks rubber hand.

* S. L. MANHART—Engineer, Steele Co., Minn. Wrist amputation.
   This is to certify that I have used an artificial hand of A. A. Marks construction for nine years. It has never caused me any discomfort. I have found it very useful in my work. The first year I was employed in a drug store, the second year I was State boiler inspector and continued for four years. Since that time I have been in the retail fuel business and frequently have to load scuttles of coal for old men, women and children who come to my yard for fuel. I can handle the shovel as well with my artificial hand as I could with my natural one.   Oct. 20, 1909.

WILLIAM MANN—Gardener, Montgomery Co., Pa. Both arms.
   I thought I would write and tell you how I am making out with my artificial arms made in 1902. I can get along very nicely. I can eat all right, and can dig garden pretty well, and write this letter with the right rubber hand   Oct. 18, 1909.

* C. A. MANSFIELD—Laborer, Rock Co., Wis. Below knee.
   The artificial leg I am now wearing was made by you in 1905. The doctor took the measurements and you made the leg by them. The leg proved to be a fine fit and I have worn it ever since. In the summer I am working over a hot range all the time and that even don't make it chafe.   Dec. 23, 1908.

* MIGUEL MARINO—Clerk, Cuba. Above knee.
   I received the artificial leg you made for me on the 30th of March. It fits perfectly and I consider it a marvelous piece of work. In four days I could walk without a crutch, cane, or limp. My friends are astonished at my good condition.   April 7, 1910.

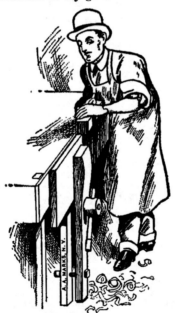

* CALVIN MARSHALL—Carpenter, Lamar Co., Tex. Below elbow.
   I take pleasure in testifying to the satisfaction I have derived from your artificial arm with rubber hand, my arm being amputated about midway between the wrist and elbow.
   I am a carpenter, and can do as much work as ever. Can use my planes and drawing knife to perfection.

EDWARD MARSHALL—New York City. Left leg below knee.

The Spanish-American War was remarkable less for its loss in killed and wounded than for its loss from disease in camp, etc. Yet a number of most astonishing wounds have been placed to its credit or debit in medical histories and reviews. For instance, in one case, a soldier—one of the Rough Riders—was shot in the middle of the outside of the left thigh. The wound of exit was in the middle of the right thigh. The natural supposition of the doctors was that the ball had penetrated both legs. An examination showed them, however, that this was not the case. The ball had entered the left thigh about midway between the knee and the hip. It had gone upward, and then across, through the lower abdomen, and finally downward to a point in the right thigh, almost exactly opposite to the point where it entered the left

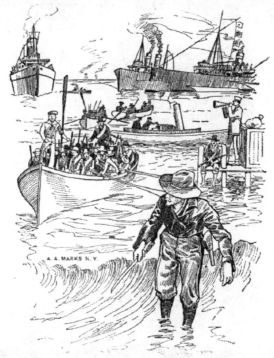

A. A. MARKS N. Y.

thigh, and passed out. Just what influenced the ball to take this course is one of those mysteries that puzzle the doctors.

The Spanish-American War was the first conflict in which small caliber bullets of great velocity were used by both sides. In the Civil War a wound in the lung from a Minie ball was almost certain to prove fatal. In the Spanish-American War with their new small caliber, high velocity Mauser and Krag-Jorgensen bullets, scarcely a single fatality came from a wound in the lungs.

Perhaps as remarkable a case as occurred during the entire war was that of Edward Marshall. Marshall was not a soldier, but a newspaper correspondent; yet, the story of his misfortune and suffering is probably as widely known as that of any soldier in the army.

He was one of the only two correspondents present at the battle of Las Guasimas, the first important land fight in which the army

took part. It will be remembered that only the marines—the
military branch of the navy— were engaged at Guantanamo.
Marshall had landed at Daiquiri with the troops the day before
the march to the front began, and learned that the Rough Riders
were likely to be engaged in battle on the twenty-fourth of June.
He marched the nineteen and a half miles through the jungle to
Siboney with the famous regiment which is so closely identified
with the name of ex-President Theodore Roosevelt, reaching that
strange little collection of Cuban shanties late at night. The next
morning at four o'clock he started to the battlefield with the regiment with which he had cast his lot. It was a fearful climb over
the precipitous hills and along the narrow jungle trails. How
cleverly the Spaniards had gauged the route over which the men
must go, and what a baptism of blood awaited them at the end of
that last trail, are now matters of history—history whose punctua-
tion marks are more than thirty graves in the National Cemetery
at Arlington.

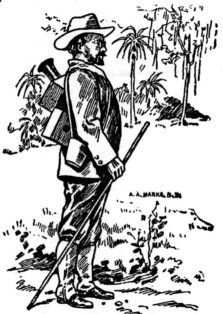

When Marshall started out on that march he was as strong a
man physically as ever had toiled along under a broiling tropical
sun. While many trained soldiers fell by the way, Marshall, a
newspaper man, carrying a burden of equipment, cameras, etc.,
probably much heavier than the kit borne by any soldier, stood
the heat almost without discomfort. Because of his business of
news-gathering he had many times to visit other regiments marching in the same direction, and to continually double back and forth
among the Rough Riders. So he probably covered at least a fourth
more ground that afternoon and night and the following morning
than any unmounted soldier in the army. When the regiment
reached Las Guasimas he was not the least fatigued. After the
regiment had reached the field of battle and he had been for an
hour at work along the firing line and among the dead and wounded
scattered about the field, he still felt no need of rest. But his
activity ceased just before the battle ended. In the advance on the

old Spanish distillery which was the temporary headquarters of the Spanish army, a Mauser bullet hit him in the spine. He fell instantly to the ground. In describing the sensation of being shot, and his later sufferings, we will use Marshall's own words:

"There was no pain as the bullet entered my body. I knew that I had been hit, because I had fallen, and because I had no power to move any part of my body. Legs, arms, fingers, toes—every member was wholly without the possibility of voluntary motion, except my eyes. I was completely paralyzed. The actual sensation of being hit was not a very different one from the sensation that I many times knew as a boy, when in a game I was struck by a base-ball.

"I am told that while four regulars were carrying me off the battlefield many hours later, convulsions seized me from time to

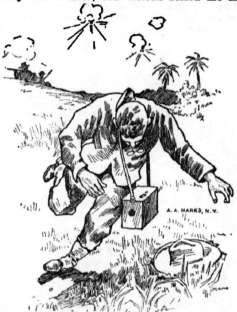

time, but I have no memory of any pain whatever until after they had placed me on the hospital ship 'Olivette.' Then I suffered, and suffered severely. The bullet had hit me in the fifth lumbar vertebra, which is near the base of the spine. If I had been marked for a target the Spaniard who shot me could not have had a chance of striking a more important nerve-center than the one which his bullet found. I have no idea, however, that the man ever saw me, much less took aim at me; for if the bullet had come from close range it would undoubtedly have passed completely through my body and killed me then and there. As it was, it struck this vertebra, and shattered it, passing upward (having been deflected by the bone) and then struck me again between the shoulders. Here again the bone changed its course and the bullet turned downward, finally lodging in the right kidney, where it remains to-day."

After a marvelous operation by the much-maligned army surgeons on board the "Olivette," Marshall was taken to New York four or five weeks later. That he reached there alive was the marvel of physicians and surgeons in all sections of the United States and Europe, and was the topic of many articles in medical journals.

For seven months he lay in St. Luke's Hospital, New York, completely paralyzed below the knees and partially affected above. Gradually, however, all signs of paralysis left him above the knees. Still, his doctors held out no hope that he would ever be able to walk. When he finally left the hospital it was necessary for him to be carried by two attendants. This state of almost complete helplessness lasted for a long time. His right leg regained some of its strength, but the nerves controlling the front muscles of the lower left leg (the tibialis anticus) were completely dead. Their support of vitality had been completely cut off by the bullet which came so near ending Marshall's life. This made it impossible for him to keep his foot from drooping or falling down. His right leg finally recovered sufficiently so that he could essay a few steps on crutches, but the dragging of the left foot made it impossible for him to do more than a few steps at a time.

Among the artists who contributed pictures to Mr. Marshall's book on the Spanish-American War was W. Frazee Strunz, well

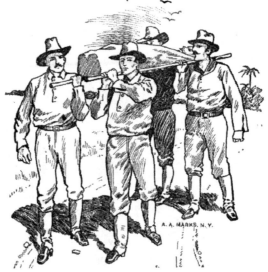

known as an illustrator. Mr. Strunz and Mr. Marshall had been associated in their professions for many years. Mr. Marshall, however, did not know that his friend and co-worker had ever met with an accident. He spoke to Strunz one night about the possibility of having that troublesome left foot amputated.

"If you do that," said Strunz, "we shall be in the same class."

"What do you mean by that?" inquired Marshall, who knew that Strunz had been celebrated as a baseball player and sprinter among the athletic set in the Quartier Latin, in Paris, when he was there as an art student, and who was familiar with the man's intense physical activity in New York. This activity went so far as climbing scene painters' scaffoldings, when he was engaged in scenic work a dozen times a day; in running up and downstairs to a studio located on the fifth floor of a building without an elevator, in long walks and in sprinting races.

"Why, didn't you know I had a wooden leg?" Strunz asked.

Marshall scarcely believed him until he proved his statement by showing the artificial limb. Strunz had his limb cut off in a railway accident when he was a child of eight. The conversation ended in Marshall's decision to see the people who had succeeded in giving his friend so perfect a substitute for a lost leg, on which he could walk without limping, run, and climb stairs and ladders with ease.

The firm which had supplied Strunz with his artificial leg was A. A. Marks, of 701 Broadway, New York, whose place of business

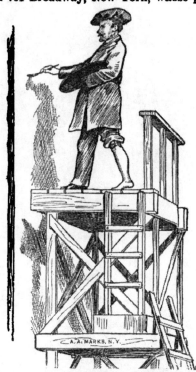

was not very far from where Marshall lived. A telephone message brought Mr. Marks himself around to Mr. Marshall's house the next morning. Upon examination, Mr. Marks found that there was no immediate necessity for amputation. Marshall's only anxiety for an amputation was that he was impeded in walking on account of the foot drooping so inconveniently. After a moment's thought Mr. Marks said he believed he could devise a scheme that would enable Mr. Marshall to walk, even if he could not properly hold up his toes.

"I shall put your foot in a sling," he said.

He did so.

He made an ingenious contrivance of straps and loops which were put on in such a way as to hold the front of the foot at the proper angle.

From that moment it became possible for Mr. Marshall to resume newspaper work. The fact that his legs were paralyzed of course made it necessary for him to use crutches, but still—he got around very conveniently. How well this contrivance served him is shown by the fact that he was enabled by it to travel with no other companions than his secretary, whom he would have taken with him in any event. He dispensed with the services of the strong valet whom his drooping foot had for months made necessary. He went nearly all over the United States on a lecturing tour and in the pursuit of his professional duties, and, in May, less than a year after he had been so terribly wounded, this broken-backed journalist sailed across the ocean and acted as the representative of the S. S. McClure Literary Syndicate at the Hague Peace Conference. His physical capacity to get around in this manner he was always

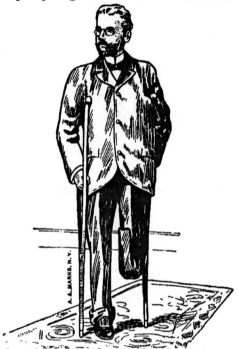

willing to acknowledge was due to Mr. Marks' happy thought of "putting his foot in a sling."

After Mr. Marshall's return to America the condition of his left leg became steadily worse, and finally, after gangrene had set in and had done its deadly work, amputation of the leg at about the calf was performed. The tissues of the stump were, of course, paralyzed, and the doctors said they did not believe Mr. Marshall would be able to wear an artificial leg in less than a year. Indeed, it was predicted that he would be in the hospital for at least three months as the result of the complication. The same vitality which had enabled him to live through his terrible Cuban experience, pulled him through again, and he returned to his desk at the offices of the S. S. McClure Company within three weeks. Not more than six weeks later Mr. Marshall stopped in to see Mr. Marks, the man who had " put his foot in a sling." Mr. Marks thoroughly understood the fact that to put an artificial leg on a paralyzed stump is a ticklish thing to do, for the paralyzed tissues, being without sensation, give no warning to their owner if injury occurred to the stump. He volunteered the belief, however, that he could make an artificial limb which should be so carefully adjusted and fitting so perfectly that there could be no possibility of injury. After consultation, Dr. Cyrus Edson, who was Mr. Marshall's physician, advised a trial.

It took Mr. Marks exactly one week to complete the artificial

limb. Marshall tried it and found it to fit perfectly. Again he
was able to go about. Again he was able to get along without
the arms of an attendant always at his shoulders. It must be
understood that the partially paralyzed condition of his other, or
right leg, had made it impossible for him to walk with two crutches
after the amputation. He had used a crutch on his left side, but
he had to be supported by an attendant on his right side.

Since the day that Mr. Marshall put on his artificial leg, no man
has been more actively engaged in journalistic work—and certainly
no field of human endeavor requires greater physical activity. He
became Sunday editor of the New York *Herald* in a few weeks,

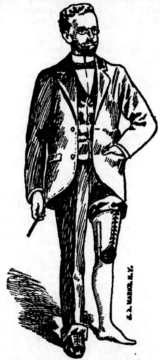

and has, since leaving that post, engaged in many enterprises
involving much traveling and physical activity,

Following is a letter which he wrote Mr. Marks not long ago
without solicitation:

My Dear Mr. Marks:

I am going away for a time and shall need some supplies. I
cannot tell you what a comfort that artificial limb has been to me.
You know that my right leg is still paralyzed from the knee down,
and that it is still somewhat beyond my control. Such is not the
case, however with the leg made by you. I can handle it almost as
well as I handle the one God made for me, and I am afraid that I
make it do far more than its fair share of work. Sometimes I
almost wish that it may be necessary to amputate the right leg, as
I can certainly handle the left one much better than I can the one
which is still flesh and blood. Very sincerely yours,

EDWARD MARSHALL.

The difficulties that were present in Mr. Marshall's case were the
partial paralysis of the motor nerves and the total paralysis of the

sensory nerves, resulting in the absence of sensation in the stump and a complication of infirmities in the opposite leg.

The artificial leg made for him was constructed upon the model of cut E 17, illustrated above. This model has a rubber foot and is suitable for short and long stumps, as well as those of medium length, as shown in the accompanying cuts.

J. W. MARSHALL—Office Work, Lauderdale Co., Miss. Below knee.

I have worn one of your artificial legs nearly ten years and find it gives satisfaction in every particular. I lost my leg in May, 1899, amputation six inches below the knee which left my limb very sensitive in front but this sensitive place is fully protected by your leg. I would not wear any other leg. My position is that of check clerk and this keeps me on my feet from morning till night.   Oct. 21, 1909.

* E. T. MARTIN—Chile, S. A. Below knee.

The fit is perfect and my son is able to use the leg with the greatest comfort.

My son begs me to tender you his most earnest and heartfelt thanks for the blessing that you have been the means of rendering to him.

J. S. MARTIN—Marion Co., S. C. Knee bearing.

I have been wearing one of your artificial legs since July, 1905, and find it satisfactory. I wear the leg without straps and use it from early morning until ten or eleven o'clock at night.

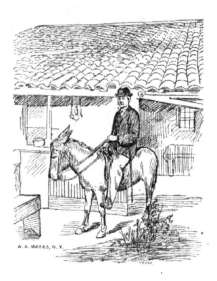

* ANTONIO PINTO MARTINO—Merchant, Natal, Rio G. del Norte,
    Brazil. Above knee.

You have permission to print my testimonial in your books as I can utter none too favorable words for the work you have done for me.

My right leg is amputated above the knee. You fitted me from measurements. I get about in a very natural manner, attend to my business, I mount and dismount my donkey and ride perfectly well. Enclosed find my photograph.   Oct. 7, 1909.

* U. E. MAST—Druggist, Lagrange Co., Indiana. Below knee.

I purchased my first artificial leg from you in 1892 and wore it every day for eleven years. My only expense in that time for repairs was $1.88. In 1903, I purchased my second limb of you which I have worn every day since without one cent of repairs or expense. My business is druggist and jeweler and I do a great deal of walking. I can easily carry two large pails of water

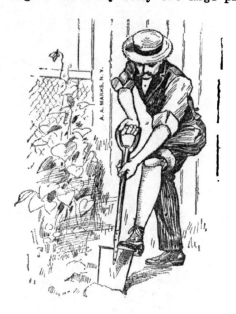

up or downstairs, spade my garden, split wood, climb a ladder, carrying fifty pounds on my shoulder. In fact I can do nearly any kind of work. The Marks limb is the best I have ever seen.

* CAMPO E. MATEUS—Chester Co., Pa. Above knee.

Having had the misfortune to lose a leg during the last civil war in Colombia, S. A., I have been using one of your artificial legs for six years. Indeed I will tell you that I am very much pleased with it. I walk without cane because I don't need it. I have written to some of my friends who have lost legs in the same war, recommending your house as the best.   Dec. 10, 1908.

* THE HON. L. MAUR—Judge, Germany. Above knee.

While at the University from 1870-1872, I suffered the amputation of my left thigh, the nerves and end of bone were insufficiently covered. Until 1894 I used the product of a local firm, which was made of leather and steel, weighing some six kilograms, with knee and ankle joints. The weight and clumsiness of this machine made it a heavy burden. This annoyance was ended by your leg. I received two from 1894-1896, which I hope to use for many years. I have never seen a better limb. The simplicity and durability of its construction recommend your limb and I repeat my sincere thanks to you.—Translated from German.   Oct. 28, 1909.

* H. N. MAYO, M.D.—Salt Lake City, Utah.

I applied one of your legs to Mr. Prongos to-day and everything to a detail was satisfactory. Thanking you for your prompt attention and care with my order.   Feb. 24, 1908.

JOHN MATTHEWS—Street Sweeper, Westchester Co., N. Y.

I bought an artificial leg of you in 1866. I wore the same until 1888, then I obtained a new one which I am now wearing. Two artificial limbs in forty-four years with practially no repairs, certainly reflects credit to the work that you do. I have always been a general utility man, have scraped the streets, shoveled,

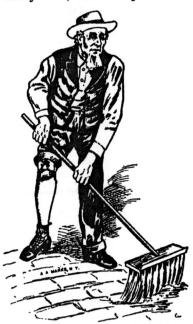

used a pick-ax, blasted rock, and carried articles of heavy weight, in fact have always been occupied with a kind of work that would put the artificial limb to the severest tests. You are at liberty to refer to me.   April 12, 1910.

* M. G. MELL—Grain Dealer, Grady Co., Okla. Ankle joint.

I don't know how to express my gratitude to you for the good you have done me in making my artificial foot. A foot without fault.

I have lived in this vicinity over seven years and very few know that I wear an artificial foot. My testimonial cannot be too strong in recommending the A. A. Marks artificial feet.   Oct. 23, 1909.

J. W. MERSHON—Undertaker, Lackawanna Co., Pa. Below knee.

The leg I got of you seven years ago is all right. I never have any trouble with it. I have worn your legs for forty years and always with comfort and satisfaction. I wore one ten years with no repairs to speak of. I have worked ten hours a day for years making furniture and undertaking.   Oct. 20, 1909.

J. W. METCALF, M.D.—Brooklyn, N. Y.

Refer to me as to the merits of the Marks limbs.

MRS. F. J. MICHAUD—Quebec. Shortened leg.

My daughter, when a child, was afflicted with hip-joint disease which left one leg shorter than the other.

The shoe which you arranged for her has made walking much easier and less tiresome. She walks with scarcely a limp. It has now been worn seven years.   Oct. 16, 1909.

* B. J. MILAM, M.D.—Macon Co., Mo.

The artificial leg you made for Mrs. Geiselman in June, 1894, has done her good service. She has worn the leg every day, doing all her own housework. She says she would not take $1,000 and do without it. She is well pleased in every respect. Oct. 18, 1909.

* N. MILDENSTEIN—Lubeck, Germany. Below elbow.

In regard to the artificial hand I got of you fourteen years ago, I can say it exceeds my expectations.

If I were compelled to work for my living the rubber hand would be of great use in any occupation. I recommend the rubber limbs to anyone who has become crippled. Oct. 29, 1909.

* ED. J. MILES—Eaton Co., Mich.

I am much pleased with the artificial leg you made for me. It is entirely satisfactory—could not do without it.

A. MILLER—Machinist, Oneida Co., N. Y. Below knee.

Several years ago my foot was amputated just above the ankle. I tried different limbs with ankle movement, and found them unsatisfactory. Have worn one of your artificial limbs for thirteen years, and am still wearing it with comfort and satisfaction. My occupation is one in which I am obliged to do a great deal of walking. Oct. 15, 1909.

ARTHUR J. MILLER—Glasgow, Scotland. Hip joint amputation.

The artificial leg with pelvic socket for hip joint amputation you made for me in 1905 is giving the utmost satisfaction. Sept. 1, 1909.

* FRANK MILLER—Driver, Cook Co., Ill. Above knee.

I had my leg amputated in 1883 on account of disease. In September, 1891, I ordered an artificial leg from you. You made it from measurement I had made at home and sent to you. The leg was received promptly and fitted acceptably. I wore it continuously for twelve years, during which time it did a great amount of hard work, and I walked long distances. I was so well pleased with the leg that in April, 1903, I ordered another of you, which I am now wearing in the most satisfactory way. Oct. 24, 1904.

* LON. MILLER—Ohio Co., Ky. Below knee.

My son has been wearing an artificial foot of your make since August, 1901. It has given perfect satisfaction, and a great many people can't tell he has an artificial foot. We are glad we got one of your make.

* ROBERT MILLIGAN—Rancher, Alberta, Canada. Wrist joint.

I purchased from you an artificial arm eight years ago which has given me the greatest satisfaction. June 3, 1909.

* CHAS. L. MILLS—Laborer, Aroostook Co., Me. Below knee.

I wish to drop you a few lines regarding your wonderful invention. I received the artificial leg you made for me from measurements about a year ago. I never expected anything could be manufactured that would so completely meet the demands. In three weeks after I got your leg I was able to go to work as well as anyone and walk as far. I have had a great many of my old friends come up and speak to me and wonder at the marvelous work your leg has done. A short time ago a friend of mine wanted me to go to the woods with him. I had not been in the woods for three years before, but I went and I found that I could go through the woods the same as he could. April 2, 1910.

LOUIS MINET—New York City, N. Y. Ankle amputation.

I am very well pleased with the foot I got from you for my son in 1902, when six years old, and find it very complete and satisfactory. The boy enjoys play with it like the rest of the boys. Oct. 20, 1909.

* AUGUST B. MODENBACH—Erie Co., N. Y. Both below knees.

I have never met with a person who could walk as well as I can, who has had both legs amputated and wearing artificial ones. There are few who believe that I'm amputated as I am. I never use a cane unless I go a great distance. I am pulling overshoes in a shoe factory and stand from 7 in the morning until 5 in the afternoon, then I go to lectures three times a week. These artificial legs have now been in use over ten years and they are still in good condition. A year ago I took the first prize at a masquerade ball. I impersonated "The Lone Fisherman," and engaged in the dances and my crippled condition was never disclosed.   Jan. 23 1910.

* PEROSHAW B. R. MODY—Manager, India. Below elbow.

It affords me great pleasure to add my testimonial to the long list you already have.

In June, 1902, I had the misfortune to lose my left arm three inches below the elbow, on account of blood poisoning. Shortly after I forwarded to you the measurements for one of your artificial arms, which arrived in due time, and which I am wearing regularly since, and am glad to say has given me great comfort and satisfaction.

My occupation is that of manager of a joint stock company, and I find the arm a great help in my duties.   Dec. 13, 1909.

GEORGE MOEHN—Plumber, Brooklyn, N. Y. Above knee.

In the year 1901 I fractured my leg, and had it amputated. I have two friends with Marks legs who surprised me by their good walking. This caused me to have Marks make me one, five weeks after the amputation. I am satisfied that I could not have done better. My stump is only six inches long, and my friends are surprised when they see me walking along the streets. Oct. 16, 1909.

* LOUIS MOHLFELDT—Farmer, Lewis Co., Mo. Above knee.

I desire to state that your artificial limbs are what they are represented. Have had two of them and consider them the best. Would recommend anyone wishing a limb to use yours. Oct. 21, 1909.

* RIGOBERTO A. MONDACA—Valparaiso, Chile. Below knee.

I have the pleasure to inform you that the last artificial leg you made for me fits me perfectly. It is so comfortable that it would be very difficult for me to enter any complaint.

As you will remember it is the third artificial leg you have manufactured for me, and I have enjoyed the benefits of your skill so much that I have absolute confidence in your ability. Every time I have ordered a new leg from you it appears to have been better than the former one.

As I am now it would be difficult to distinguish which is the lame leg and which is the natural. I would recommend anybody who has been so unfortunate to lose their limbs to try one of your manufacture; it will be sure to give them complete satisfaction.   Dec. 29, 1909.

* MRS. NELLIE MONTAGUE—New Zealand. Hip amputation.

The artificial leg you made for me was received and is found to be a splendid fit. I am able to walk admirably.   Nov. 21, 1907.

MRS. MOORE—Brooklyn, N. Y.

My boy Christopher, aged twelve, obtained an artificial leg for thigh amputation from you and is using it nicely and goes to school every day and walks back and forth, which is a good distance from home. He doesn't use a cane. He is as happy as he can be. He was playing football Saturday and played as rough as any of the boys. I will highly recommend you to anyone, and if you wish to send anyone here to interview my boy, I will be glad to have you do so.   Nov. 25, 1907.

* ARTHUR MOORE—Tinsmith, New Zealand. Below knee.

The leg I received from you is giving me great satisfaction. It is amputated below the knee. I find I can get about well. I walk two miles every morning and return at night. I go out at night without feeling the least exhaustion. I am a tinsmith by trade, and work without trouble.

* FRANCIS M. MOORE—Ford Co., Kas. Above knee.

On the 18th of September, 1903, I received the artificial leg that I ordered from measurements, to take the place of the limb I lost on account of varicose veins in 1889. You will thus see that fourteen years elapsed since the amputation and the application of an artificial leg. I get around very well, my only regret is that I did not get the leg long before. Going about so many years on crutches got me into habits, and a peculiar way of carrying my stump that has occasioned me some little trouble, which, however, is disappearing gradually. If I had obtained my leg six months after the amputation I am sure I would to-day be walking as well as any person in possession of their natural legs. As it is, I would not take anything for the artificial leg, it is a source of great comfort, relief, and help to me.   Oct. 24, 1909.

* FELICIAMO de LEON MORALES—Telegrapher, Guatemala. Above knee.

Thirteen years ago I received an artificial leg from you. It has been of great use to me. The leg is well constructed. Although warranted for five years it has already lasted more than twice that and I believe will last for a good many more years. I feel it a public duty in making this fact known. March 12, 1910.

* THOMAS MORAN—Worcester Co., Mass. Above knee.

In 1907 you constructed an artificial leg for me. I have had no trouble with it whatever. I hardly realize that I am using one. My stump is above the knee, only six inches from the body. I shall be pleased to communicate with anyone looking for information pertaining to artificial limbs.

Meeting a young lady the other day, she kept looking at me. Finally she said, "I have been looking at your nether limbs for some time, as I saw in the paper that one of them had been amputated. Did you really lose one? You certainly do not look like one who had." I told her I did, but had an artificial limb made by A. A. Marks, of New York. "Well," said she, "Mr. Marks must be a grand man to imitate nature so perfectly. He deserves the homage of all." To elicit such comments—and they are made frequently—shows how well you have succeeded in overcoming obstacles which appear almost insurmountable in your field of endeavor.   Feb. 11, 1908.

* FRANCISCO SOLERNO MOREIRA—Soldier, Brazil. Below knee.

In 1897, as ensign of the 39th battalion of infantry of the Invincible Brazilian Army, composed of heroes and giants, I received a bullet wound in the joint of my right foot in battle, which necessitated the amputation of the leg a little below the knee. I had no thought or hope of a further military career. I graduated from the military school at Ocara, with every promise of a successful and brilliant career, but alas, the injury I received in the battle shattered my hopes, and left me almost without ambition. In my most bitter moments of depression, I chanced to get possession of your descriptive catalogue. After looking it over very carefully, I procured from you an artificial leg. I have had it now five years. I walk with such perfection that only my most intimate friends, those who are acquainted with my affliction, know that one of my limbs is artificial. My good friend and illustrious benefactor of suffering humanity, accept my thanks for the perfection of the apparatus you have given me, which has permitted me to resume the military duties which I so love. Of the various limbs which I have seen, French, German and English, those of your make are the most perfect.—Translated from Portuguese.

BYRON MORFOOT—Printer, Erie Co., Ohio. Below knee.

The artificial leg you made for me is still in use. I have worn it continually now for fourteen years and have not spent fifty cents for repairs on it. I consider a Marks leg the only one manufactured that will fill the requirements. I have traveled in every state and territory, over mountains and in fact all kinds of places, and the leg has never failed me once. I will do all I can for your firm.   April 18, 1910.

* F. MORGADO—Machinist, Vera Cruz, Mexico. Below knee.

It is with pleasure I inform you that the artificial leg I ordered of you in 1904 for Alberto Paredes, amputation below the knee, for which I took and sent you measurements and diagrams, has been received and worn with perfect satisfaction. The limb is so perfect and well finished that in less than ten days after putting it on Mr. Paredes returned to his work, the same that he was engaged in before amputation. The work is very hard, as he is foreman of the loading of steamers in the bay. Every time Paredes meets me he repeats his gratitude for having told him about your house. He says that the only way he could be improved is to have his natural leg back again. The leg you made and sent to him fits perfectly.

In regard to the artificial leg you made for me in 1902, I take pleasure in saying that I use it constantly. I am also engaged in hard work, I am a machinist. The leg will undoubtedly last many years longer. In regard to perfection and workmanship, I sent a voluntary testimonial some months ago, and the thought expressed in the same is repeated now.—Translated from Spanish.
                                              Oct. 23, 1909.

* J. H. MORGAN—Laborer, Columbia Co., Ga. Below knee.

I am now using my second artificial limb purchased from you.

I was working in the R. R. yard at Waycross, Ga., when the accident happened which necessitated the amputation of my left foot, about midway between knee and ankle. I commenced using my first artificial limb in December, 1896, using it continuously until February, 1904. I am now using my second limb with entire satisfaction, it fits perfectly. I can see no room for improvement.
                                              Oct. 20, 1909.

* THOS. H. MORGAN—Porter, Philadelphia, Pa. Below elbow.

I wish to express my appreciation for the hand you made me in 1895. It has and is giving excellent satisfaction.   May 6, 1909.

* EDWARD E. MORRIS—Clerk, Oneida Co., N. Y.—Above knee.

I am wearing the leg you made for me in 1904 every day and would not be without it. The leg is still in fine shape. It gives me great pleasure to show my leg to anyone who is thinking of getting one.   Nov. 21, 1907.

* MURDOCK MORRISON—Cape Breton, Nova Scotia. Below elbow.

I purchased an artificial arm from your firm in January, 1904, and may say that it gave entire satisfaction.   Feb. 29, 1908.

PERLEY N. MUDGETT—Farmer, Lamoille Co., Vt. Above knee.

My artificial leg works nicely. It enables me to get about my farm, and do considerable work. It is much better than the one I had with an ankle joint; it is easier for the stump and more comfortable in walking.   Oct. 19, 1909.

* KEVORK MUNCHERIAN—Missionary, Turkey.　Below knee.
THE ARMENIAN MASSACRE—An artificial leg sold into captivity.

It seems to be the strange order of things that, periodically the world is to witness scenes of exceptional horror.　Christians are fed to lions in the Colosseum; or in shirts of tar, burned like candles to illuminate the gardens of a Roman Emperor.　A French Revolu-

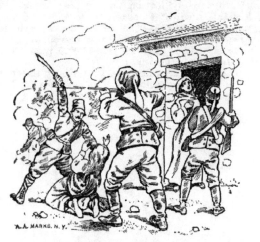

tion with its guillotine and "days of terror" deluges a land in blood; and, in our own day, in the full blaze of the nineteenth century, the most shocking of all appears in the Armenian massacres.

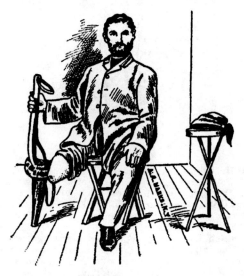

For six hundred years the Armenians were the most submissive servants of the Ottoman Empire, and the most prosperous of the non-Mohammedan races, Christians and Jews, who paid tribute as a penalty for not accepting Islam.

The accession of the present Sultan marked a change in their condition. He had not been long on the throne before a constantly increasing series of oppressions were begun.

The reason for this course of action is not hard to seek.

Sultan Abdul Hamid lost Bulgaria, a valuable part of his dominion, because of its prosperity and spread of European ideas of liberty, and European civilization among the people. Fearing he would lose Armenia also, if it became as enlightened as Bulgaria; and, giving "fear of rebellion" as an excuse, he entered on that course of persecution beginning with a merciless taxation, and ending with the slaughter of more than 30,000 persons, under circumstances of incredible horror.

Among those who, while escaping with life, "suffered the loss of all things," is a native missionary, the Rev. Kevork Muncherian.

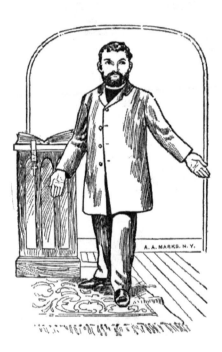

Having lost his right leg by reason of a snake bite, he managed to get about on a peg leg of local manufacture for a number of years, when through the kindness of a brother missionary, he procured an artificial leg from A. A. Marks, of New York, which he used with great comfort and assistance in his missionary labors.

Mr. Muncherian writes:

"The leg which I got from you nine years ago was very satisfactory, and I wore it with comfort for seven years, but during the massacre two years ago my house was burned, and all my possessions carried off by the Turkish soldiers.

"Among other things, they took my artificial leg, and sold it into captivity. Since that time, after having been saved from death in a wonderful way, I have been obliged to use my old wooden peg leg.

"Although I am a native of Marash, Turkey, for ten years I had been living and engaged in business in the small town of Anderin, preaching the Christian gospel in a little church on Sundays, and

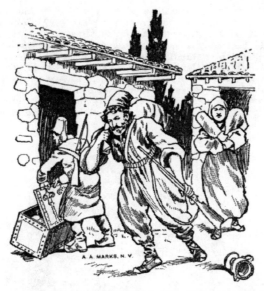

occupying my spare moments in the interest of the Christian faith. At the time of the massacre my wife and children were in Marash, while I was in Anderin. The greater number of the inhabitants of Anderin are Moslems. At the time of the massacre I had fifty liras ($220) worth of goods in my shop, and 100 liras ($440) worth of

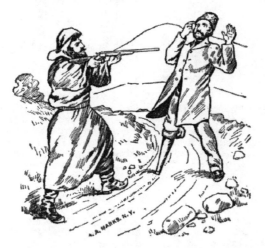

wheat, barley, corn, and other grains. All of these were carried off by Moslem robbers in the course of a few days; on several occasions I barely escaped death. Suddenly one day without any warning a company of Armenians from Zeitoon, having tired of Turkish oppression and tyranny, made an attack on the town, and after a short but sharp contest took possession, and proceeded to plunder the houses of the Moslems, and to kill all the Turks they could lay their hands on.

"In that terrible scene, the way in which I was saved was wonderful; when I came out from my place of hiding those that caught sight of me mistook me for a Moslem and attempted to kill me, and I escaped only by crying out, 'I am a Christian, I am a Christian,' at the same time making the sign of the cross.

"I was in greatest danger when spied by a Gregorian monk. I made the sign of the cross just in time to escape being pierced by a bullet which he was about to fire at me.

"The goods and grain I have already mentioned, and also the artificial leg I got from you, had been stolen by the Moslems.

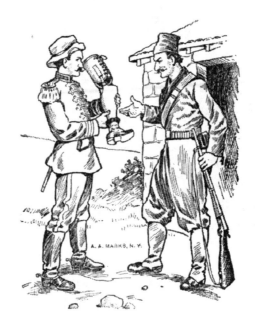

"Having lost everything, saving only my life, I joined the Armenians when they were leaving the place, and that night, hungry and destitute, I traveled a large part of the way on foot and peg leg to the village Geben, five hours distant. The third day after my arrival I happened to see my artificial leg, which the Armenians had brought with them. The Turks had thrown it away as a thing of no possible use, and so it had been picked up and brought to Geben by the Armenians. Just at this time the Osmanli army attacked Geben, and I was forced to flee to Zeitoon; my journey lasted fifteen hours, and was through a wild, mountainous country. I had to walk most of the way on my antiquated peg leg; the journey would not have been half as arduous if I had had my artificial leg instead of this crude peg affair.

"According to investigations I made afterwards, the leg I left in Geben was captured by the Osmanli soldiers, and sent as a prisoner to the headquarters of the army corps, and there sold and held into captivity.

"A few days after my arrival in Zeitoon, the Turkish army made an attack on the town. On the third day of the conflict I climbed up a steep mountain and hid in a cave, sheltered by a great rock. I stayed in this cave without food or water for three days and nights, after which I went back to Zeitoon. There I got on a horse with the intention of riding up to the Turkish lines to see if I could get through to Marash, to my home and family; but no sooner had I set out from the town (two miles from the Turkish lines) than the Turkish soldiers began to rain bullets on me. I succeeded in reaching the outworks of the defences of Zeitoon, but could go no further so I turned back to re-enter Zeitoon, still under a murderous fire, but praise God not one of the bullets hit me. I was obliged to remain about three months in besieged Zeitoon, in the midst of a terrible and continuous battle—without a cent,

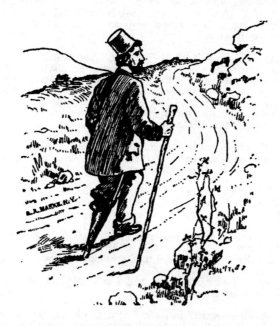

hungry, and in great sorrow and fear. Finally, through the mediation of the great powers the war ceased, Zeitoon was saved, and I returned to my native city, Marash. As soon as I reached the site of my home I found that during my absence one of my little girls had been killed, all my household furniture was stolen, and my house burned down.

"Since those terrible times I have been working in this and surrounding villages, under the direction of missionaries of the American Board, as a relief agent and preacher, at a salary of $5.28 a month, while my wife is engaged in Marash at a salary of $3.52; you will thus see that we have to live in a most economical and exceedingly uncomfortable way. I hope to receive my new leg, when I will be in better shape to work and travel.

"Yours sincerely,
"KEVORK MUNCHERIAN,
Armenian Missionary."

* MRS. C. W. MUNDEN—Calcutta, India. Above knee.

I have worn a Marks artificial leg for twelve years. I wore an English made one before that. My experience with both has taught me that the Marks leg is far better. I shall always speak highly of it. I shall always be pleased to recommend your legs to anyone requiring them.   March 24, 1910.

* MRS. MARY MUNELLY—Essex Co., N. J. Below knee.

I am very much pleased with the artificial leg you made for me ten years ago. I go around and do not use any cane and the leg is still in good condition, although it has seen ten years of hard service. You are at liberty to use this letter any time you see fit.   Jan. 27, 1910.

* HUGH W. MUNSON—Student, Dixon Co., Neb. Below knee.

My leg works fine. I would not have an ankle joint of any kind now. I outran two fellows lately that did not know I had an artificial leg. Your limbs are and shall always be highly recommended by me.   Jan. 9, 1908.

* WILLIAM MURDOCK—New Zealand. Above knee.

Seventeen years ago my leg was amputated above the knee, and I got an artificial leg. It did not turn out suitable, so ten years ago I forwarded measurements to you for one of your legs. I am glad to say this has proved in every way satisfactory. The rubber foot with spring mattress in particular being very comfortable—there not being the slightest jar when walking.

* WALTER MUSE—Laborer, Sumter Co., Ga. Below knee.

Have been wearing your artificial leg since I got it and I am glad to say that it pleases me very much.   Nov. 25, 1907.

* A .M. MYERS—Teacher, Lee Co., Va. Below knee.

With pleasure I endorse your rubber foot. My leg is amputated below the knee, and I have worn one of your artificial limbs over six years.

I was fitted from measurements, and I find the leg to be in every particular what you represented. I am a teacher, and am on my feet a great deal. I can run, jump, and skip almost as if I had two natural feet.

I have walked as high as ten miles in a day. I have not had to pay out one cent for repairs.   Oct. 19, 1909.

E. A. NELLIS—Sheriff, Litchfield Co., Conn. Below knee.

In 1864 I lost my leg by amputation below the knee. In 1865 I procured, as I supposed, one of the best artificial legs in use, the wearing of which gave me much pain, and I was often obliged to go back on crutches until the irritated and swollen stump was again in condition to wear the leg. It also annoyed me very much by frequent rattling at the ankle joint. Repair bills were from $6 to $8 a year. I was oblged to use a cane when walking. I wore this leg about two years. I met a great many wearing artificial legs made by various firms, all of whom were laboring under difficulties similar to my own. I think it was in 1867 or 1868, while in Watertown, N. Y., I met a gentleman wearing one of your artificial legs with rubber foot. I was surprised to see this man go up and downstairs actually on a run. He also moved about among the guests at the hotel noiselessly and quietly, with the grace and ease of natural motion; he advised me to get one of your artificial legs with rubber foot. I at once wrote to you, requesting you to send me instructions and blanks for taking measurements.

I received a prompt reply, and ordered a leg. I have worn your legs constantly from the time I first received one, never having lost an hour's time from its use.

I go up and downstairs, up and downhill, through the brush, hunting and fishing. In fact, I go when and where I please with ease and comfort.

ROBT. NEWBERY—Mechanic, Brooklyn, N. Y. Below knee.

It gives me pleasure to tell you that the artificial leg you made for me six years ago last June is as good as ever. I work twelve hours a day at hard work. Your limb cannot be beat for workmanship and material. I am seventy years old.   Oct. 18, 1909.

* GEORGE NEWMAN—Barber, Chase Co., Kas. Ankle amputation.

I was hurt thirteen years ago, run over by railroad cars, which caused amputation at ankle joint of right leg. Have worn your artificial limb ever since, and am doing well. I don't think there is any other that can beat it. I have worn it with comfort, and strangers can't tell the difference, or which foot is off. I am a barber by trade, and have to be on my feet frequently half a night around my chair, and walk a mile every day from shop to home, besides that I ride horseback every day. Couldn't get along without your rubber foot.   Oct. 20, 1909.

* BENJAMIN J. NICKERSON—Laborer, Harris Co., Texas. Both below knees.

The pair of artificial legs you made for me in 1886 is still in use. They have certainly done good work for me and I have taken pains to show their merits to others in need of limbs.
          Dec. 23, 1907.

* SYDNEY NICHOLLS—Tunnel Worker, England. Above knee.

I am very much pleased to say that I have been a wearer of the Marks artificial leg for the past eleven years, and I for one can speak as regards its success as a leg. It has had nothing done to it in the way of repairs since I have had it. I can walk twenty miles on it with comfort and without feeling any bad effects.
          July 23, 1908.

* MRS. BERTHA NICHOLS—Clay Co., Neb. Below knee.

I am glad to say that I am well pleased with the artificial leg. I have worn it a great many years and do my own housework and walk a great deal. I ride horseback, dance and ride a bicycle.
          Jan. 15, 1908.

* MRS. THOS. NICHOLSON—Skagit Co., Wash. Below elbow.

I want a new arm and I want it made as much like the old one as possible. I am still wearing the arm made for me sixteen years ago, and I cannot do without it, but will order a new one for fear that I may not be able to wear the former one much longer. It never gave me any trouble. I have five children and I do all my own housework, and the artificial arm helps me wonderfully in every way.   Nov. 20, 1906.

R. J. NIDDRIE, M.D.—Simcoe Co., Ontario.

When considering the question of artificial limbs, you may be sure that with me it is "Marks" first, last and all the time. You have furnished my patients in the most skillful way, always giving the best of results.   Oct. 19, 1909.

* MRS. J. A. NILSON—Sweden. Below knee.

I am a little over fifty years of age. I lost my leg below the knee some years ago. Everybody thinks I am a wonder that knows that I am wearing a leg. I can walk and carry as much as I please, and I have had the leg on now every day for fifteen years. I handle it perfectly.   May 27, 1906.

* EDWARD NOONAN—Operator, Dubuque Co., Iowa. Below elbow.
If you look over your books you will find I purchased one of
your artificial arms over four years ago. I have been using it every

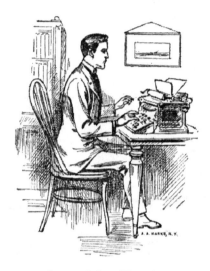

day since on a typewriter and handling from 350 to 500 messages
daily. To say I am satisfied with the arm is putting it mildly.
Dec. 18, 1908.

* MRS. H. E. NOORDUYN-CHURCHILL—Holland, Europe. Above
knee.
At last I am able to send you a photograph of my son and I am
sure you will be pleased at his appearance with your artificial leg.
He wears the leg constantly and it is remarkable how quickly he
has gotten used to it.   May 6, 1909.

* A. NOSEWORTHY—Fisherman, Newfoundland. Above knee.
I had my leg amputated in February, 1902. I purchased one of
your artificial legs in 1903. Since then I get around with ease
and comfort and I never use a stick and have never stumbled.
I find the rubber foot and knee joint to work perfectly. I am
a fisherman and can get about in a boat with very little difficulty.
Nov. 2, 1909.

* A. OGLESBEE—Screven Co., Ga. Right arm above elbow.
It gives me great pleasure to add my testimonial to the long list
of those who are using your artificial limbs. Two years ago I
had the misfortune to have my right arm cut off above the elbow
in a cotton gin. When I sent for an arm I had very little faith in
my ability to use it. However, since I have worn your arm I find
myself able to perform nearly all the work that is necessary to
be done on the farm. I can drive, plow, or hoe, with very little
inconvenience, and I certainly consider that in my case your limb
has been a Godsend.

* MIGUEL PEREZ ORTIZ—Tinsmith, Mayaguez, Porto Rico. Below knee and below elbow.
I wish to inform you that I am very much pleased with your
invention, as the leg and arm you made for me have and are
both giving the greatest satisfaction. I use both in a very natural
way and feel very much indebted to you.   Jan. 24, 1908.

JACOB ORKEN—Washington, D. C. Above knee.

I have received the artificial leg in good condition and am well pleased with the knee joint; it works naturally and perfectly.

I have worn for the last twelve years several other makes, but I have come to the conclusion that yours is the best of all.

People are surprised at how well I walk, they cannot tell that I have an artificial leg. Have always used a cane, but with your leg I have no occasion to use one.　　　　Jan. 25, 1910.

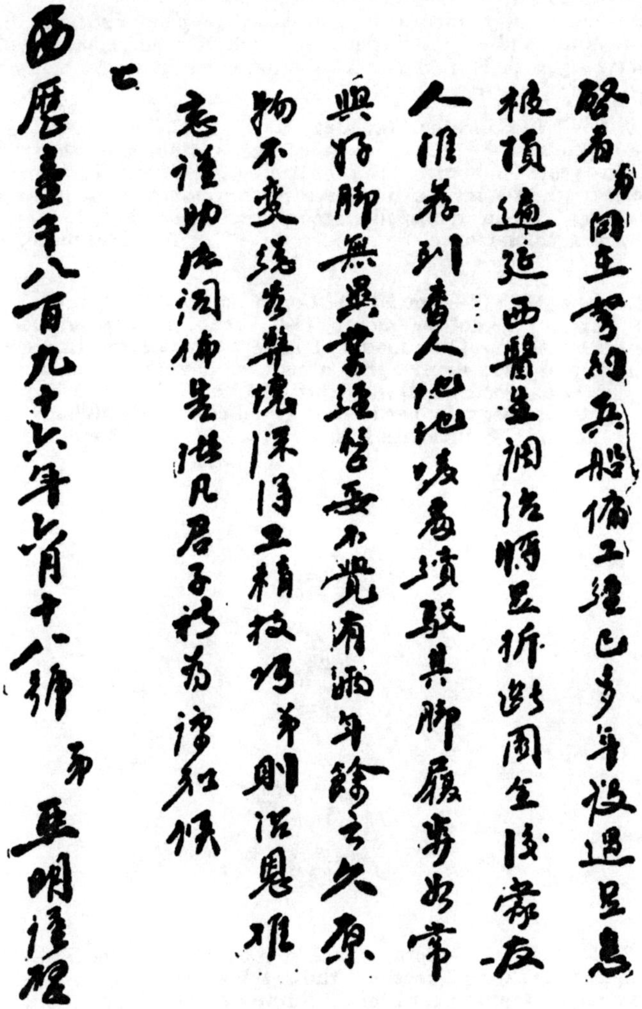

啓者 為同至雪的兵船備工理已多年後過呈惠
被頃遍延西醫生調治惜呈折斷周全後密友
人谁若到貴人地也岌為惧致其脚履步如常
興好脚無異業運営垂不覚有淌年餘玄久原
物不变送当荤塊深得工精技巧弟則洸恩難
忘谨此洞佈芳惟凡君子行為诸知候

西歴壹千八百九十六年七月十八日
亜明隆煜

* HIS EXCELLENCY THE COUNT OKUMA OF JAPAN—Waseda, Tokio, Japan. Above knee.

I am desired by His Excellency Count Okuma to inform you that the artificial leg which you made for him reached here some time ago in good condition. The Count is exceedingly gratified with the admirable workmanship of the leg.　　　　T. KATO.

HARRY P. OSBORN—Stenographer, Essex Co., N. J. Below knee.
I have been wearing legs made by you for over eighteen years and would wear no other as no other leg would give satisfaction.
Both of my feet were deformed from birth. At the age of eight years it became necessary to amputate my right foot about six inches above the ankle. A few months later I received one of your legs and have never missed a day wearing it from early morning until late at night.   Nov. 2, 1909.

V. C. OVERTON, M.D.—Jefferson Co., Texas.
I can cheerfully and willingly say that your artificial limbs have no equal and all the patients that I have recommended you to are perfectly satisfied; in fact I have never had a single complaint.
                                                          Oct. 15, 1909.

* J. C. OWEN—Collector, Jamaica, B. W. I. Below knee.
The artificial leg received from you some time ago when I was fourteen years old gives me entire satisfaction. My work is collector and this makes it necessary for me to do a great deal of walking. I can truthfully recommend your legs to anybody requiring artificial ones.   March 13, 1909.

* SUSANO S. ORTIZ—San Miguel Co., N. Mex. Below knee.
The leg you made for me in 1899 has given me satisfaction. I know it is the best leg made. I have worn it every day since I bought it and have never spent a cent on having it repaired, and to-day it is as good as new. I will be very glad to recommend your leg to anybody in need, and if you know of anybody, refer him to me and I will write him.   Sept. 22, 1913.

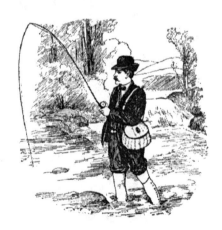

* LESLIE PALMER—Clerk, Franklin Co., Me. Above knee.
In December, 1902, I received the artificial leg you made for me, it was just seven weeks after the amputation. I applied the leg the day it arrived, and it has not been off my stump since except at night. I am able to dance, which I enjoy very much. I do not use a cane, and have walked five miles on one stretch. The limb has been perfectly satisfactory, and I am able to stand the strain of an athletic life in Maine with great enjoyment, such as hunting, brook fishing, and mountain climbing.

* H. PACKER—Farmer, New Zealand. Below knee.

I received the leg and am very well satisfied with it. I can get about splendidly. I do almost the same sort of work I used to do.

When I lost my leg I never thought I would be able to get about very well again, but I. find that I can get about as well as ever I could. All my friends tell me that I have gotten on wonderfully well. I have had every satisfaction and I think I have given it a good trial as I have had it eight years and have done some very rough work in a very rough country. I build fences, cut firewood, and work in the gravel pit, and also shear sheep. Dec. 14, 1909.

WM. H. PALMER—Hampden Co., Mass. Both below knees.

I see in your catalogue that there are many feats which persons on pairs of artificial limbs are able to perform. I have been wearing a pair of yours for nearly eleven years and I stand to-day ready to challenge any man who is amputated the same as I am to run a train of cars as I do when they are going twenty-five or thirty miles an hour. I have done this and can prove it right here. July 28, 1908.

* A. F. PANKNIN, M.D.—Charleston Co., S. C.

The pair of artificial legs you made for Mr. Grooms some years ago have suited him admirably. He paid me a visit about a month ago, walking all the distance (about a mile) with only the aid of a cane. I don't think he could have had a more satisfactory fit. You made the legs from measurements that I sent you, and Grooms did not leave his home.

* MRS. MILDRED M. PARLIN—Kennebec Co., Me. Knee joint.

I have worn an artificial leg of your make since 1903, thigh amputation. I have been doing the greater part of the housework on a farm for my family of five. Oct. 21, 1909.

MANUEL A. PARRAGA—San Salvador, C. A. Above knee.

It is nineteen years since I obtained an artificial leg from you. During this period I have not had an opportunity to find the least fault with it. I walk very much, and without a cane or support. I suffer no pain or uneasiness.

Since I have returned to Central America I find it necessary to make long journeys on horseback. In this the leg has assisted me very much. I pride myself on my easy and graceful movements, and the facility with which I mount and dismount.

The India-rubber foot is a most excellent invention; without it I question my ability to walk with safety in this country, the streets are so very rough and stony.

* GEO. H. PARREN—Laborer, Norfolk Co., Mass. Knee joint.

My leg is standing it very good; I got it from you in 1891. I do a great deal of walking and work very hard. All I need now is a new set of suspenders and the leg will doubtless last me a great many years longer. Oct. 11, 1909.

* G. E. PARSONS—Time Keeper, Shannon Co., Mo. Wrist amp.

The artificial hand purchased from you six years ago is in perfect repair, and has given all the satisfaction promised by you.

I find it especially helpful in my office work, in telegraphing, handling books, papers, etc. Jan. 27, 1910.

* AMBROSE Z. PARVIN—Tailor, Lancaster Co., Pa. Below knee.

The first artificial leg I bought of you was in 1894 and the second in 1906. I would not wish a better one. They are strong, light, and I can always depend upon them. I know of many around here wearing the complicated kind and I walk much better than any one of them.

D. J. PATTERSON—Worcester Co., Mass. Below elbow.
The artificial arm that I received from you in 1903 is all that I expected. I have worn it every day, and find it a great help.
Jan. 22, 1909.

* FRANK R. PATTERSON—Tel. Operator, Blair Co., Pa. Ankle-joint amputation.
I received the new foot and have been wearing it all the time since. It fits O. K. and seems to be satisfactory in every way.
March 9, 1909.

* FRED H. PAUL—Dentist, Hamburg, Germany. Ankle amputat'n.
I am to-day, as I have always been, convinced of the excellence of your appliances. I shall certainly never wear any other kind than yours. I have worn one since 1897 and have up to the present time never found the slightest cause for complaint.   Nov. 11, 1909.

* W. E. PAWSON—Porter, Wellington, New Zealand.   Knee.
As the result of an accident I lost my right leg in the knee joint. I have had four years' experience of wearing one of your artificial limbs, and have no hesitation in saying that they are unsurpassed. I may state that I could not have been better fitted had I been measured and fitted in New York personally. I have not once had occasion to leave the limb off on account of soreness of any kind whatever, and consequently do not feel the loss of my own limb to the extent I at first thought.
The rubber foot is the invention of the age, being every bit as flexible as the human foot. In ascending hills it affords every facility. In fact, my friends express surprise at the easy manner with which I negotiate this task; but the rubber foot does it all. I am quite satisfied. I have recommended several to you for limbs, and have no hesitation in doing so, as I feel sure I am doing the right thing in their best interests.

* PEDRO G. PAZ—Honduras, Central America. Below elbow.
About a year ago I received an artificial arm which you made for me. It has turned out so well that I do not miss the natural one. Please accept my thanks for your meritorious work.
May 14, 1908.

* YSIDRO PENAFIEL—Student, Cumberland Co., Me. Below elbow.
I recognize the good results of your artificial limbs. I have been using one of your artificial arms for now two years, and it has given me perfect satisfaction and it is still in perfect condition.
Dec. 12, 1908.

* ADOLFO PEREZ—Zacualtipan, Mexico. Above knee.
I beg to say the leg you made me is much more satisfactory than the one I used before. I can walk perfectly with it, although the ground is very uneven here. I feel very grateful to you, as all should be who have been relieved by you as I have been, after so much suffering. Translated from Spanish.

* JOAQUIN PEREZ—Railroad Employee, Uruguay. Above knee.
Recognizing the value of the artificial limbs invented by you, especially the leg you sent me, I am pleased to state that I wear it every day without any difficulty, although the stump is only three inches in length below the body. I feel grateful to you for having enabled me to walk naturally again.—Translated from Spanish.

ROBERT H. PERRY—Painter, Hudson Co., N. J. Above knee.

I am still wearing the leg you furnished eighteen years ago. I have worn it comfortably with less than six dollars cost for repairs. My occupation (house painter) gives it a good test. I can

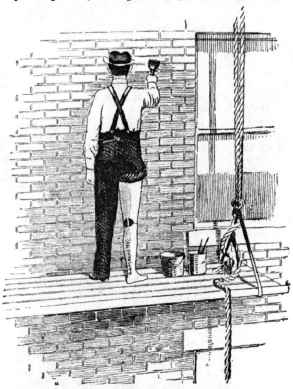

and do work on scaffolds, ladders—in fact, anywhere. I have but a three-inch stump. I am well satisfied.   Oct. 16, 1909.

* AUGUST PETERSON—Kane Co., Ill. Below elbow.

I am the boy who got an artificial arm from you four years ago, and I am well pleased with it.   Jan. 29, 1908.

* H. E. PERKINS—Truckman, Oxford Co., Me. Below knee.

I am a truckman. Have worn artificial limbs for seventeen years. I consider your artificial limbs superior to others. I find I can walk as fast as anyone who has two good feet.   Oct. 18, 1909.

* ALICE PFOHL—South Africa. Below knee.

You may think me ungrateful for not acknowledging the receipt of the leg, and letting you know how I am getting on with it. I received the leg a few days before Christmas, and have been wearing it ever since, and am glad to say it gives me every satisfaction, both in comfort and efficiency.

E. F. PHILLIPS, M.D.—Schuylkill Co., Pa.

Allow me to congratulate you on the perfect fit you have made for Mr. Jacob Ball, whose measurements and diagrams I took and sent you for an artificial leg. The people here who do not know that he lost a limb have not detected it in his walking. Mr. Ball is certainly a walking advertisement for you.

* J. B. PHILLIPS—Tools, Contra Costa Co., Cal. Above elbow.
    The artificial arm, above elbow amputation, fits and works perfectly. My brother put it on as soon as it came and has not had it off since. He has found many uses for it and would not be without it. You may refer anyone to me or to him.
                                                    March 21, 1908.

* RAFAEL MARINO PINTO—Merchant, Bogota, Colombia. Above
    knee.
    I have been using the artificial leg which I obtained of you in 1904 through Dr. Alejandro Herrera of this city, and I take pleasure in manifesting to you that I am completely satisfied with it, as it has turned out so well I can manage it with the greatest ease and amongst a great many in this city wearing artificial limbs I believe I walk the best.   Nov. 24, 1909.

* JOHN PITTMAN—Farmer, Scott Co., Ark. Below knee.
    It affords me great pleasure to add my testimonial to the great number of letters you receive. I bought a leg style E-17. It has the rubber foot with spring mattress. It is satisfactory in every way. I ride horseback, can mount and dismount with as great ease as I formerly did.   Aug. 17, 1909.

* S. M. PLATT—Chittenden Co., Vt. Below knee.
    I have now one of your legs, I think, eighteen years. It has not cost me $1.00 for repairs. I give you a good recommend.
                                                    Nov. 8, 1907.

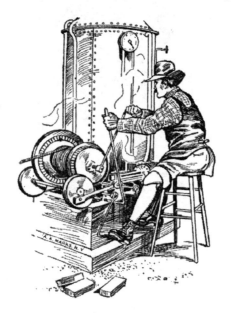

HOMER F. PORTER—New Haven Co., Conn. Above knee.
    I have been employed by the R. R. as a hoisting engineer for the past year.
    I have to work two brakes, one with my artificial limb and one with my natural, and also two levers with my hands. I have to climb a sixty-foot pole every morning. I do my own firing and all the work about the engine room.

* A. S. POTTER, M.D.—Parry Sound, Ontario.
Dennis is using the arm you made for him on his farm, brushing, logging, plowing, etc.; has found it very satisfactory and a perfect fit.   June 8, 1908.

* ERIC A. A. POTTER—Hairdresser, New Zealand. Above knee.
I received the artificial leg you made for me about six years ago, and have had no trouble in walking about with ease and comfort.
I have seen several makes of artificial legs, and I consider the "Marks" with the patent rubber foot the best. I take much pleasure in recommending the "Marks."   Dec. 9, 1909.

J. DENSMORE POTTER, M.D.—Onondaga Co., N. Y.
Mrs. K. E. Cardner's leg works to a charm. She can get about without even a walking-cane, on the Marks leg. She does her housework without any difficulty.

* REV. J. WESLEY POTTER—Perry Co., Pa. Above elbow.
I purchased an arm for right humerus amputation in September, 1906. If I could not have another I would not sell this one at any price. I never thought it would be so helpful to me.   May 5, 1908.

WM. POTTS—Window Dresser, Quebec, Can. Above knee.
As for myself I have never looked back since I purchased the leg. You warned me not to wear it longer than two hours at a stretch at the beginning, but as a matter of fact I have worn it every day since the deal several months ago from 7 a. m till 11:30 p. m., sometimes into the next morning. I am following my daily work which is window dressing and attend to sales during the day.   March 15, 1910.

C. W. POWELL—Bookkeeper, Missoula Co., Mont. Above knee.
I would say that I have worn an artificial leg made by your firm for eight years. My leg was amputated above the knee and since wearing your limb I have experienced no difficulty in getting about and attending to business. Wearing the leg is attended with no discomfort, and I would be pleased to recommend your house to persons so afflicted as to need your services.   Oct. 19, 1909.

* W. O. POWELL—Farmer, Clarke Co., Wash. Below knee.
You constructed an artificial leg for me in 1891 and another in 1899.
You will thus see that for nineteen years I have only had two artificial legs and when I need a new one it will be from you, as I feel that my experience with your work would compel me to continue my patronage with you.   Dec. 4, 1909.

* CHARLES PRICE—Hotel Keeper, Galveston Co., Texas. Partial foot.
The artificial leg you made for me is a perfect fit and I walk without a cane and without the slightest limp. I have worn several limbs made by other companies, but none of them gave me the satisfaction that yours does.   Dec. 12, 1908.

* E. T. PRINTZ, M.D.—Appanoose Co., Iowa. Below knee.
The artificial leg you recently made from measurements for me is very satisfactory. I like it very much and do my work as well as ever. I run my automobile, using the artificial foot to manage the foot brake.   March 31, 1910.

* MISS MARION BLANCHE PRINCE—Teacher, Newfoundland.
Wrist amputation.

Nearly ten years ago I had to have my left arm amputated.
It affords me great pleasure to state that having obtained one
of your artificial hands, I am more than pleased with the results.
It is all that can be desired.

The rubber hand is indeed something to be proud of, and enables me, as a school teacher, to handle all the work with ease.

I would not be without it for anything.   Oct. 29, 1909.

* JAMES W. PRITCHETT—Saw Filer, Gibson Co., Ind. Above knee.

I have to say that the artificial leg you made me from measurements fits as perfectly as possible.

If I had come to the shop and you had taken the measurements
yourself, I doubt that results would have been better.

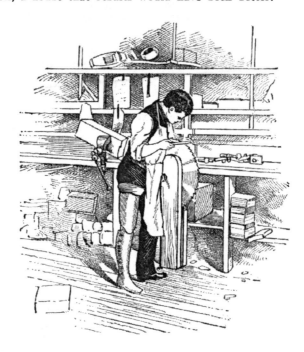

I have worn it for about eight years. I put it on the next day
after I got it, and have worn it every day since, from early in the
morning until late at night. My occupation is circular and band
saw filer; I keep up all the saws for a large circular and band sawmill. I have to be on my feet most all day. I get around almost
anywhere without a stick. As to the rubber foot, I think it is the
finest thing out. It does not jar me when I make a misstep. I
only have six inches of a stump, and I get around better than
others I see that have worn other makes of legs.

* CARL PROHL—New Zealand. Ankle amputation.

I had my foot taken off at the ankle joint when I was seven
years of age, when I reached the age of nineteen I had an artificial
foot made by you. Ever since then I have had every satisfaction
with it. I can ride a bike, and have done some very heavy work
with it.

* GEORGE H. PURCHASE—Student, Billings Co., N. D. Below elbow.

I think my arm in every particular is a grand success, and I will always be pleased to speak in its praise to my fellow-unfortunates. No doubt you will be greatly surprised to know that I wrote this entire letter and addressed envelope with my artificial

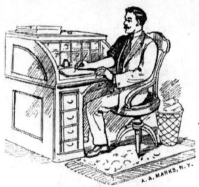

hand. I think if you will compare this with former letters of mine you will pronounce this the best writing. Oct. 30, 1909.

* GEO. W. PURDY—Lighthouse Keeper, Dukes Co., Mass. Shoulder joint amputation.

In reference to the artificial arm I purchased of you seven years ago, I wish to state that I have found it extremely useful. I used to be a sailor on board a steamship, but now I am a lighthouse keeper. I can do anything that is required of men and without the arm I could not fill the position. I use the hand in carrying oil up to the tower, it aids me in filling the lamp. I use the arm when I paint and I do considerable of that. I also use it in pushing a wheel-barrow. Remember this lighthouse is not a bug-light, it is one of the first lights on the coast, first order, the one everyone depends on in making into Vineyard Sound. Oct. 18, 1900.

SAMUEL RAPP, M.D.—New York City. Below elbow.

I well know that Edward Wiley, who is now absent, is satisfied with his hand; he is able to drive a team of horses, and do other farm work.

* W. B. L. REAGAN—Farmer, Monroe Co., Tenn. Above knee.

I am delighted with the ease with which I walk on the artificial leg you made for me. I can handle it so much better than I could the old one. Sept. 24, 1908.

* A M. REDDING—Salt Lake Co., Utah. Below knee.

The leg I purchased from you in December, 1898, has proved entirely satisfactory. It is in good condition, and I've never had one cent expense with it. I was only sixteen years old when I began wearing your leg, and having grown considerably since, the leg has been lengthened to meet this growth. Sept. 3, 1907.

W. S. REDDY—Notary Public, Montreal, Can. Both legs at knees.

I wish to express to you my heartfelt thanks for the comfort I experience in the new pair of artificial legs. They are certainly a credit to your noble firm, one that has done so much to relieve the afflicted and sore-distressed. Dec. 12, 1908.

FRANK REED—Freight Agent, Allegheny Co., Pa. Partial hand.

I purchased a hand for partial hand amputation from you some years ago and I find everything satisfactory. Jan. 30, 1908.

* MRS. CLEMENT QUINN—Wright Co., Quebec. Above knee.

Having worn one of your artificial legs, with a rubber foot, for the past thirteen months, I take pleasure in letting you know how well I am getting along. My stump is a little over six

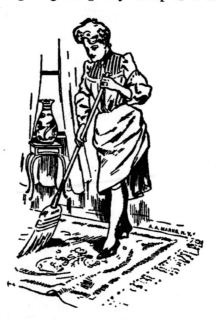

inches from the body. (Amputation caused by tuberculosis in the knee joint.) I can walk without the aid of a cane and do all my housework.

* GEO. H. REID—Coal Miner, Perry Co., Ohio. Below knee.

In 1901 I began to wear one of your artificial legs. Your make is far above all others that I have ever seen. It does not get out of order and is reliable.   Feb. 28, 1908.

* WARD REID—Fireman, Northumberland Co., Nova Scotia, Can. Above and below knee.

The pair of artificial legs, one for amputation above the knee and the other for amputation below, which you made for me nine years ago, have been worn right along. They have given me great service and benefit. I have been acting as fireman on board a steam boat for the last two summers.   Sept. 30, 1907.

* C. A. REIDER—Lawyer, Wayne Co., Ohio. Above knee.

My artificial leg is now over three years old. It has given me great satisfaction. I take pleasure in giving you a good recommendation.   May 20, 1909.

F. E. REINWALD—Farmer, Tioga Co., Pa. Shortened leg.

Having worn an appliance for a deformed limb since last fall, I can positively assure all my unfortunate friends that they do not comprehend the advantages of an artificial limb until they have used one of yours.

Since I have worn the appliance I can get around much better and do more work, and meet the demands of my vocation much better than before.

* JOSE MONGE REYES—Lawyer, Costa Rica. Above elbow.

I have the pleasure of stating that immediately after having sent you the measurements for my left arm, amputated two inches below the shoulder, I received from you in the month of January, an artificial one, which fits me perfectly well, and served me up till now without any repairs at all. By reason of my occupation necessitating my frequent appearance in public places, I can fully appreciate what a boon your work is doing to humanity.

A. E. RICHARDSON—Mechanic, Tolland Co., Conn. Instep amp.

I take great comfort in wearing the foot you made me in 1903. I could not be without it a day. I can walk any distance without the least discomfort.   Oct. 27, 1909.

* JOAQUIN RICALO—Teacher, Oriente, Cuba. Knee bearing.

The artificial leg manufactured by you and which I have been wearing since 1885 is superior to any other appliance I have ever seen. I am never tired of recommending your estimable firm to persons who may have had the misfortune to lose any of their members.   Feb. 18, 1909.

* CYRUS RIDENOUR—Shoemaker, Washington Co., Md. Below knee.

I am wearing your artificial leg every day, and I get along very well. I don't think there is any other leg made as good as the rubber foot leg. I am a shoemaker by trade, but can do all kinds of laboring. I can plow, dig, saw and cut wood, and in fact everything that is to be done on a country farm.   Oct. 18, 1909.

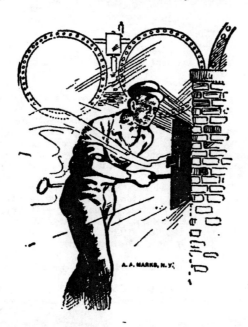

* H. D. RINEHART—Fireman, Lewis Co., W. Va. Below elbow.

I received my artificial arm in good condition, and am much pleased with the rubber hand. My arm is amputated three and one-half inches below the elbow. I am a fireman stationed in the mill. I can perform my work all right. I would not do without my arm.

* GEORGE RISDON—Beadle Co., S. Dak. Both insteps.

I am very much pleased with my feet; I walk first rate with them. Last week I walked from Huron out to my farm, a distance

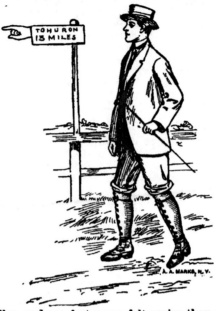

of thirteen miles, and my feet never felt easier than when I got to the end of my journey.

* C. H. RIST—Farmer, Erath Co., Tex. Above knee.

About nine years ago, I got one of your artificial limbs, and have been wearing it all that time. It fits just splendid, and is so easy to wear I can't praise your limbs too highly. I recommend them to all who are in need of them. They are the best artificial limbs in the market. That I might have a reserve leg in case of an accident, I got a new one five years ago, and have worn it enough to know that it cannot be beat. It fits perfectly in every way, and is very easy to wear.   Oct. 25, 1909.

* VICENTE RIVERA—Winchman, Chile. Above knee.

The artificial leg for amputation above the knee you made for me last fall was promptly received. I have worn it from the start with the greatest of satisfaction. I walk better and much lighter than I ever did with the leg I obtained from France. I shall certainly tell everyone in need of an artificial limb the excellence of your invention.   Feb. 28, 1910.

DAN. E. ROBINSON—Merchant, Otsego Co., New York. Both below knees.

I am still wearing the pair of artificial legs I got from you seventeen years ago. I weigh 185 pounds and use the legs continually.
                              June 4, 1908.

* W. A. ROCK—Engineer, Madison Co., La. Below elbow.

Eleven years ago I lost my right hand, one month later I purchased of you an artificial hand, which I have worn constantly for nine years. The work performed by this hand is of the most severe kind, being an engineer in charge of an oil mill, doing all kinds of repairing, etc. The hand is valuable far beyond any estimate I could put on it.   Oct. 19, 1908.

K. SAIGO—Japanese Legation, Washington, D. C.   Below knee.

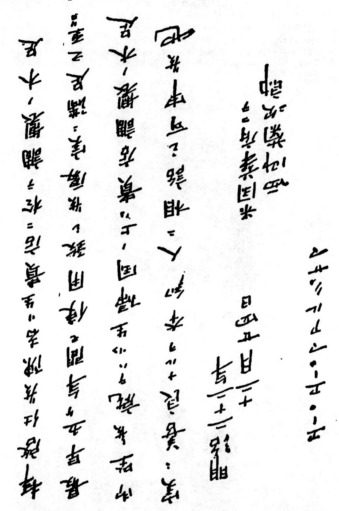

Translation.   I have worn an artificial leg with rubber foot made by you for the past five years, and assure you it has given me the best of satisfaction.   I heartily recommend your work.   I shall gladly speak well of it to all my countrymen afflicted as I am, when I return to Japan.

* S. J. SAVERINSKI—Tailor, Winona Co., Minn.   Above knee.
Having worn one of your artificial legs since 1887 I have no hesitation in saying it is the best leg in use.   It is simple and durable.   April 15, 1909.

LEWIS A. SAYRE, M.D.—New York.
I have had frequent occasion to apply A. A. Marks most valuable Patent Artificial Leg, in cases where I have unfortunately been compelled to mutilate my patients by amputation, and the admir-

able imitation which that substitute has given of the original limb, and the perfect satisfaction to the wearer, is the highest possible commendation that I can give it.

JOHN SCHARFF—Newsboy, Westchester Co., N. Y. Ankle amp.

I sell morning papers on the R. R. trains, get on and off while the train is in motion, and wear one of your rubber feet; very few of my friends know of the fact, and those who do regard me as the

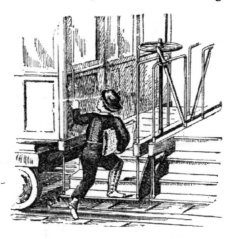

possessor of a remarkable foot. I experience no inconvenience; I heartily recommend your leg as the best made.

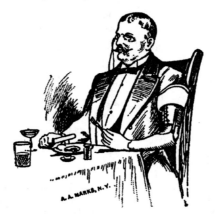

* A. B. SCOTT—Railroading, New Brunswick. Below elbow.

I purchased an artificial arm from you over seven years ago, and up to the present time it has proved a perfect success. It is a help to me in many ways. If I had not had it, I could not have done near as much work on the farm as I have, and feel greatly obliged to you for the prompt attention that you have given to me, and will always work in your interest. I take pleasure in recommending your work to others, and hope that if you publish this letter it will have some effect in influencing persons in need of artificial limbs to patronize you.   Oct. 25, 1909.

VALENTINE SCHICK—Farmer, Sullivan Co., N. Y. Knee bearing.

I am wearing one of your knee-bearing legs with comfort and satisfaction. I can do all farm work. December, 1904, I lost my house by fire. The next spring I built a new one. I climbed all over the scaffold and a forty foot ladder. Always paint the house myself, which is quite a job. I will recommend your limbs to anyone that is in need of any.   Oct. 20, 1909.

* **HEINRICH SCHLENZ**—Saddler, Espirito-Santo, Brazil. Hip-joint amputation.

In April last I received a leg made by you especially designed for a hip-joint amputation. I am pleased with it. Your limb is well manufactured and cannot be excelled. I assure you I will recommend your house with pleasure when opportunity affords.
                                                June 25, 1909.

* **A. J. SCOTT**—Farmer, Caddo Co., La. Below elbow.

I am very well pleased with your hand. It is a great deal of help to me. I use a fork to advantage in eating. Dec. 15, 1909.

* **ROBERT SCHELDON**—Clerk, Lehigh Co., Pa. Below elbow.

My rubber hand is very satisfactory. I work ever day, and frequently drive fast horses, and ride my bicycle.   Oct. 16, 1909,

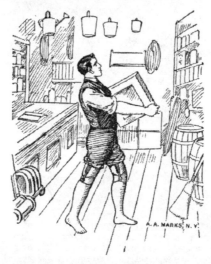

* **E. B. S——** Store, Arapahoe Co., Col. Both below knees.

I received my artificial legs July 31st, and put them on at once. Wore them that evening and all the following day, working in the store from six o'clock in the morning until ten o'clock at night. I must say that I am well pleased with them. The fittings are as good as could be made under any circumstances. My limbs are lighter than I expected, as I wrote you in ordering them that I wanted them extra strong, as my work was heavy.

LOUIS W. SELIG—Albany Co., N.Y. Knee Joint Amputation, age 13.

It is with great satisfaction that I write you, it is just one month to-day that I began to wear the artificial leg you made for me, should I be in need of my crutch or cane, I would not be able to find them, as I do not know where I placed them a month ago, since your leg came. I think your leg is the best substitute for the natural leg in the market. I have learned to ride a bicycle and next winter I expect to go skating.   June 15, 1910.

I. L. SECOR—Farmer, Bradford Co., Pa. Below knee.

Nine years ago you fitted an artificial leg to me, which I have worn continuously with perfect satisfaction. Feb. 8, 1909.

GEORGE SHAFER—Farmer, Bergen Co., N. J. Below knee.

My left leg was amputated about six inches below the knee. Your leg suits me very well.

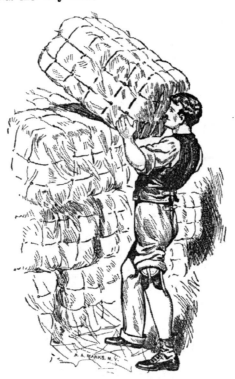

I can do most anything a farmer is required to do, plow, cultivate, and help in a feed store, carrying anything that comes in bags, and store away a carload of hay in one day, bales weighing from 130 to 160 pounds, and pile them up six feet high. There is a great improvement in the last foot which is now seven years ago.   Oct. 19, 1909.

* MISS ELLA C. SHANNON—Housekeeper, Coffey Co., Kas. Wrist.

About eight months ago I purchased an artificial hand of Marks. I have worn it ever since, and think it is fine. I would not be without it for anything. I am a young housekeeper, and find my hand a great aid in helping me with my work. I can write with my hand and can carry many small things.

* J. E. SHANNON—Store Keeper, Telfair Co., Ga. Below elbow.

The artificial arm I bought of your four years ago has given me entire satisfaction.   Feb. 14, 1908.

P. L. SHANNON—Farmer, Spottsylvania Co., Va. Knee amputation.

Have received one of your artificial limbs and have worn it constantly. It gives entire satisfaction in every particular. I can do any kind of work connected with the farm. I have not used cane or crutch since I began wearing it six years ago. Oct. 18, 1909,

* **JAMES W. SHAW**—Teacher, Ozark Co., Mo. Above knee.

I am thinking that you would like to know my opinion of your ability as a manufacturer of artificial limbs, and my appreciation of the leg purchased of you in 1900. I have worn the leg ever since I received it. I walk well, and without a stick or crutch. I am highly pleased with the leg, and expect to purchase another from you when necessary. The leg seems to be solid, and full of vim yet. Oct. 21, 1909.

* **LEO G. SHELBY**—Laborer, Bernalillo Co., N. M. Below elbow.

The artificial arm you made for me ten years ago has given perfect satisfaction. I still wear it. Jan. 1, 1908.

* **JOHN SHIELDS**—Wire Weaver, Australia. Below knee.

The artificial limb you supplied for me is giving every satisfaction. With other makes I used to have blisters on my stump, causing much pain, as well as inconvenience, especially in hot weather. It is a great comfort. I wish you every success in the completion of patched up humanity, as we say here. Dec. 5, 1909.

* **PAUL E. SHIPP**—Farmer, Fayette Co., Ky. Knee amputation.

My leg is off at the knee with patella on end. The artificial limb you made for me in 1902 has given satisfaction. I walk without a limp. Have never used a cane or crutch. Sept. 16, 1907.

* **J. G. SHIRK**—Laborer, Dickinson Co., Kas. Below knee.

The limb fits me all right. I have been wearing it ever since 1870, am getting old, but get along good. Do all kinds of farm work. Would recommend them to anyone in need of limbs. Nov. 5, 1909.

* **MRS. JOHN SHULTZ**—Baltimore Co., Md. Below knee.

I am wearing one of your artificial limbs with rubber foot, made from measurements, and find it entirely satisfactory. Oct. 16, 1909.

* **DAVID C. SHOEMAKER**—Mill Hand, Columbia Co., Pa. Wrist.

The artificial hand you made for me is a perfect fit, and I would not know how to get along without it. It has exceeded my expectations. I can turn and do all kinds of bench work the same as I did before. Nov. 10, 1909.

* **L. C. SHOEMAKER**—Undertaker, York Co., Pa. Below knee.

I suppose you think the leg you made for me January, 1891, was worn out long ago. Well, not much. The leg is in use every day and has been for seventeen years. It has never cost me ten cents for repairs, and does not show any signs of giving out. I am an undertaker and furniture man and am on my feet all the time. The stump has never been sore or even chafed. Anything I can do for you here I will cheerfully do. Feb. 18, 1908.

* **G. B. SILLIMAN**—Farmer, Otsego Co., N. Y. Below knee.

I have worn one of your artificial legs for over eighteen years every day and have not paid out anything for repairs. Nov. 14, 1907.

* **GREGOIRE SIMMELIDY**—Manufacturer, Egypt. Below knee.

Your inventions from technical as well as industrial points prove you to be a real benefactor of humanity.

In spite of long travels and voyages made by land and sea, the artificial leg that you made for me in 1902 is still serviceable and well preserved, promising to last a great many years longer.

Congratulating you, my friend, for enjoying universal recognition which I know you so worthily deserve, I beg you to accept the expressions of my sincere friendship and greetings. Nov. 11, 1909.

* BENJAMIN SIMMONDS—Accountant, Newfoundland. Above knee.

I have now worn one of your legs for some time, and I am very glad to say that I am quite satisfied with it. I was fitted from measurements taken at home. The amputation is four inches above the right knee. I do a lot of walking, and last winter I had to go through snow over three feet deep, and I walked it with no trouble.

It is quite common to listen to people asking which leg is off. I went to a party the other night and there was a dance. Many who saw me dancing did not know that I wore an artificial leg, and would not believe it when told.   Dec. 27, 1909.

* L. SIMPSON—Merchant, England. Below knee.

The artificial leg I got from you now nine years ago is as good as ever, and I can walk, for an old man, very well with it. It has cost me nothing in repairs, except what you have kindly done for me, a very different matter to the London legs, of which I have had two at L:38-0-0 each, and which were always wanting some repairs, but there is really nothing to wear out in the Marks leg, and I can confidently recommend them to anyone who requires one. In addition to this they are so "light" and that is where also I found a great difference, as Marks legs are pounds lighter than the London legs, and this also applies to the legs I had made for me at Bradford. I really think there is not a better maker in the world, and that is saying a great deal. Mr. Barstow measured me and ordered the leg.   April 6, 1908.

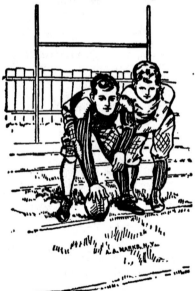

* ANTONIO SIRACUSA—Atlantic Co., N. J. Above knee.

I had the misfortune of losing my right limb two inches above the knee. It happened on April 15, 1900, when I was six years old. About a year after I got one of your artificial limbs. I cannot praise your artificial legs enough. I would not want to be without mine for anything. I do a great deal of walking, and running, play football without any trouble, and just as good as many other boys that have their natural legs.

* ANDREW SINCLAIR—Tailor, Edinburgh, Scotland. Below knee.

The limb I last obtained from you is comfortable and in every way a complete success. Quite recently I did one hundred miles walking in four days, doing thirty-six in the first. July 31, 1909.

* P. D. SLOAN—Cigars, Hocking Co., Ohio. Knee amputation.

I have worn your artificial limb about eleven years; can do any kind of work, ride a horse as good as anyone. I run a stogie factory, do all my own selling, and travel through five different counties. I live in a very hilly country, go hunting right along with other hunters in season, and travel over the roughest ground. There is nothing like your rubber foot. I have tried several other makes, and they were all failures. Oct. 18, 1909.

* R. H. SMEAD—Fireman, Lucas Co., Ohio. Below elbow.

I find the arm you recently made for me a great help. I can perform almost any kind of work with the hook. It gives me great pleasure to praise your work. March 6, 1910.

* CLAY SMITH—Porter, Franklin Co., Tenn. Below knee.

I haven't lost a day from work. I walk about two miles every day putting out switch lights, those that do not know that I have lost a foot cannot tell it in my walking. My depot agent is as well pleased with my limb as I am myself. I have been his porter for nine years, and am still able to do the same work. My doctor says it is remarkable the way I carry heavy articles. Oct. 20, 1909.

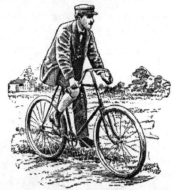

FRANK H. SMITH—Hampden Co., Mass. Below knee.

I have mailed you a photograph of myself on a wheel. I have worn a Marks leg for a great many years, and can do most anything with it. I ride from fifteen to twenty miles almost every day on the wheel, and have ridden forty. I have walked thirteen miles with hardly a stop. Have used a leg with an ankle-joint, but find the Marks leg the best. I have worn the present one for eighteen years. Oct. 19, 1909.

* JOSEPH SMITH—Laborer, Marion Co., Texas. Above knee.

The artificial leg you made for me in 1888 is still in good service. I have worn it continuously for the last twenty-two years. I pray God's blessing on you as you have done so much good for the crippled. Jan. 25, 1910.

* RUSSELL E. SMITH—Mill Hand, Bristol Co., Mass. Ankle amputation.

I am wearing one of your artificial limbs for over nine years. I work in a grain mill all day with ease and comfort. I can ride a wheel and play ball as well as if I had my own two feet. Oct. 19, 1909.

* FRANK SNOW—Railway Clerk, Cape Colony, Africa. Below knee.
You may remember making an artificial leg for me twelve months ago. I have much pleasure in informing you that it has given me every satisfaction. I would not care to wear the old type of leg now. It is a pleasure to walk on this one. Dec. 21, 1907.

* JOHN W. SOMERS—Laborer, Nova Scotia. Below knee.
I must tell you that I never had so much comfort with any artificial as I have had with the one I have now, made by you in 1906.   Nov. 10, 1909.

MRS. G. P. SPALDING—Suffolk Co., Mass. Below knee.
I take great pleasure in stating that the leg is satisfactory in every particular. I experienced very little difficulty in becoming accustomed to wearing it and am able to walk with scarcely any limp.   Oct. 16, 1909.

* FRED SPARKS—Mail Carrier, Union Co., Ohio. Below knee.
The limb I got of you is a wonder. I have had it seven years. You or anybody else couldn't perceive that I have an artificial limb. Even my nearest friends didn't know it till I made it known and then you ought to see them. I wouldn't take $25,000 and do without it, that is saying a good deal. It is a great boon to mankind. I am a United States mail carrier and perform my duties with the greatest ease.   Oct. 23, 1909.

* FREDERICK SPARROW—Farmer, Nelson, New Zealand. Above knee.
My son Stephen wishes me to tell you that the leg fits well and is satisfactory in every way. You have made a good solid job of it. Your artificial limbs are well known in this country and I shall lose no opportunity in adding to your reputation. Dec. 27, 1907.

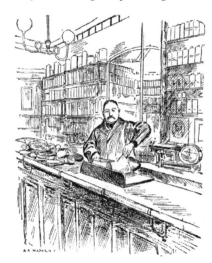

GEO. W. STEINMETZ—Delicatessen, Mt. Vernon, N. Y. Below elbow.
The artificial arm made for me fifteen years ago has been satisfactory and enables me to sell goods from my own counter, and I herewith submit a picture showing the use I put the artificial arm to. A large fork will be seen which is inserted in the palm lock and held so that I can hold a ham while it is being carved.   Dec. 12, 1909.

WILLIAM WALLACE STEWART—Druggist, Passaic Co., N. J.
Above knee.

Shortly after graduating, while visiting some relatives, I had the
misfortune to be struck on the knee-cap by a rock, which resulted
in the loss of my left leg above the knee. I despaired of ever being
able to engage in my chosen profession, that of a druggist. I was
told by my physician that my case was by no means desperate,
and that I should be able to walk almost as well as ever if I tried

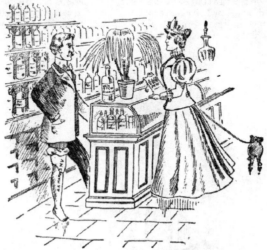

one of Marks legs. As soon as my stump healed, I went to
see Mr. Marks, who provided me with the leg I have worn for six
years, and with which I can walk easily and comfortably, attend
to my duties as prescription and sales clerk in a busy pharmacy.
Mr. Marks deserves unceasing thanks for his skill, care and attention to my case.

* DR. STOREY—Middlesex Co., Mass.

The leg you sent Mr. Porter was immediately applied; found to
fit excellently. He gets in and out of a carriage; never uses a
cane. He drives a horse, fixes his garden, and in fact everything
he ever did before he lost his leg.

* JOS. STRANGEWAY—Laborer, St. Louis Co., Mo. Above knee.

I bought an artificial leg for thigh amputation of you in 1898
and I want to say right now that this will be the first penny I
have spent on it and this for a new set of shoulder straps. I have
worn the leg every day for eleven years and have not missed a day
of hard work during that time.   April 5, 1910.

* GEORGE W. STRAUCH—Telegraph Operator, Schuylkill Co., Pa.
Above knee.

The leg I purchased of you in 1903 is giving the best of satisfaction, indeed, I often wonder if I have it on. A glove on the
hand is not more comfortable. I wear it on an average of eighteen
hours out of every twenty-four. As a railroad operator it is meeting every requirement in addition to the work of a large garden.

It is thirty years since I purchased my first leg of you, and
wore the leg continuously and gave it hard usage. The cost of
repairs for all that time was $8.00. I could have worn it much
longer, but it got too small, owing to my increasing weight.
December, 1903, I purchased the second one.   Oct. 16, 1909,

CHARLES SUDDARD—Carpenter, Toronto, Canada. Both knee amputations.

You supplied me with a pair of artificial legs for knee joint amputations a year ago last August. The legs have given me the best of satisfaction. I have worn them all the time and walk considerably. Am an upholsterer and stand at my work for ten hours and often walk to my boarding-house, which is quite a little distance.	Feb. 13, 1908.

* R. L. SUMMERSGILL—Stone Cutter, Greene Co., Pa. Below knee.

Received artificial limb from you about seven years ago and it is giving good satisfaction. My leg is amputated about ten inches below the knee. Wear your limb every day.

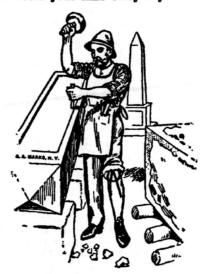

I am a stone cutter, handle marble and granite monuments, flag stone, etc., so you see my work is very hard on any person with two good feet. Will add I don't suppose there is any person gets around much better than I do.	Oct. 23, 1909.

* W. B. SUMNER—Farmer, Lawrence Co., Mo. Below knee.

The artificial leg I got from you is a nice fit and is all right. I lost my leg December 24, 1902, and in three months got the leg. I am well pleased with it. I plowed and attended to ten acres of corn the first year, and last fall plowed and sowed twenty acres of wheat, so you see the leg is very helpful.	Oct. 20, 1909.

* J. H. SWARTZEL—Merchant, Augusta Co., Va. Below elbow.

I received the last hand you made for me in 1903. I have been wearing it every day since I got it with perfect satisfaction. I am in the general mercantile business and it is a great help to me. In fact I can't see how I could get along without it.	Oct. 19, 1909.

* A. L. SWENSON—Student, Nicollet Co., Minn. Below elbow.

The arm I received from you has delighted me. It has given me several agreeable surprises. I find it much handier than I expected to. I have worn it constantly without any inconvenience. That such a perfect fit was possible from measurements is a surprise and the rubber hand is certainly a marvel, flexible and yet stable enough to hold my Homer for me when I look up a word in the lexicon.	April 23, 1909.

* W. R. SWINK—Laborer, Marion Co., Ore. Above knee.
I have been for a long time desirous of writing you and expressing my continued satisfaction with the artificial leg you made for
me in 1893, and now avail myself of the opportunity since I ob-

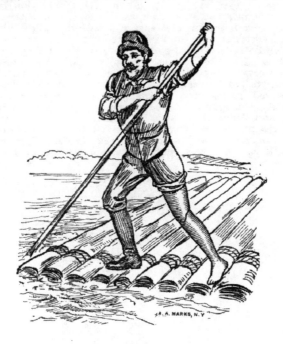

tained it. I have walked much and without a cane or support.
I suffer no pain or uneasiness from it. I do considerable rafting.
My artificial leg is my best friend; without it my life would be
miserable.

* JOSEPH H. SYLVESTER—Hotel, Suffolk Co., Mass. Below knee.
I am pleased to state that I have worn your artificial leg with
rubber foot for thirty years. I have worn legs with wooden
feet, but never got the comfort out of them as I have from your
make. Have induced quite a number of my friends to wear your
rubber foot leg. They are pleased and satisfied. Will be glad to
interview anybody. My work requires me to stand on my feet
all day.   Nov. 8, 1908.

* DR. R. F. TAGGART—Dentist, Hillsborough Co., Florida.
I have worn A. A. Marks make of artificial legs since May, 1868.
The first one I wore continually for thirty years. The one I am
now using I have had six years, stump only five inches long. I
have practiced dentistry for the last twenty-five years. I walk
with ease.   Oct. 6, 1910.

F. M. TALBOT—Contractor, Essex Co., N. J. Below knee.
In the fall of 1890 I met with a railroad accident which crushed
my leg and amputation was made below the knee, leaving a stump
three inches in length. My first experience with an artificial limb

was with a Wood Socket, after wearing it for eighteen months I
had one made with Slip Socket in preference to having the old one
refitted, as my stump had changed considerably and I thought that
the trouble was caused from the ill-fit. After wearing the second
one for over a year, my stump got in such a condition that my
life was in danger and it was impossible for me to attend to my
duties. I think it was in 1894 that I called on you and after you
had examined my stump, you pronounced it a case of strangulation,
and you said you could make me a limb that would relieve me of
that trouble. I ordered the leg of you and have been wearing it
for eleven years with perfect comfort and ease. As you will recall
I called on you a few weeks since and had you fit a new limb with
the improved rubber-foot, which is proving very satisfactory.
I am in the contracting business, principally constructing large
elevators and foundation work and attend to the outside work,
which keeps me on my feet constantly, this I do with as much
ease and comfort as any man could that is obliged to wear an
artificial limb. Your new rubber foot is a great improvement on
the old one.   May 17, 1909.

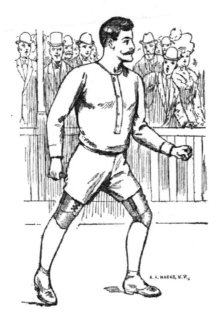

* ARTHUR G. TAYLOR—Pedestrian, Warwickshire, England. Both
  below knees.
   When a lad sixteen years old, I had both of my legs cut off in
a shuttle train accident, and my life was despaired of, but my
robust constitution carried me through. Six months after the
company procured a pair of legs for me made by a local leg-maker,
but bad fitting and construction rendered them of little use.
My fellow workers took up a subscription and bought a pair of
American legs, Marks patent, with which I can do almost anything. I am now twenty-six years old and engage in all kinds
of sports. Recently I walked a match against time and made a
mile in twenty minutes. My stumps are hard as nails. All of
which I have to thank Marks for.

* COLIN M. TAYLOR—Clerk, New Zealand. Below knee.

I have worn your rubber feet for nine years, the one I am now wearing being fitted with the "Spring Mattress," which I find a great improvement. It gives more spring to the walk, enables me to stand on a sloping surface, such as the deck of a ship at sea, and almost entirely does away with the thumping sound which always accompanies artificial feet.

My occupation at present is that of a bank clerk, but I was three years on a farm and did all the usual rough work attached to that industry without suffering any inconvenience. I can run and jump and play tennis. I go in for rowing, and find the foot in no way interferes with the sliding seat. I also ride a bicycle as well as if I were quite sound.

W. H. TAYLOR, M.D.—Jefferson Co., Tenn.

In matter of finish, durability, simplicity of construction, completeness of action, and perfect adaptation to stump, the Marks artificial limbs are far superior to anything I have ever seen.
Oct. 15, 1909.

* JOHN TENNANT—Jeweler, Greymouth, New Zealand. Below knee.

I have just had an inquiry as to where a young fellow should go to get a leg. Being one of your enthusiastic patients, I immediately wrote MARKS.

My leg is giving me every satisfaction and I am getting on splendidly. Have been wearing it for eight years. I tell those who, like myself, have been unfortunate, your legs are worth their weight in gold.
Dec. 26, 1907.

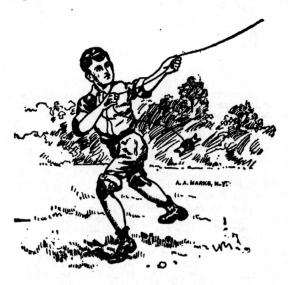

FRANK TRIACCA—Schoolboy, Fairfield Co., Conn. Below knees.

I am going to school every day and walk both ways. My artificial legs give the best of satisfaction in every way and have proved a great benefit to me. I walk, run, and play as well as most boys. When I tell persons that both of my legs are artificial, they will not believe me until they examine them.
June 10, 1909.

* J. W. VAUGHN—Bartow Co., Ga. Partial hand.

My right hand was mangled and amputated September, 1889, and in March following you made me one of your patent rubber hands, since that time I have had the second one made, and

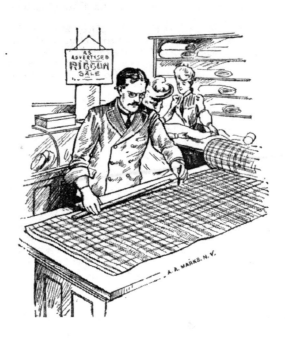

between the two wear and use them constantly. I can use mine almost as well as the natural hand. I can drive, use knife at table, write rapidly, as I am now doing, measure goods by the yard, or most any other work. I was fortunate in having my hand amputated below the wrist, leaving thumb and wrist bones, which enables me to secure the artificial hand around the wrist like a glove.   Oct. 18, 1909.

* REV. ALEXANDRO VILLA—Missionery, Mexico.   Wrist amp.

In 1903 I received my artificial hand, which is such a blessing that I am unable to express in this letter how satisfied I am.

As I am a well-known person throughout the state of Sonora, Mexico, and having lost my left hand, I was very much observed by the people. I endured the loss for twelve years, deprived of the privileges of which I am now master. I received a catalogue of your firm, saw the advertisements, but I did not believe that they were exactly as represented until I decided to have a hand made by you. It is useful in eating, in holding many things, especially my Bible, which I hold with my left hand, and turn the leaves with the right, and as I am so well known in the villages, where I preach the Holy Gospel, many ignorant persons who have seen me gesticulate thought that it was supernatural. Formerly I lacked the movement of my arm, now I move it naturally.—Translated from Spanish.   Oct. 25, 1909.

JOHN VEILLEUX—Shoemaker, Quebec. Above knee.

The artificial leg made for me in 1902 gives complete satisfaction. I am a shoemaker by trade and ever since I have my artificial leg I have not lost an hour's work. Previously I could only work

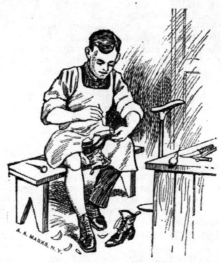

six or seven months in the year. I have walked three miles and a half and have not suffered any pain in my stump, which is only four inches long on the outside of the thigh and three inches on the inside. I now walk as easily as before my amputation as well as going up and downstairs. Jan. 3, 1910.

* G. C. WABY—Farmer, New Zealand. Knee amputation.

I beg to say that the leg I received from you, made and fitted by measurements, is very satisfactory. I have worn it about eight years. I am a retired farmer, in my seventy-first year, and I find the leg invaluable as it enables me to take sufficient exercise to keep in health. Dec. 7, 1909.

SIDNEY WACHTER—Salesman, New York City, N. Y. Below knee.

My leg was amputated about fourteen years ago; I was eight years old then. I commenced wearing artificial legs six months after the amputation and will say that your artificial leg comes as near to the natural as it is possible for a substitute. I have been playing baseball nearly every day in summer and could cover almost any position and now I have a position where I am constantly on my feet in the store or walking to different parts of the city selling goods. Oct. 16, 1909.

* J. T. WADE—Engineer, Gibson Co., Tenn. Below knee.

I had the misfortune to lose my right foot about twenty-six years ago, and have worn one of your artificial feet for fifteen years. It has given perfect satisfaction and I am wearing the second one, which is as satisfactory as the first. I am an engineer and I can get about to do my work without any difficulty. Oct. 24, 1909.

* G. E. WAITE—Merchant, Bedford Co., Tenn. Below elbow.

The arm and hand you made for me ten years ago has given perfect satisfaction. It has not cost me anything for repairs. I believe it to be the best arm made. This is the second you have supplied me, the first one was made about twenty years ago. Jan. 20, 1910.

* MISS MARY WALKER—Heckmondwike, England. Below knee.

The Marks artificial leg ordered by Mr. Barstow has proved to be a perfect fit, and I can walk splendidly. I walked two miles before I had worn it five weeks. I am so thankful. Dr. Broughton of Heckmondwike and I will always speak highly of Mr. Barstow's ability in taking measurements for artificial limbs as mine were taken accurately. Dr. Broughton says that at any time you may refer anyone to him, when he will be pleased to speak of your care and ability in such cases.   June 19, 1908.

* JOHN WALL, JR.—Farmer, Lee Co., Ill. Below elbow.

The artificial arm I got from you through Dr. E. F. Lark, is a fine piece of workmanship. I would not part with it for any price. I am well satisfied with it in every way. I could not get along without it now.   Jan. 13, 1909.

* THOMAS WARD—Engine Driver, New Zealand. Above knee.

I am very much pleased to be able to say that the leg I received from you is giving every satisfaction. As you are aware, my leg was amputated above the knee, leaving only seven inches of a stump. I drive a log-hauling engine in the bush, and can get about without the aid of a stick, and can ride on horseback with ease, in fact I can get about almost as well as I could before I had my leg amputated.   Dec. 13, 1909.

* GRADY WASHINGTON—Mill Hand, Webster Co., La. Below knee.

I am getting along alright and my leg has given me good satisfaction and is a good fit in every way.   Oct. 23, 1909.

* JAMES M. WEAVER—Clerk, Montgomery Co., Va. Above knee.

The leg you made for me in 1904 I am wearing without any trouble. It fits nicely, and I am pleased with it. Oct. 18, 1909.

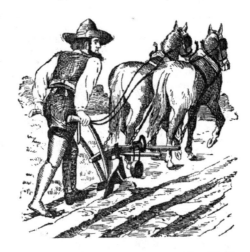

* CHARLES E. WEBB—Farmer, Chenango Co., N. Y. Above knee.

I have worn one of your artificial legs for nearly thirteen years, and am exceedingly well pleased with it.

The rubber foot is a grand invention, no squeaking or getting out of order. It can be depended upon, and the knee-joint is the strongest and best I ever saw. I am farming, and do all of my work, such as plowing, sowing, cradling, and everything that a farmer has to do.

I was never able to wear it constantly, as it hurt me very much and the springs were always breaking, leaving me almost helpless on the street.

When I came to my home in Ireland my friends hearing about a man named McKee, who was wearing one of your make with rubber foot, advised me to try one. I sent you measurements, from which you made my leg, and I never regretted having done so. The change was marvelous. I am still wearing it, although ten years old.

This leg cannot be beaten for ease and comfort. I am a clerk and timekeeper in a large foundry, and have a great deal of walking from one department to another, but I find no difficulty whatever in going about.

A young man here, who had his leg amputated above the knee, got one from you lately through my recommendation, and can go to dances and otherwise enjoy himself as well as ever he could before losing his leg.   Nov. 6, 1909.

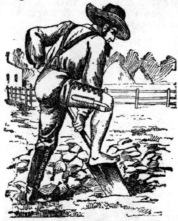

* J. H. WILLARD—Farmer, Buckingham Co., Va. Below knee.
Have worn your leg for nineteen years with great comfort. My occupation is a farmer. I can do most any work a farmer is called to do, such as plowing, harrowing, etc. My leg is amputated four inches below the knee. I am highly pleased with my leg; it was fitted from measurements.   June 6, 1908.
* JOHN B. WILLIAMS—Mail Carrier, Floyd Co., Ga. Above knee.
In April, 1904, I received one of your artificial limbs. The finest piece of work I ever saw. I had been on my crutches for ten years. I am about twenty-eight years old. Lost my leg in falling from a wagon, my leg was amputated three and one-half inches from hip. I never dreamed of ever walking without a crutch. After seeing your book on artificial limbs, and guarantee, I decided to buy a limb made from measurements, as per your directions. When I got the limb it was a perfect fit. The second day I threw away my crutches, and am now going about and doing my work well. I am a rural mail carrier. Can harness my horse, roll buggy in and out of stable.   Nov. 1, 1909.
* PHILIP WILLIAMS—Washington Co., Miss. Below knee.
I desire to let you know of the comfort I have had in wearing the artificial leg made for me in August, 1902. I would not be without the leg for anything. It not only enables me to walk naturally, but enables me to perform my work. It is thoroughly comfortable to wear.   Oct. 18, 1909.

* S. P. WILLIAMS—Sawmill, Alexander Co., N. C. Above knee.

I lost my leg May, 1891, and applied one of your artificial limbs the first of September following, and have been wearing it ever since until recently I sent a new measure and had another of the same kind made. It is all right, and fits all right. I was running a sawmill.   Oct. 24, 1909.

* WALTER A. WILLIAMS—Montgomery Co., Pa. Below knee.

The leg I received from you proved very satisfactory. I have been wearing it every day since I received it. I shall recommend your leg every chance I get.   Oct. 18, 1909.

* W. C. WILLIAMS—Conductor, Colleton Co., S. C. Below knee.

I have worn the artificial leg you made for me from measurements I sent you three years ago continually and it has given perfect satisfaction. My amputation is below the knee. May 1, 1909.

* HORACE WILLISON—Butcher, Brandon Co., Manitoba. Below elbow.

I do not know what I would do without the artificial arm you made for me. I do not think there is anything I cannot do that I did before the amputation.   Nov. 21, 1909.

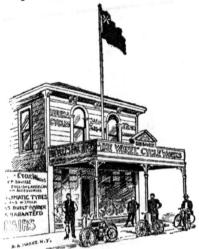

* ROBERT ALFRED WILLIAMSON—New Zealand. Above knee.

The leg you made from the measurements I sent you eight years ago fits admirably, and from the very first I was able to walk with comfort, and with no rattling of joints. I think the rubber foot is a great improvement over the ankle joint.

I work at the bicycle trade, and find the leg a great help to me in every respect, and never have to leave it off on account of soreness. I can thoroughly recommend your leg to all who are afflicted to be the next best to nature's.   Jan. 19, 1910.

DAVID C. WILSON—Foreman in Foundry, Jersey City, N. J. Below knee.

On the first of September, 1902, I suffered the loss of my right foot above the ankle. I was measured and fitted with an artificial by you nine weeks and a half after the accident, and received the foot at my home in the middle of the eleventh week, and I have worn it right along since then. I am foreman of a foundry in Jersey City, and I am as competent, with the aid of my rubber foot, to fill my position as I was previous to the accident. Am on

my feet from six o'clock in the morning until late at night, and
find no difficulty in getting along.

I take great pleasure in recommending your rubber feet to any
who may need them.   Oct. 25, 1909.

JOHN J. WILSON—Inspector, New York City. Below knee.

Have worn your patent artificial legs for nearly fourteen years,
and will make application for a new one from the Government
just as soon as the time comes. I have only about three inches
below the knee. I am on my leg twelve hours every day.

* HERBERT WRIGHT—Farmer, New Zealand. Below knee.

I take pleasure in testifying to the satisfaction I have derived
from the use of your artificial limb. It is nearly seven years ago
since I received it from you. I am a farmer, and have done all
kinds of rough farm work successfully. At times I have severely

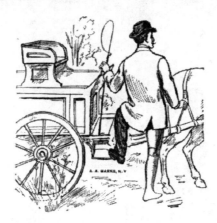

tested the rubber foot in lifting heavy weights, and it has stood
the work remarkably well. I shall always remain grateful, and
I would say to all who unfortunately need an artificial limb, "by
all means secure one from A. A. Marks."

* JOHN WINDSOR—Laborer, Wellington, New Zealand. Below
    knee.

I shall recommend your firm to anyone in need of artificial
limbs.   Feb. 4, 1909.

ST. CLAIR A. WODELL—Dental Student, Boston, Mass. Below
    knee.

The word "wonderfully" inadequately expresses the satisfaction
I received from the artificial leg you made for me. I have worn
limbs for many years with ankle joints but I have never before
known how to walk naturally on an artificial leg. The stiff ankle
and rubber foot is the thing. I am a dental student and find that
the rubber foot with spring mattress is of inestimable value. At
the end of the day I now feel as though I can walk home and
not have the help of somebody to carry me home. Last night I
attended a dance, for the first time in my life I attempted to
dance the gliding dance in which I was successful. After the
dance I went home and walked four miles and felt good for
another.   Feb. 13, 1909.

inches above the right knee, but I can say that I have not lost any time, with the assistance of the artificial leg constructed in your factory, the merits of which are strength and ease in walking, I know no better. To everybody in need of an artificial limb I recommend him to apply to your factory.   Nov. 26, 1909.

* ABSOLON M. YGLESIAS—Lima, Peru, South America.

I take great pleasure in assuring you that the artificial leg which I ordered of you to replace the one I lost in the engagement of August 27, 1884, has proved to my entire satisfaction. It is just that I should recommend your work, since I have been enabled to avail myself of it to such advantage.

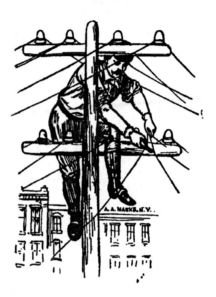

ALVAH YOUNG—Wireman, Boston, Mass. Below knee.

Alvah Young, employed by the Edison General Electric Co., New England Division, 38 Pearl Street, Boston, Mass., as a lineman, is a living example of the remarkable degree to which rubber feet restore lost members. He lost one of his legs some years ago in a railroad accident. He had a Marks rubber foot and artificial leg applied, and since then has engaged in active manual labor, earning his livelihood. He will climb a pole as dexterously as any of his associates, hold himself on the cross-bar with his artificial, and place the wires in a thorough workmanlike way.

* ALVA J. ZABRISKE—Beaver Co., Utah. Knee amputation.

I am wearing the leg I ordered from you sometime ago satisfactorily, and think the Marks leg all right. I advise everyone that needs one to buy of you. You can beat the world on artificial limbs.

* ANGEL ZEVALA Y MADERO—Mexico. Below knee.

I have the pleasure to state that the artificial leg constructed by you for me, for amputation below the knee, is so natural that persons who were not aware of the operation which I underwent scarcely believe I am lame. I have returned to my former employment and I only experience natural fatigue.—Translated from Spanish.

THE PANAMA CANAL

The Panama Canal, by which vessels pass from the Atlantic to the Pacific through Central America, is looked upon as the most

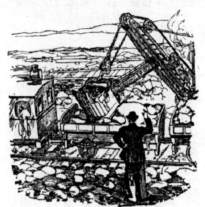

Steam Shovel at Work.

stupendous engineering achievement of the age. The work has employed from 30,000 to 50,000 persons daily. The blasting and moving of rock, the operations of dredgers and steam shovels, the building of railroads and the moving of trains, have been the call

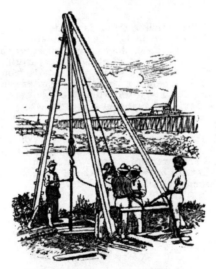

Wash Drill Gang at Work.

for the surgeons' skill in removing mangled and lacerated legs and arms.

The Isthmian Canal Commission has generously furnished their maimed employees with artificial legs and arms of the best and most suitable construction, irrespective of cost; the type of limb to be that most suited to the climate and conditions of the locality. Most of the laborers were natives of the tropics, and after being equipped with artificial limbs went to their homes or returned to their work on the Canal. Marks waterproof legs and arms were the only kind manufactured that would meet the demands. It must be

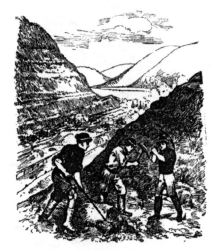

Culebra Cut.

remembered that the Panama Canal is located in the tropics. The temperature varies but little between Summer and Winter. It is very hot at midday and moderately cool at night all the year round. During the winter months the weather is dry; during the summer months the tropical rains set in and water falls from the skies in torrents without a moment's warning. An employee with an artificial leg starts for his work when there is every indication of a clear and dry day; before he has a chance to get under cover, rain comes in torrents and he is drenched to the skin, even his artificial leg is soaked. An artificial leg of the usual construction will not stand this treatment. But the Marks Waterproof leg cannot possibly be hurt by any amount of such exposure. For this reason the Marks waterproof leg was found to be adaptable to the conditions that prevailed in the Canal Zone and was therefore preferred and procured in large numbers.

CHAPTER XXXVIII

STUMP SOCKS. FOR ARTIFICIAL LIMB WEARERS

COTTON, WOOL, AND SILKATEEN

A stump bears the same relation to an artificial leg that a natural foot does to a shoe. Comfort and cleanliness demand that a sock should be worn on the stump, the same as on the foot.

A sock in either case provides a medium for collecting and absorbing the particles of waste and moisture that are thrown off from the skin, and by removing the socks, airing, and frequently washing them, the stump will be kept in a more healthy condition, and the socket of the leg will be better cared for.

There are persons who do not use socks, but wear their artificial limbs directly to their stumps, and permit the sockets to collect and absorb the excretions of the skin, and when the sockets become foul with the collection of effete matter, they are scraped out and

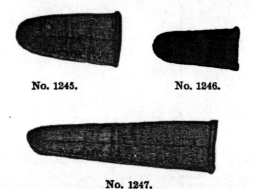

No. 1245.　　　　No. 1246.

No. 1247.

revarnished. This method cannot be condemned too strongly. The stump, as well as the artificial leg, suffers from such treatment.

Every wearer of an artificial limb should be provided with an ample supply of socks, so that frequent changes can be made. The same regard should be given to the stump as is given to the natural foot. If a stump perspires excessively, changes should be made more frequently.

We manufacture our own socks, and keep a large stock on hand and are able to fill orders promptly.

Our socks are ma_ ; of cotton, wool, and silkateen.

Cotton socks are knit of choice staple, they are durable and pleasant to wear; they are preferred by those who cannot endure wool.

Woolen socks are knit from yarn especially prepared for the purpose; the yarn is the best and softest that can be procured, with only enough twist to make it wear well. It is absolutely free from cotton or any foreign fiber.

Silkateen socks are made from exceptionally fine thread, they are knit on a machine constructed for the purpose; meshes are small, sixteen stitches to the inch, much finer than socks made from cotton or wool. These socks are especially suitable for tender and delicate stumps. Silkateen is a comparatively new thread; it is strong and will stand the effects of wear a great length of time. It has a luster resembling silk; it is very smooth and soft to the touch.

Cotton and woolen socks are made in two colors, white or brown, silkateen socks are of a natural grayish tint.

Our stock consists of eleven different sizes, ranging from ten to thirty-six inches in length, and in width to fit any ordinary limb.

In ordering socks the following measurements should be given:

Length of Sock. Circumference at top of Stump, 4 inches from top, 8 inches from top, 12 inches from top, 16 inches from top, 20 inches from top, 24 inches from top, 28 inches from top.

Some persons use a long sock to cover the stump to the body, and a shorter one to cover the stump to the joint (knee or elbow).

When a short one is needed, give only the length and circumferences of that part of the limb that is to be covered.

The following schedule will enable anyone to determine the sizes and the prices of the socks required.

No.	Length of sock.	Circumference at largest part of stump.	Cotton.		Woolen.		Silkateen.	
			Price each.	Price per dozen.	Price each.	Price per dozen.	Price each.	Price per dozen.
0.	1 to 10	Under 15	$0.20	$2.00	$0.40	$4.00	$0.60	$6.00
1.	10 to 15	" 15	.30	3.00	.50	5.00	.70	7.00
2.	10 to 15	Over 15	.40	4.00	.60	6.00	.80	8.00
3.	15 to 20	Under 15	.40	4.00	.60	6.00	.80	8.00
4.	15 to 20	Over 15	.50	5.00	.70	7.00	.90	9.00
5.	20 to 25	Under 15	.50	5.00	.70	7.00	.90	9.00
6.	20 to 25	Over 15	.60	6.00	.80	8.00	1.00	10.00
7.	25 to 30	Under 15	.60	6.00	.80	8.00	1.00	10.00
8.	25 to 30	Over 15	.70	7.00	.90	9.00	1.10	11.00
9.	30 to 35	Under 15	.70	7.00	.90	9.00	1.10	11.00
10.	30 to 35	Over 15	.80	8.00	1.00	10.00	1.20	12.00

One-quarter or one-half dozen of the same kind and size sold at dozen rates.

When a short sock in addition to a full-length one to come only to the knee-joint is desired Nos. 0, 1, or 3 will be suitable.

In determining the number of size, five inches should be added to the length of the stump to allow for turning over the top of leg and the shortening caused by the stretch in drawing on the stump.

Elastic Webbings, 2 inches wide, 60c. per yard; 1½ inch wide, 50c. per yard; 1 inch wide, 40c. per yard.

Non-Elastic Webbings, 2 inches wide, 30c. per yard; 1½ inch wide, 25c. per yard; 1 inch wide, 20c. per yard.

Clamp Buckles with Snap, 1½ and 2 inches, 25c. each; Snaps, 1½ and 2 inches, 15c. each.

Socks and Supplies will be sent postpaid if remittance accompanies the order.

Remittance can be made by postage stamps, money order, registered letter, express, or draft on New York. No goods will be sent C. O. D. unless one-half the price is enclosed with the order.

Address: A. A. MARKS, 701 Broadway, New York City.

CHAPTER XXXIX

HOW TO REACH OUR ESTABLISHMENT

We have endeavored to impress the fact that personal fittings for simple amputations are as a rule unnecessary, and that we do not advise anyone to go to the expense and annoyance incident to coming to us without first making an attempt to obtain a suitable artificial limb by measurements. In order to place the matter on a basis of safety to the wearer, we obligate ourselves to make all alterations and refittings (should they be necessary) without charge.

It is also emphatically stated that amputations leaving the stump with abnormal conditions, incapable of being explained either by drawings, descriptions or casts, are exceptions, fittings in such cases should be personal. Those who decide to come to us for personal attention will be welcomed and promptly attended to on their arrival.

WHERE WE ARE LOCATED.—We are located at 701 Broadway, one door north of Fourth Street, a distance of less than two miles from every railroad and steamboat terminal. $1.00 or $1.50 is the most that can legally be charged for carriage or taxicab to convey a person to our door. Any person can, however, take a car at the point at which they arrive and be conveyed to Broadway and there transferred to a car that will stop at our door. Five cents will pay the fare. The system of transfers in New York is very convenient and accommodating.

WE MEET PATRONS.—We will meet any person on arrival, if we are made acquainted with particulars a day or two in advance, provided the arrival occurs during the day. If it occurs after business hours, it will be well for the person to go immediately to some reputable hotel near by and remain there overnight, or go to the Broadway Central Hotel, 671 Broadway, which is within 300 feet of our establishment.

BUSINESS HOURS.—Our establishment is open for business from eight o'clock in the morning to five o'clock in the afternoon, except Saturdays when we close at one o'clock. We are not open Sundays or holidays.

BOARDING AND LODGING.—Accommodations can be obtained at reasonable rates in New York City. Furnished rooms in private houses can be had for from $2.00 to $5.00 per week, table board can be had from $3.00 to $5.00 per week. Rooms in hotels vary from fifty cents to $2.00 per night, with board from $2.00 to $5.00 per day. A person coming to New York expecting to remain a week or more, and wishing to keep expenses down, can engage a furnished room and eat in restaurants, living expenses while here can thus be kept within narrow limits. The Mills House, located at 164 Bleecker Street, is within one-half a mile of us. This is one of a chain of hotels conducted for the accommodation of respectable men of small means. A room can be had for twenty cents per night and meals at fifteen cents each.

WHERE TO HAVE YOUR MAIL ADDRESSED.—Upon leaving home, instructions should be given to address letters and telegrams to the care of A. A. Marks, 701 Broadway, New York City.

Patrons have the liberty of our premises while in New York, and if they are shopping, they can have their goods delivered at our store. They can make engagements to meet parties here and have the exclusive use of private rooms for private interviews.

CALLS MADE TO RESIDENCES.—Persons will be attended to at their residences, no matter where they may reside, if expenses and extra time are paid for.

WOMEN IN ATTENDANCE.—Women who prefer to be waited upon by one of their own sex, will find women in our office for their accommodation.

BRANCHES.—We have no manufacturing branches. Our factory is located in New York City and in no other place. Our skill and judgment cannot be relegated to one in charge of a manufacturing branch. If we were to establish branches we would have to place them under the management of others and would, more or less, jeopardize the welfare of our patrons. As substitutes for branches, our system of fitting from measurements has been devised and found adequate.

If the reader desires to order a limb and does not care to take measurements himself, he can call upon his physician or druggist, or upon one whom we will designate, and have measurements taken.

INTERIOR OF THE LARGEST ARTIFICIAL LIMB MANUFACTORY IN THE WORLD.

(Seven Floors of 25x100 feet each.)

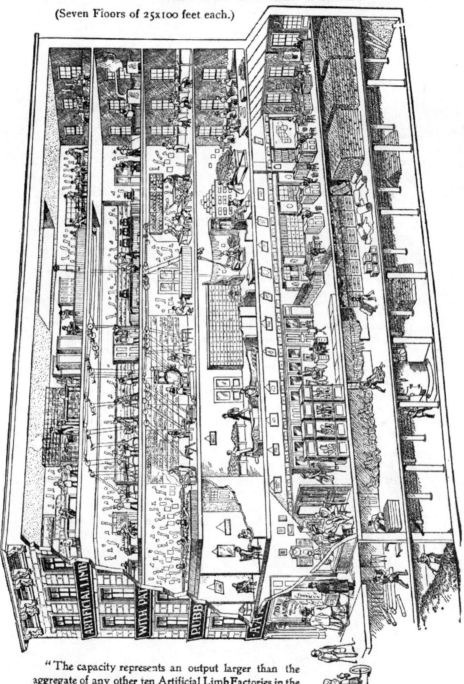

"The capacity represents an output larger than the aggregate of any other ten Artificial Limb Factories in the World."—SCIENTIFIC AMERICAN.

A. A. MARKS, 701 Broadway, NEW YORK CITY.

CAUTION

———

Artificial limbs with rubber hands and feet are the inventions of A. A. Marks and the members of the firm bearing that name.

The patents that are owned by the firm have the following dates:

March 7, 1854.	July 12, 1887.
December 1, 1863.	March 8, 1892.
March 7, 1865.	January 3, 1893.
November 16, 1880 (First).	September 17, 1895.
November 16, 1880 (Second).	July 9, 1912.
March 30, 1886.	

These patents not only cover the original inventions, but the more important improvements that have been made upon them.

The limbs have proved a blessing to the maimed. They stand peerless before the world. Over 44,000 have been put in use, and the verdict is overwhelmingly in their favor.

The large and increasing demand for Marks inventions has excited the envy of our competitors. Discarded inventions and expired patents of a quarter of a century ago have been more or less mutilated and offered as rubber feet, rubber ankles, rubber toes, pneumatic pads, etc., etc.

We advise all persons who are in need of artificial limbs to deal directly with us, and obtain the genuine and not submit to doubtful experiments.

Order should state that none but Marks artificial leg or arm will be accepted. The genuine bear the name of the firm and the dates of patents.

A. A. MARKS,

Established 61 years.   701 Broadway, New York, U. S. A.

Date Due

CPSIA information can be obtained at www.ICGtesting.com
Printed in the USA
LVOW11s0036111213

364800LV00008B/165/P